The Quest for a Child

The Quest for a Child

Two Small Wings

Hana Konečná

Anshan

The Quest for a Child

International edition published 2008 by

ANSHAN LTD
6 Newlands Road,
Tunbridge Wells,
Kent.
TN4 9AT. UK
Tel +44 (0) 1892 557767
Fax: +44 (0) 1892 530358
e-mail: info@anshan.co.uk
Website: www.anshan.co.uk

Cover design – Graham Rich

Language editor – Katerina Prajznerová, Madeleine Štulíková

Reviewers:
Prof. PhDr. Ivo Čermák, DrSc.
Prof. MUDr. Ladislav Pilka, DrSc.
Doc. MUDr. Tonko Mardešić, CSc.
Doc. PhDr. Michal Miovský, PhD.

Typeset by Vikatan Publishing Solutions, Chennai, India
Printed and bound in India by Replika Press Pvt. Ltd.

British Library Cataloguing in Publication Data
A catalogue record for this book is available from the British Library

ISBN 978 1905740 772

Contents

Preface

The potter, Sher Muhammad, was a master of his trade. His speciality was making pots as large as a human being, called khumas, used for the preservation of water… From these pots Sher Muhammad made large profits…and yet he still considered himself an unhappy man who had been betrayed by life because in his house there were no children. Sher Muhammad had tried everything. He prayed, for years he gave donations to the mosque, he even invited exorcists and magicians, but all that proved useless; his wife did not become pregnant and they were both growing old.

The house was always in good order and filled with a dignified calm. For years, the same dishes stood in the alcoves, not a single cup was broken, and the silk blankets looked as good as new. But such dignity is pleasing only for hard hearts, and that was something Sher Muhammad did not have. How he would have rejoiced if one lovely day all the dishes up to the last little pot got broken by a carelessly thrown ball, if the silk mats got dirty from curious little hands using them as toys!

He used to talk with his wife about children and they used to mourn together. But when they became old, when all their hopes had disappeared, they stopped talking about it. Each felt guilty before the other and each suffered alone, in silence.

Once he unwittingly broke the tacit agreement not to speak about children, 'Do you know what I dreamt about?' he said, 'I dreamt that we had a son, a strong and screaming little boy!' The old woman got her hackles up, hunched over, and looked at him with an imploring look, as though she were saying, 'Forgive me!' He sighed and turned away. Perhaps, he thought, it was he who should have begged for forgiveness. The evening passed in quiet sadness…

That night he woke up and saw the old woman kneeling in front of an open window. The moon lit her up to the last wrinkle. She was praying and he began to listen. She was asking Allah for a child—what nonsense at 60 years of age! Her whisper was passionate, she was not conscious of what she was saying as she reproached Allah. In her voice were many years of hardship, unfulfilled desire for motherhood, loneliness and sadness of frustrated hopes. But there was also belief despite everything: despite reason, despite reality.

'All-powerful!' she tore at her grey hair, fell face down to the floor, tightened her bent back under her white shirt awkwardly, and, having run out of words, she wailed gloomily.

The old man was overcome with a wave of pity. He lay on the bed quietly and bit the pillow so that the tears would not spill from his eyes. He felt deep tenderness towards his wife.

After a while, the old woman lay down in her place next to him. She lay without moving and so did Sher Muhammad. They both knew well that the other was awake but out of consideration for each other, they feigned sleep, pretending to believe this simple lie. They did not exchange a single word all night, but in their thoughts they said much, and they forgave each other because they understood that they lived one life together. He lived for her, she for him —they had lost their own private lives long ago.

It was a hard night for Sher Muhammad. With relief he welcomed the morning, and he looked forward to forgetting the sorrowful thoughts in his usual daily worries. It was very early, the morning light had not yet lost its bluish shade and the day was just beginning. There were two hours left before leaving for the bazaar. Sher Muhammad started to examine his pots again. He knocked on the first five pots and there was a clear sound. He knocked on the sixth one and there was a peep…there was a child in the pot. He knew it was the boy from his dream. There had been a miracle in the house. Both the potter and his wife understood this: 'I knew it would happen, I expected it all the time. I just did not know when and how,' said the old woman.

According to the regional law at that time, a child could be adopted only if its parents had not presented themselves after three months. For Sher Muhammad the three months were endless and his wife in constant torment. Every day she spent in fear that someone would come and take the child away. But all her fears proved unfounded. The last day passed and nobody had claimed the foundling. On the ninety-first day, in the presence of the required number of witnesses, the clergyman carried out the ceremony of adoption and Hajj Nasreddin passed into the potter's house.

Nasreddin's Adventures, L. Soloviov

Foreword

It seems natural: you have known each other long enough and you are beginning to think about having a child, so you decide to get married. You send out wedding announcements. Your friends suspect that you, the husband to be, have to get married because you got your partner pregnant. When you insist that is not the case, they make it clear they fear you have lost your senses. Your girlfriends whisper about you, the wife to be. In a conspiratorial way and often with a poorly concealed envy, they wonder, 'in what month is she due?'

The wedding march has ended, you have furnished the apartment, and you have gained a good position at work, precisely according to the plan. Simply, the time is right for the arrival of a child. You no longer pass shops with children's goods without interest. Now you examine in detail what they have to offer. You, the newly wed husband, inspect the buggies and estimate how much a child's football kit would cost. You, the newly wed wife, curiously peep into prams; you discover that there are beautiful maternity outfits in the city centre, exactly your style. You calculate the best month to conceive so that you won't need to carry the baby during the summer heat and, of course, you stop using contraception. You eagerly expect the arrival of the two small wings of the stork.

After the first month, you are surprised that you were not successful right away, but there are still so many chances. The second month you become unsure, and after three months you begin to lose your patience. For years, you had scrupulously protected yourselves against pregnancy. Was there, after all, no reason for that? Your lovemaking becomes a pragmatic relationship, directed by the thermometer and the calendar.

Before the wedding, you learned to answer questions about children with wit. Now you are no good at being on top of things, when you have to deal with well-meant advice: 'you mustn't think about *It* when you are doing *It*,' 'go for a holiday to the sea and you'll bring back a baby for sure', 'go and socialise to get your mind off it,' 'you mustn't stress yourself so much,' 'be glad you have no children, you don't know how much work they are, this way you can at least enjoy yourself.' Your parents start asking about grandchildren and they assume you are not trying hard enough. At work, the boss keeps postponing your promotion, since a wedding is usually followed by maternity leave.

Menstruation becomes a regularly occurring horror. The thermometer, an unwanted witness to your failures, goes back to the bottom of the first aid kit. On the way back from work, you choose streets without any children's shops, even if it means a long detour. When you happen to see pregnant women or mothers with prams, you break into tears. TV ads for diapers bring on fits of crying. The two small wings have still not come.

There is a flash in your mind—this is the end. The end? No, my friends, it is the beginning! You can now set out on a quest for a child! Yes, at this moment, it may be a quest into the unknown. It may seem difficult, demanding, and full of traps. However, it also promises to be a quest full of discoveries and exciting adventures—like that holiday when there was all that rain at the beginning and you lost your way. You didn't reach the planned destination, but still you are filled with happy memories and good experiences, precisely because you followed a somewhat different direction from that planned.

To make your quest for a child as smooth as possible and to help you navigate the hills, precipices, and dark corners along the way, I have created a basic map and travel guide for you. It took me some time; the territory is much larger than I initially expected. I have read a hill of books—both ancient and new. During my investigation, I discovered many established scholars in various fields who sometimes do not know about each other's work. I have also met many people who got lost on their quest. I have roughly charted this path, thanks to the experts and their patients who have been willing to talk with me, as well as to the many other more or less accidental travellers I met along the way.

> There is a lot that I could tell you about, doctor, that could perhaps help others as others have helped me: the decision to conceive a child; the influence of the family on our infertility treatment—illnesses, deaths, adoption and foster care, the disabilities of our family members; our friends' children; twins, triplets; the reaction of the wider community; employer's attitude; time demands—examinations, sick leave, injections; communications with doctors; listening to other couples' stories; sharing information with other infertile couples; reading articles and watching TV programmes about

> infertility; the relationship with my husband and the effects on our lovemaking; the gradual understanding of the whole area of infertility treatment; the art of articulating what one wants, of deciding which doctor one wants, what to tell to which friend, whom to ask for advice; the dim view of the future; the life values and priorities... (f)

The map is somewhat different from the ones you may be used to. It is a collage of ancient stories, expert texts and pieces from the locals' and the travellers' drawings. Instead of the dry statement that the fountain is 100 metres away, I prefer the more authentic description, 'and then you'll hear the falling drops.' Since it is important to differentiate who says what, for example, 'it is at a stone's throw away,' or 'it is right next to the hat shop,' I indicate in parentheses whether it is a woman's observation (f) or a man's (m), or that the advice, 'don't drink the water' comes from the local physician (p). Throughout the book I have inserted these verbatim quotes into explanatory paragraphs to help you better understand the subject and your feelings.

Whenever I travel, whether the trip is joyful, sad, too long, or frightening, I usually sing. Perhaps that is why, as I was writing, my ears resonated with tunes from various songs. In the end, I decided to use excerpts from these songs as the chapter titles and as the book title. I hope that on your quest for a child you will feel like singing.

Have a good trip!

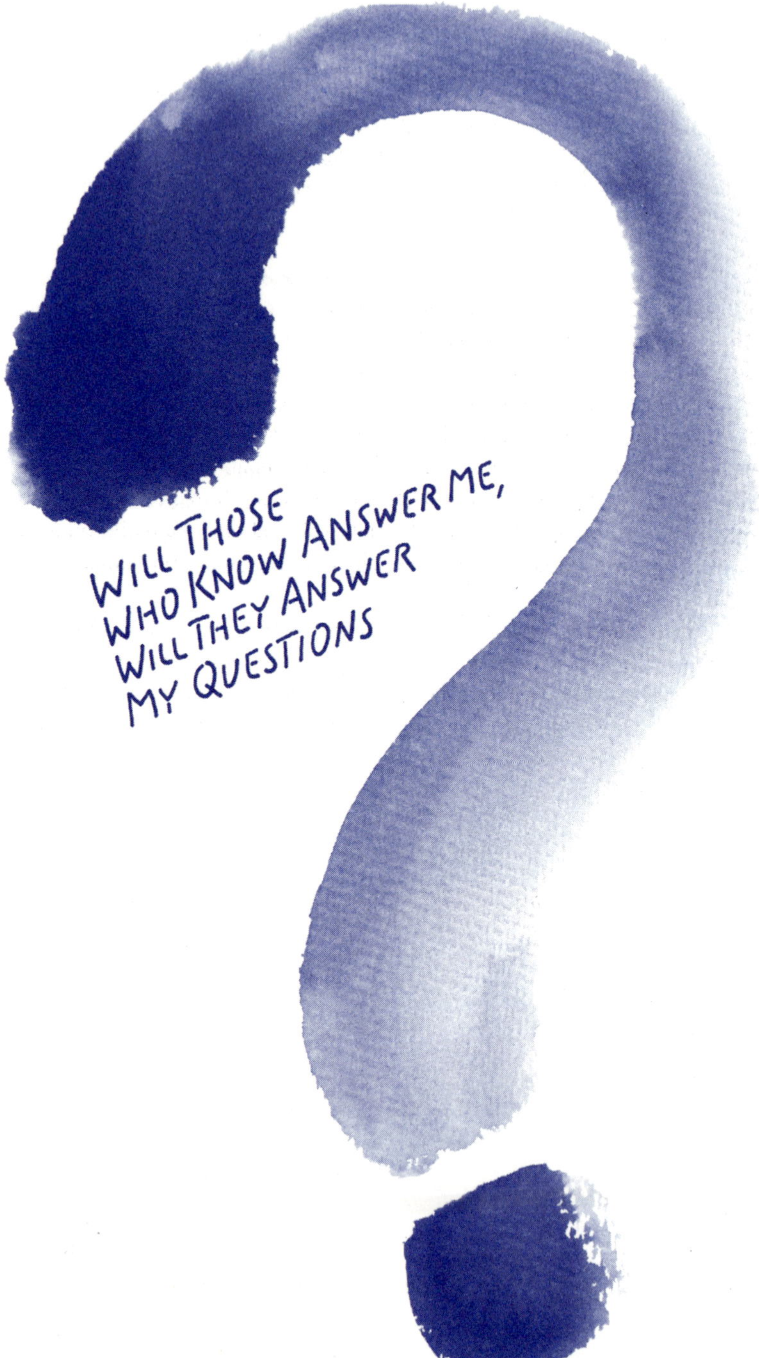
WILL THOSE
WHO KNOW ANSWER ME,
WILL THEY ANSWER
MY QUESTIONS

Will Those Who Know Answer Me, Will They Answer My Questions

What is Hidden in the Word Sterility?

When you first see a doctor with the complaint that you have been trying to get pregnant for several months and nothing happens, you will probably hear the words 'sterility' or 'infertility'. What do they mean? All terms designate the same thing and there is no unity in their usage. Sometimes sterility refers to a couple's inability to get the woman pregnant after a year or more of unprotected sex, while infertility refers to the tendency to miscarry, that is, to the inability to carry a child for the full term of pregnancy or give birth to a live infant. Generally, it is estimated that 80% of all impregnated eggs end up being miscarried 20% of the time, and the rest of them perish of their own accord in the next cyclical bleeding, without the woman noticing anything. It is estimated that 4% of women of reproductive age are women who miscarry. However, sometimes the term infertility broadly refers to a couple's inability to get the woman pregnant after a year or more of unprotected sex, to the tendency in women to miscarry, as well as to infertility in men. This broader usage makes sense: since most of the time we do not know whether the egg did not become fertilised or whether it did become fertilised but perished in menstruation, a strict distinction between sterility and infertility may not be accurate.

Sometimes a distinction is made between primary infertility (pregnancy has never occurred) and secondary infertility (pregnancy occurred in the past but now it has not occurred after a year of effort). Again, the question comes up as to whether pregnancy really did not occur or whether it was just not detected. The term 'idiopathic infertility' is used when there is no cause detected after gynaecological, andrological, endocrine, microbiological, genetic, immunological, and many other examinations.

All the above terms are medical, but some are also commonly used in everyday life. Particularly the word sterile brings up the idea of something completely barren, with no sign of life, something that smells of disinfectant. When we label people infertile, we may seem to indicate that they have never done anything good and they should not be counted on in the future, either. A new term, 'involuntarily childless' has recently been introduced in an effort to express the psychological aspect of the matter. This term can be difficult to understand, and it is also somewhat misleading, but we do not have a better one at the moment. Involuntarily childless refers to people who do not have children although they would like to have them. This situation can be caused by a fertility problem, but also, for example, by the lack of a partner or by a failure in the adoption screening process. Therefore, another positive aspect of the psychological term involuntarily childless is that it takes into consideration the biological as well as psychosocial causes of unfulfilled parenthood.

> I didn't have a child for a long time, I didn't feel it as something negative. My partner did want children. After eight years of our relationship I (without planning on my side) got pregnant, and, at the age of 37, I gave birth to a son. When he turned one, my partner left me and has shown no interest in his son since then. I don't regret it at all, I am happy that I have the little boy. I am sad about my partner's leaving mainly because I won't have any more children. When I see pregnant women and mothers with prams, I envy them. If I am born a second time, I'll start having children earlier and will have three. (f)

This woman would like to have a child but she has no partner. She is involuntarily childless. It is paradoxical that she is involuntarily childless although she already has a child. In this sense, the term is misleading. It does not take into account the frequent situation in which a person wants to have more children. There are quite a few couples who already have a child or children but their quest for another child is unsuccessful, if, for example, they have a fertility problem. I would like to draw attention to this term and recommend it for use instead of infertility. Infertility should not be used even in medicine, since it suggests something final and hopeless. Infertility should be replaced by the term fertility problem, which is more fitting because it suggests hope: a problem can be corrected; only a very few are irreparable.

Is Infertility an Illness?

When we hear the word ill, we imagine someone who is limping, coughing, in pain, on a special diet, bandaged, simply someone who is in some way visibly physically suffering. A couple who cannot have a child do not limp or cough and they often look better than a couple raising three small children. If the childless couple suffer at all, then it is 'only' mentally.

Based on the World Health Organization (WHO) definition and the logic of the argument that lack of health corresponds to a disease, infertility can be considered a disease. Since it has been established as an illness, infertile people should undergo treatment.

All this may sound a little bureaucratic, like a useless play on words. However, the official status of infertility as an illness has had far-reaching consequences, for example for the financial participation of the government in treatment, as well as for the research and training opportunities in this area. As a psychologist, I would especially like to emphasise the psychosocial aspect of this matter. Someone who is legitimately ill is regarded with much more respect than someone who only complains and has no officially accepted reason to do so.

Moreover, infertility is a special illness, for it is an illness of couples. Whether the cause is gynaecological or andrological (the male equivalent), the effects are borne by both partners. In addition, without the other partner's informed agreement, it is impossible even to start some of the therapeutic procedures. While problems of couples are common in psychotherapy, in medicine such cases are rare.

Are We an Exception?

Most women's magazines devote some space to contraception, that is, advice on how to prevent the arrival of a child. Fortunately, modern humans have at their disposal many means of avoiding an unwanted pregnancy. But this may, with some level of exaggeration, create the impression that, unless a couple ingeniously protect themselves, the woman might get pregnant just by affectionately thinking about her partner.

But that is a mistake! Humans are beings with reduced fertility and even for a completely healthy couple the probability of pregnancy in one menstrual cycle is only 25%. You may not want to believe this since you probably know many couples who only once and... But according to the statistics, 60% of couples conceive within 6 months, 80% after 9 months, and 85% after 12 months of intensive efforts. The remaining 15% have more or less serious problems. If you have become worried after the first unsuccessful attempt and this information has set your mind at ease, then I am glad.

Is the Infertility Rate Increasing?

There is no simple answer to this question. It is true that the media keep bombarding us with threatening data about decreasing fertility, especially in males. According to these reports, the average sperm concentration in males has fallen by half and the number of infertile males has doubled in the last 50 years. Some specialists claim that this decrease in fertility has been brought on by pollution and stress. However, others point out that these numbers are valid only for certain geographical areas and that the causes have not been clearly established. They claim that the infertility rate remained the same, only human behaviour has changed. Women want to have children at a higher age when their fertility is biologically lower. Moreover, thanks to the extraordinary developments in this area of medicine in recent years, more couples actively seek help when they have problems, and so more people get into the official statistical data. While, in the past, physicians could mostly just advise patience, people often did not go to them with their fertility problems. Today available medical treatment consists of a large range of diagnostic and therapeutic methods and can offer couples much more hope.

What's the Story About the Women's Age?

When to become a mother is a dilemma of the 21st century. According to the statistics in the United States, the number of women who have their first child after the age of 30 has quadrupled since 1970. People live longer and women postpone motherhood, as they believe that later on they will be more mature, live in a stable marital relationship, and will be financially secure. These reasons are understandable and certainly praiseworthy, but the female body simply ignores them.

> I can only sigh about how unjust nature is. I would feel ready to have a child now, at the age of 52, after I have accomplished a lot and experienced a lot. Now I am finally sufficiently calm. But I guess it was supposed to turn out this way. When I was 30, I was flying around the world, photographing like mad, and I did not want to miss anything. At that time I would have left the child with someone for half a year, then I would have returned and what then? Poured gifts on him or her? Told the child how I loved him or her? It's always something for something. (f)

With increasing age, women's ability to have children decreases. It starts to drop slowly around age 30 and at age 40, the probability of pregnancy is low. Additionally, the probability of miscarriage rises; statistics speak about 40% likelihood in a 40-year-old woman. But women often do not know this.

The contraceptive pill has brought along the feeling of a free 'decision about children'. It is a false feeling because it offers only half the freedom, when not to have a child. The decision when to have a child is not fully in our hands. Women keep themselves in good mental and physical health and they assume that their ovaries will remain in the same condition. However, ovaries grow old much faster than other organs. The media churn out information about advances in reproduction technologies and they create the deceptive impression that science can do anything. Everything seems so easy; in California, even a 63-year-old woman became a first-time mother. But this woman is an exception.

Many methods are still in the experimental phase. Moreover, given the ethical problems, there remains the open question of whether such methods will actually be introduced. More and more 40-year-old women seek out specialists in reproductive medicine, and many are caught unaware of the fact that their chances are small. You cannot put your biological clock on pause. The situation has gained such dimensions that many professional and patient organisations have decided to launch public information campaigns.

The previous paragraphs were certainly not intended to horrify any woman above 30 and deprive her of her hope in a good ending. (I myself had children after 30 and the third and the fourth ones even after 40.) But I am convinced that it is better to be truthfully informed, and act and plan for the future accordingly, than to live on idle hopes and then be desperate.

For those who are not planning to have a child yet and so far have just been seeking an answer to the question whether to have a child and when, I offer a part of an excellent editorial from a women's magazine:

> I remember the time when I was myself pregnant for the first time. I was 22, studying at university, single, living in a dormitory, and it is obvious that I was without money. Alas, my plan for a three-month internship at the radio station, which was supposed to ensure a great position for me later on, was shattered. When I announced the news, in my opinion terrible, to the editor-in-chief, she gave me a hug and said: 'My dear, pregnancy always comes at an inconvenient time. Either you don't have a job, or you do have it and are worried about losing it. Either you have no apartment at all, or

you have it so perfectly furnished that you would rather not disturb its style. One woman has no father for the child, another one has three at the same time. Do you want a child? So have it. The rest is going to take care of itself.' She was right. My child was in such a rush to get out into the world that in the end it lived in it just a few minutes. What was left was a huge abyss: an individual study plan, thanks to which I would have been able to graduate even with a child. An old house that I'd come by miraculously during the pregnancy. The man who had wanted to be its father, and the playsuit that I'd bought... I had thought that the baby would be too much in my life, but now I missed it. Since then I've known that the time for a child is any time. Any time when you yourself want it. (f)

What are the Causes of Infertility?

Until recently, people assumed that the cause of infertility lies almost always in the woman. As long as the man was potent, he was automatically considered fertile. But potency is not a sure guarantee of success. Many of Casanova's successors are taken aback at the result of their sperm examinations. Male impotency is one of the many possible reasons why a couple remain without a child.

Medical research has proved that both partners share in the failure of the woman to become pregnant almost to an equal degree. According to the latest information, a slightly higher fraction is due to andrological causes (the man's side). Dysfunction in both partners occurs in roughly 20% of cases and hence it is a major and, unfortunately, frequent mistake that, when a cause is found in one partner, the other is not examined.

It is the man (or the woman) who is to blame; it is the man's (or the woman's) fault, I often hear, even from doctors. It is necessary to emphasise that nobody is to blame for fertility dysfunction. The word cause, not blame, should be used when it is necessary to identify the reason for a couple's fertility problem. Frankly, where else but at the doctor's should we look for causes on the male (or female) side. Alternatively, the medical terms andrological fertility problem and gynaecological fertility problem should be used as they are emotionally neutral and suggest that the matter is strictly medical.

What are the Prerequisites for a Successful Quest for a Child?

There was once a woman who did so want to have a wee child of her own, but she had no idea where she was to get it. So she went off to an old witch

> *and said to her, 'I would so dearly like to have a little child. Do please tell me where I can find one.' 'Oh that!' said the witch, 'Nothing easier. Take this barleycorn—mind you, it's not the kind that grows out in the fields or that the fowls are fed with. Put it in a flower-pot, and see what happens!' 'Thank you very much,' said the woman, giving the witch a shilling. She went straight home and planted the barleycorn, and in no time there came up a lovely great flower that looked just like a tulip, only the petals were shut tight as though it were still in bud. 'It is a pretty flower,' said the woman, and she gave the lovely red and yellow petals a kiss; but directly she kissed it, the flower burst open with a pop. It was a real tulip—that was plain enough now—but, sitting on the green pistil in the middle of the flower, was a tiny little girl. She was delicately pretty and no taller than your thumb, so she was given the name of Thumbelina.*
>
> 'Thumbelina', Hans Christian Andersen, *Fairy Tales*

A beautiful and poetic piece of advice, isn't it? It also mentions kissing and planting a seed, and so it is a much more progressive explanation than the classic story about the stork or the crow. However, I am afraid that today even pre-school children would not fully believe Andersen's description. On the other hand, does Andersen's 'Thumbelina' not anticipate the latest methods in reproductive medicine? We go to a special place, something is placed somewhere apart from us, we pay with a golden coin, and, after some time, there appears a child. Before we get to these latest methods, let me first discuss a more conservative, but also a more pleasant and cheaper procedure.

The essential prerequisite in this procedure is that only a heterosexual couple can have their own biological child. The introductory fairy-tale explanation may be progressive, but not even the witch goes so far as to remind the woman of the necessity to have a partner. Or the fairy tale is, in fact, so progressive and timeless that it envisions future possibilities. But the quest for their own biological child remains blocked for a number of people who have either not found a heterosexual partner with whom they would like to have children, or they lost their partner before their desire for a certain number of children had been fulfilled (divorced, widowed).

A heterosexual couple is not yet out of the woods, because consent and capability are also necessary for fertilisation. As with the availability of a heterosexual partner, consent and capability are not matter-of-course for everyone. If one partner lacks the will or capability and the couple have no sexual intercourse, we have a case called apparent sterility. This situation can occur for several reasons. First, the couple are not aware that without sex, pregnancy will not occur or they have not yet mastered the technique. In this situation, it is usually recommended that the couple see a sexologist or a psychologist. Second, the man has problems with erection or ejaculation or the woman has trouble with dyspareunia (painful sexual intercourse). In this case, the cooperation of a gynaecologist, sexologist, and urologist or andrologist is necessary, since the cause of these problems is not always mental, as is generally assumed.

Not even the most ingenious lovemaking techniques will always suffice in the quest for a child. Certain mysterious inner processes must function as well. Therefore, another prerequisite is maintaining good physical and mental health. Infertility or reduced fertility are often either the side effects or the symptoms of other illnesses, for example of various thyroid dysfunctions or tumour growths. Smoking, drinking, taking drugs, dietary extremities (obesity, anorexia) and other violations of a healthy lifestyle certainly do not make the quest for a child easier. The influence of mental health on fertility deserves a chapter of its own and will be dealt with later in more detail.

The normal development and function of the genital organs are part of the prerequisite for physical and mental health. However, given the central subject of this study, it is necessary to devote more space to this issue. Most people generally know how to tackle things and they do not lack good will or capability. But since we are usually not interested in this area, most of us have only a vague idea as to how things function inside us. But things change when we are taken aback by our failures and when doctors start inundating us with names of organs we did not even know existed. Then we must review and relearn our biology. The next section is meant to serve as a 'cheat sheet'.

What Did they Teach us at School?

The female reproductive organs fulfil five functions: they create female gametes (eggs or oocytes), produce female sexual hormones, enable inner fertilisation, ensure the development of an embryo and fetus, and, finally, they ensure the birth of a human being.

All of the female reproductive organs are inside the body. The vagina links the body surface with the cervix uteri, which leads into the womb (the uterus). The womb is an organ the size and shape of a pear, formed by muscles. In the womb, the fertilised egg settles and then grows. The womb is covered by a lining (endometrium), which is richly supplied with the blood that is necessary for the development and nourishment of the fetus. From the upper part of the womb protrude the fallopian tubes, where the

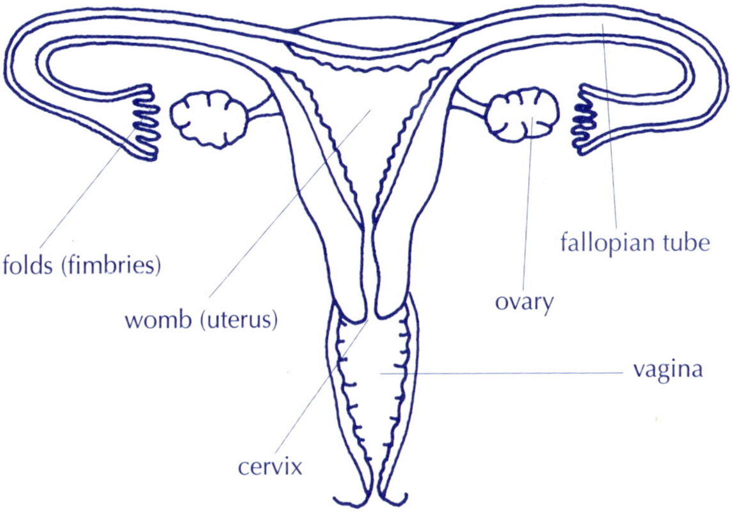

Figure 1.1: Female reproductive organs.

fertilisation of an egg by a sperm usually occurs. The fallopian tubes are on both sides of the womb, reaching backward and downward to the ovaries. The eggs are stored and mature in the ovaries. The ovaries are gonads with hormonal secretion and cycles. Hormones from the ovaries influence the womb, milk glands and vagina. A woman is usually born with 400,000 immature eggs.

The menstrual cycle is a hormonally governed process in which areas of the brain (especially the hypothalamus and the pituitary gland) and the target gonads collaborate. The hypothalamus produces, as a result of outer and inner influences, a hormone that releases gonadotropin (GnRH). This then stimulates, in the pituitary gland, the production of two basic gonadotropins—the follicle-stimulating hormone (FSH) and the luteinising hormone (LH)—which control the whole process leading toward the release of an egg (oocyte).

The amount and the specific function of both FSH and LH change in the course of the menstrual cycle. There are three phases:

1. The follicular phase-FSH stimulates the growth of the follicle, in which the egg develops and matures until the ovulation phase. Oestrogens also develop in the follicle at this time. Around the middle of the menstrual cycle, these oestrogens, among their other effects,

cause a change in the cervical mucus that makes it possible for sperm to develop and move in the mucus.

2. The ovular phase: after a pronounced increase in the level of LH, which is about the 14th day after the first day of menstruation, ovulation occurs. A mature egg is released from the follicle and, prepared for fertilisation, it travels toward the womb. A human egg can be fertilised about 24 hours after ovulation.
3. The luteal phase: after ovulation, the follicle changes into the so-called yellow body (corpus luteum) which, in addition to oestrogens, also produces the hormone progesterone. Both of these hormones affect the lining of the womb (endometrium) so that it is prepared to accept the fertilised egg and support its further development.

When fertilisation does not occur, the corpus luteum stops functioning around the 26th day of the cycle. During menstrual bleeding, parts of the endometrium leave the womb along with the unfertilised egg.

The male reproductive organs create male gametes (sperm), produce male sexual hormones, and enable fertilisation. The male reproductive organs are inside as well as outside of the body. The testicles are located within the scrotum. The sperm and the hormone testosterone are produced in the testicles. From the testicles, the sperm move into the complex channels of the epididymis (a tube attached to the back of the testicle) where they remain until they have completely matured. Then they travel through the gonaduct (vas deferens) into the gonecysts where they are preserved. The whole process of the creation and maturation of sperm takes about 10 weeks. In ejaculation, the sperm are released from the gonecysts and are mixed with a thick liquid from the prostate; this forms the semen, which passes into the vagina during sexual intercourse.

The creation of sperm is controlled by a hormonal process in which parts of the brain and the target gonads collaborate, similar to the menstrual cycle of women. As a result of external and internal influences, the hypothalamus produces a hormone that releases gonadotropin. This then stimulates the production of two basic gonadotropins: follicle-stimulating hormone (FSH) and luteinising hormone (LH). FSH and LH affect the function of testicles: FSH stimulates the production of sperm in the Sertoli cells, and LH influences the creation of testosterone in the Leydig cells. In the Sertoli cells, the immature sperm change into mature forms, called spermatozoa, which gain the ability to move actively in the channels of the epididymis.

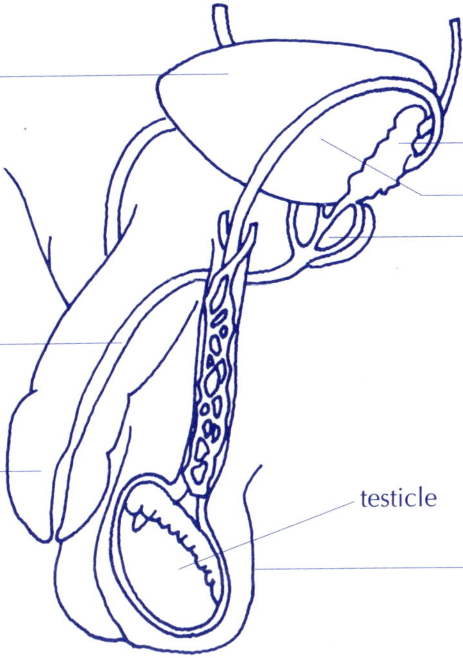

Figure 1.2: Male reproductive organs.

Only when all of the factors described above work well and cooperate can a successful fertilisation, pregnancy and birth take place. If a dysfunction occurs in any part of these processes or in the cooperation of the various factors, the likelihood of a positive result is greatly diminished.

To Sum Up

Let's review the things that are necessary for a human being on the quest for a child:

1. A heterosexual partner. Modern medicine can bypass this requirement on the quest for a biological child. This may also depend on ethical and legal norms in your area. In some countries, it is possible for a single or homosexual person to undergo assisted reproductive technologies (ART), in others the condition for this therapy is a heterosexual couple and, in others, it is essential to be heterosexual and married.

> After about four years of being in a relationship, we agreed that we would widen our family. When my girlfriend was not successful in getting pregnant, she went to see her doctor. After an examination, the doctor sent us to a specialist who examined us both, and, since we learned that it is necessary to be married for procedures like artificial fertilisation, we organised a wedding. (m)

On the quest for an adopted child, the customs are also different around the world. Often a single person can apply for adoptive parenting, but applicants must fulfil other conditions, which will be discussed in a separate chapter.

2. The capability of and consent to fertilisation. Medicine can bypass the condition of capability of fertilisation and whether it may do this depends on ethical and legal norms in a particular area. Consent is a different matter. Sometimes one of the partners is not interested in having a child.

> We want a brother and so does Mom. She keeps telling Dad that nature is calling. But Dad always replies that he can't hear anything. (f)

Even though medicine can bypass the lack of interest of one of the partners, it may not do so for ethical reasons in some countries.

> A beautiful young woman came into the infertility clinic and asked for 'artificial fertilisation'. The interview revealed that her husband is so busy that he isn't at home much, and if he is, he is so exhausted that he isn't interested in sex. She excluded the possibility that her husband didn't want a child or that he had a lover. (p)

For the latest technological treatments, a medical indication is necessary in many countries.

3. Sperm capable of fertilisation. When a man has a reduced sperm count, reduced sperm motility or sperm shape abnormalities, or when the sperm are clustered together, specialists speak about pathosperm. If there is no mature sperm in the ejaculate, then the physician will write the term azoospermia in the medical report. This dysfunction is caused by a problem either in the creation or in the transport of sperm. This is a condition that medicine can treat and, when this is not successful, can bypass. It is technically possible to use sperm from a donor. Whether this is also permissible depends on the ethical and legal norms in your area.

4. An egg capable of fertilisation. Some women suffer from an irregular behaviour of the ovaries, caused by a dysfunction of the hormonal, nervous or immunological systems. Modern medicine can treat and/or bypass this condition. It is technically possible to use eggs from donor women. Whether this is also permissible depends on the ethical and legal norms in your area.
5. Unobstructed, correctly functioning genital passageways. The sperm has a long way to travel towards an egg. It has to get from the testicles to the vagina, pass through the cervix and the womb into the fallopian tubes, where it is to meet the egg. Thc complicated pathway can be made difficult or obstructed by, for example, a problematic environment in the vagina. The motility of the sperm can be reduced, they may become immobile or completely annihilated. Finally, if the fallopian tube is blocked, the sperm will not meet the egg at all. Modern medicine can treat or bypass this condition, as well. The egg can be fertilized by the sperm outside the body and the embryo can be implanted in the woman's uterus. Whether this is also permissible depends on the ethical and legal norms in your area.
6. Suitable conditions for the implantation and development of an egg. According to statistics, 15–20% of detected pregnancies end within the first 20 weeks by a spontaneous miscarriage. The cause of the tendency to miscarry may be on the side of the foetus—usually it is a genetic cause—or on the side of the mother, who does not have suitable conditions for the implantation of the fertilised egg and its further development in the endometrium.

This is also a condition that medicine can treat and, if necessary, bypass. It is technically possible to implant the embryo in the womb of another woman. Whether this is also permissible depends on the ethical and legal norms in your area.

Do Nerves Play a Role?

Many people consider the first and second criteria listed in the previous section to be the only conditions for achieving pregnancy: a heterosexual partner and both partners' capability of and consent to fertilisation. Infertility is then considered a special illness: not an illness in the classic sense, but an illness in the sense of incapability, especially in men, or in the sense of unwillingness, even if subconscious, especially in women.

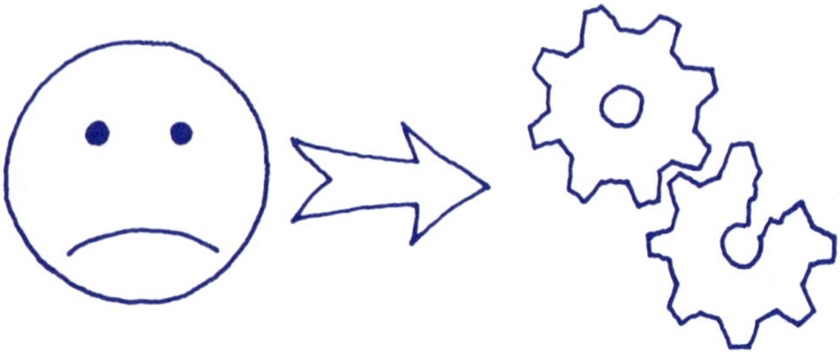

Figure 1.3: Mental causes of infertility problems.

Some kind of mental health problem is considered one of the main causes of infertility by many therapists, researchers, and patients. Sufficient evidence for this view is usually provided, for example, by fertilisation after adoption, fertilisation after the first visit to the clinic, after a change of physician, after making an appointment for a new therapeutic procedure, after psychotherapy, placebotherapy or medication. Some also point to disturbances of the previously regular ovular cycle after arranging in vitro fertilisation. This is a view that corresponds with what is called linear causality. When the psychological cause disappears, the problem disappears as well. You could imagine it would look something like this:

What Kind of Problem could it Possibly Be?

Perhaps I am not patient enough and we want it too much. (f)

I think that mental block is the cause in my case. (f)

The physicians didn't find anything in particular that could be a serious obstacle in getting pregnant. A possible reason could be stress. (f)

Unfortunately, I suffered from mental block. My menstruation, which I had lost after the wedding (and which was the reason I was undergoing treatment), returned after we adopted. (f)

It may have been partly a mental problem. (f)

I think that the subconscious is very strong. Even though, on a rational level, you try to suppress your feelings, for example when it is necessary to relax and not get stressed, subconsciously you still feel tension, doubt. (f)

We were not successful because of my attitude 'we must have a child now or never' and my partner's reaction 'I won't be forced into anything.' (f)

Subconscious ambivalence of intellectual women who are interested in their career. On top of that the pressure from the family. (p)

A female client in the *in vitro* fertilisation ward, the last opportunity before the permanent closure of the ward. She got pregnant because of the stress. (p)

A colleague can't get pregnant. She has lost weight, she looks 20 years older, she is stressed because of it. That must be the cause. (f)

A friend of mine got married late, she is not very pretty, not very assertive. With her, it must be mental. Her mother keeps saying: 'I am so much looking forward to grandchildren and still nothing.' It must be depressing for my friend. (f)

With them it was mainly her husband who was responsible for the failures because he was really mean to her. He put too much pressure on her, she got too fixated on the child. (f)

A friend's husband hasn't allowed adoption, it must stress her, and that's why the hope for success is lower. (f)

She miscarried from stress. (m)

For her sixth birthday we bought a dog for our first child and gave up our attempts to conceive (I had miscarried twice). After the party, I did not get my menstruation, now I have a second child. (f)

I got pregnant after I gave notice I would go back to work and enrolled my child in day care. (f)

I am convinced that, with me, it was a mental reason. I was too fixated on the child. After I decided to forget it and finally gave up, we were successful. (f)

Stimulation before the IVF was not successful (I didn't have a single egg) because my mother-in-law humiliated me, even though she knew that I was preparing for the IVF. (f)

I got naturally pregnant once but I miscarried. Now I keep failing, not even the IVFs were successful. It was a mental thing. (f)

With me it is a mental cause because the physicians haven't found anything and my husband is also fine. (f)

When I went the third time (for the IVF) I was completely relaxed, I even fell asleep there. I recalled how we'd been on a holiday at the sea, and that calmed me down. Everybody was convinced—now it was okay, now it must be a success—and it wasn't. (f)

My healer told me that the infertility was my husband's fault, that he feared subconsciously that he would lose his wife's affection. (f)

My wife miscarried out of joy, and her high fever was also out of joy. (m)

Mental reasons; now my wife got pregnant thanks to her happiness that we'd applied for adoption. (m)

Because we were putting it off—we were building up the nest—I've missed my chance. Now I am too fixated on the idea of becoming pregnant. (f)

[The intrauterine insemination] was under terrible conditions and the medical personnel behaved terribly, too (I was there seven times), I told myself, I don't want it this way. That must be why it wasn't successful. (f)

I was postponing children for after my career, now I know that I shouldn't have done that. (f)

I can't get pregnant because of a bad mother, the lack of love in childhood. (f)
People tell me that my miscarriages are due to stress, because I want the child too much and I worry that it's not going to turn out well. They tell me to 'relax, you shouldn't think about it,' etc. (f)
I have the impression that assisted reproduction is more successful in women who are currently under a lot of stress: a close relation has died, they have lost their job, they are moving, and so on. I also think that it is better if they continue to go to work after insemination or embryo transfer, when they are involved in their routines, than if they stay at home and try to take it easy. (p)
I am also stressed by the physicians, they have a significant share in it. (f)

It is interesting to look at why people think that the causes of infertility problems are mental factors. Those who are not personally affected designate the psyche as a reason because of their lack of knowledge and because they need to somehow rationalise the problem. Most other people confuse the idiopathic sterility, which is the case when the cause is not known, with psychogenic sterility. On the one hand, the designation of a mental cause offers some hope for recovery because treatment (for example psychotherapy) is available. On the other hand, as with any other illness, it is usually difficult for people to come to terms with the designation of a mental cause.

According to the testimonies, it is possible to divide the mental causes of infertility dysfunction into two groups. The first group considers the cause to be some kind of inner conflict. The second group assumes that the cause is some kind of outside pressure or stress that is too much for the particular person to handle. Stress is socially more acceptable.

The main inner conflict is supposed to be ambivalence toward motherhood ('Because we were putting it off—we were building up the nest—I've missed my chance' 'I was postponing children for after my career, now I know that I shouldn't have done that'), or ambivalence toward fatherhood ('He feared subconsciously that he would lose his wife's caring'), which is often blamed, for instance, on bad upbringing ('Because of a bad mother, the lack of love in childhood').

The source of stress can be the therapist ('I am also stressed by the physicians, they have a significant share in it'), the performance of the therapeutic procedure ('At the IUI—which was under terrible conditions and the medical personnel behaved terribly, too, I told myself, I don't want it this way. That must be why it wasn't successful'), the partner ('With them it was mainly her husband who was responsible for the failures because he was really mean to her' 'A friend's husband hasn't allowed adoption, it must stress her, and that's why the hope for success is lower'), the family ('Her mother keeps saying: "I am so much looking forward to grandchildren and still nothing." It must be depressing for my friend' 'Stimulation before the IVF was not successful (I didn't have a single egg) because my mother-in-law humiliated me') the situation ('A female client in the artificial fertilisation ward, the last opportunity before the permanent closure of the ward. She got pregnant because of the stress'), but also the woman herself ('We were not successful because of my attitude: we must have a child now or never' 'My wife miscarried out of joy, and her high fever was also out of joy' 'Now I am too fixated on the idea of becoming pregnant'). After the removal of the stress factor and despite expectations of good results, pregnancy does not necessarily follow ('Everybody was convinced—so now it was okay, now it must be a success—and it wasn't'), but it may follow ('My menstruation, which I had lost after the wedding (and which was the reason I was undergoing treatment), returned after we adopted,' 'We bought a dog for our first child and gave up out attempts to conceive (I had miscarried twice).' 'After the party, I did not get my menstruation, now I have a second child,' 'I got pregnant after I gave notice I would go back to work and enrolled my child in day-care,' 'I was too fixated on the child. After I decided to forget it and finally gave up, we were successful,' 'My wife got pregnant thanks to her happiness that we'd applied for adoption'), and, paradoxically, even a completely opposite effect of stress is mentioned ('A female client in the in vitro fertilisation ward, the last opportunity before the permanent closure of the ward. She got pregnant because of the stress,' 'Assisted reproduction is more successful in women who are at the moment under a lot of stress: a close relation has died, they have lost their job, they are moving, and so on'). I would like to emphasise that even a lot of joy is considered to be a stress factor ('My wife miscarried out of joy, and her high fever was also out of joy')!

The opinions of specialists can be divided into two main groups: the dynamically oriented and the stress oriented. The specialists' ways of interpreting the contextual circumstances parallel those of the general public.

Among the dynamically oriented group, it is said that women who suffer from functional sterility have subconscious anxieties and feelings of hostility concerning the birth of a child. These anxieties and feelings then affect the function of the ovaries or the fallopian tubes or they can suppress the women's interest in having sexual intercourse during her fertile period. The cause of infertility is considered the women's lack of acceptance of their own womanhood. 'If a woman does not get pregnant even though she wants to, she is either subconsciously defensive or her desire is not honestly motivated. A dishonest motivation is, for example, the effort to keep a partner or move marital problems into the background. In such cases the body responds more honestly and perspicuously,' say psychoanalysts[1]. Other psychological factors that are often linked with infertility are: emotional immaturity, the aggressive masculine type, the feminine erotic type, identification with a hostile mother, not the mothering type. It is necessary to emphasise that attempts to support these opinions with objective evidence have so far failed.

Is stress to blame for infertility? The defenders of the stress oriented group say 'yes'. To support their theories, they cite the disruption of the menstrual cycle of flight attendants, students who study too much, women far away from home, women who have arranged to undergo IVF, or 'war amenorrhoea'. There are studies that show that infertile women have a higher anxiety level than women who already have children. Another study shows that functional infertility is linked with higher anxiety levels than organic infertility.

I believe that studies devoted to providing evidence of psychogenic sterility have methodological errors. First, it is difficult to differentiate the effects from the causes, a difficulty these studies fail to address. I think that when psychological examinations of infertile women find problems with their acceptance of the feminine or mothering role, it is mainly the consequence of a difficult situation. How can a woman who is denied motherhood be reconciled with the mothering role? Similarly, research that compares the neurotic indexes in infertile women and in women who have children confuses causes with effects. It is entirely understandable that people who live with a chronic illness (such as infertility), without successful treatment, are mentally exhausted. It is difficult then to compare these people with a group of healthy people (and, moreover, happy parents). It is also likely that a person who knows the exact cause of his or her illness and has a way of solving the problem will be mentally better off than a person who does not have an idea of what is going to happen.

Second, these studies do not include discrepancies and negative examples. The theory that only suitable people in suitable circumstances will have children does not explain the fact that women get pregnant after rape or during war, that there are many abused and lonely children, and that there are so many abortions.

Finally, they forget about the time factor[2]. Very few couples have zero chance of the women becoming pregnant; mostly their fertility is more or less reduced. Thus, according to the probability theory, they are not completely without hope and it is a question of time and the number of attempts

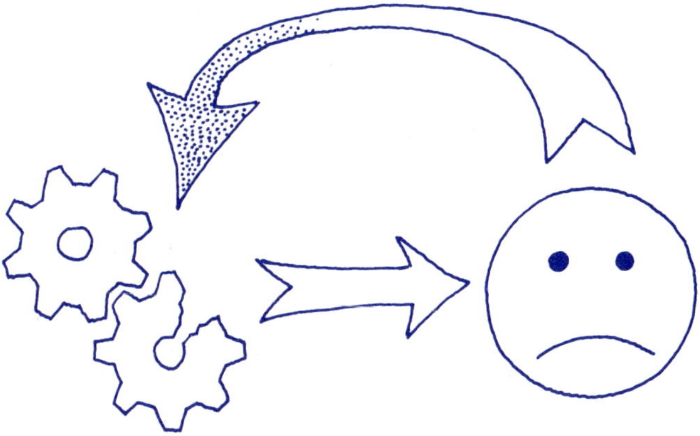

Figure 1.4: Mental consequences of infertility problems.

(and luck) where and when the chance will be lucky. Consequently, unexpected pregnancy following adoption need not necessarily be caused by a change in the psychological conditions, but only a 'factor of time'.

I suggest that the previous picture be changed to reflect this:

And there is one more aspect of psychogenic infertility. Psychological processes do not only include emotions; psychological processes include our knowledge, thinking and decision making. For example, if we decide to smoke, this is a psychological process. Smoking reduces fertility and should be considered one of the psychogenic causes of fertility disorders. However, traditionally, psychogenic causes are considered only some strange, mysterious processes converting negative emotions into illness.

Trying to resolve personal problems and learning how to handle stressful situations with a dispassionate attitude are generally beneficial efforts that should be recommended. In view of the complexity of the relationship between the psyche and infertility and in view of the level of contemporary knowledge, it is necessary to reject the speculative designation of mental disharmony as a cause of infertility[3]. First, we must exclude all of the well-known and proven causes of infertility; only then can we look at mental disharmony as one of the possible causes.

> When I told my friends that I cannot get pregnant, they said it was because of stress. So I was stressed that I get stressed. Then I thought about it and told myself that this was nonsense. I was not stressed at the beginning at all! I knew very well that one cannot become pregnant on the first attempt

and I was doing quite alright for the first three-quarters of the year. Only now I am so nervous! (f)

Is There any Meaning to All of This?

'And when He closes a womb, it is only that He may open it wondrously later.'

The Gospel of the Nativity of Mary

When we find ourselves in a difficult situation, we wonder how we got into it (causality). Sometimes we even meditate about the meaning of this situation (finality). Only a few people think that infertility can have a certain purpose, and even fewer can imagine what that purpose might be. My interest in this viewpoint has been prompted by the testimony of a man who said that he did not have a child because he did not deserve it yet. I asked him if the situation occurred so that he could improve himself and deserve a child, he replied yes. Does anyone else have a similar opinion?

So far I haven't discovered the 'why'. There must be some purpose, but I have no idea what that might be. (f)
So that I would not spoil the child. So that I could devote myself to something else, but to what? (m)
I think that everything has its reasons. (f)
I've come to the conclusion that if I am unable to have my own children, it is so that I can devote myself better to those entrusted to me (I am a teacher). (f)
I am a believer, I believe that there is a meaning to it (four miscarriages), perhaps I'm not mature enough yet. (f)

If people see any meaning in having to undergo the quest for a child, it is as an opportunity for their personal growth or for the fulfilment of some other tasks.

SOMEWHERE THE JOURNEY WILL END,
BUT THE WAY WILL STAY HIDDEN
UNTIL YOU GET THERE

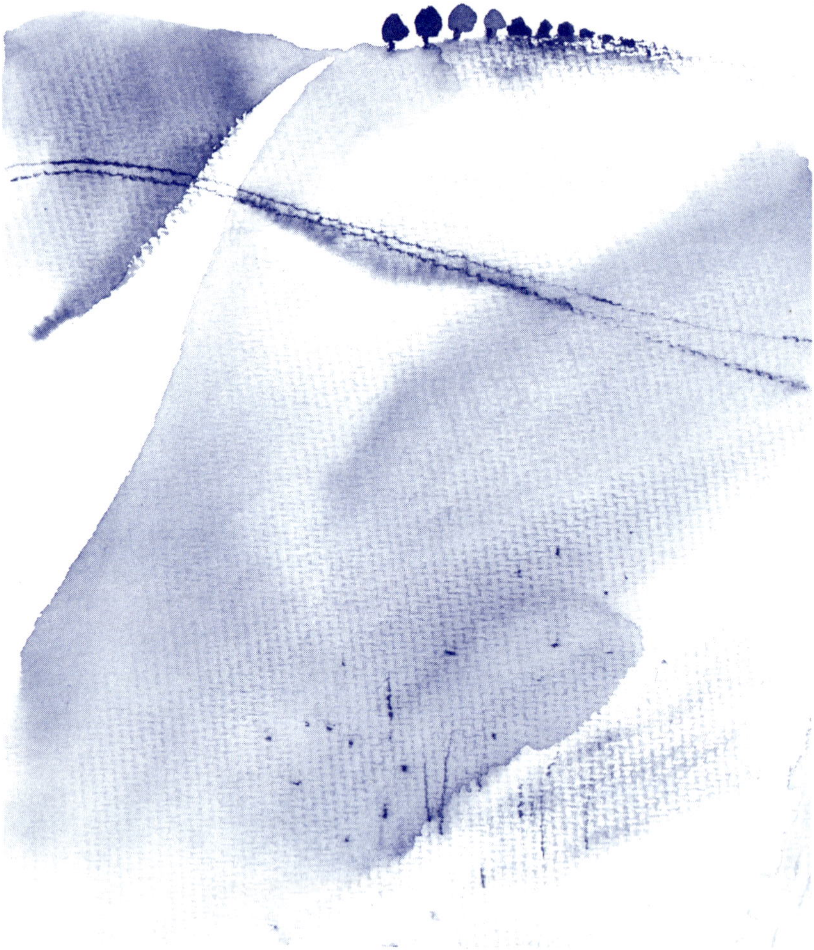

Somewhere the Journey Will End, But the Way Will Stay Hidden Until You Get There

Once upon a time, there was a man, his name was Bukhur, and everything he touched came to life and blossomed. And when Bukhur got married and brought Mara to his home, and she brought with her all she knew, you would not find a prettier house and farm than theirs in the whole area. But there is no winter without frost and no human without suffering! Time flew by and Bukhur's whitewashed house and Mara's garden that was like a brightly woven carpet suddenly seemed under a spell. Everything was swept, there was not a speck of dust anywhere, and the silence—not even a little cry! If only there were someone here to cry and bring some mud over the threshold, and break and throw things around, what shall I say, you know well what I mean. I'll say only so much that a godsend descended on Bukhur and Mara out of the blue and that Mara's two arms were not enough to hold it.

One afternoon, when Bukhur was on his way to get something in the neighbouring village, just a few steps behind the backyards he saw a tiny old man sitting by the road. Right away Bukhur knew that the old man was a stranger. He greeted him politely and said, 'If you are going far, grandfather, and if you need a bit of rest, just go down the hill a little ways, and in the first house you'll find my wife. Mara will serve you as it suits a guest.'

'Thank you, son, thank you,' replied the old man, 'I look frail, don't I, but I have no pain and I do not need anything. But you look like you could pull up trees and yet I can see that you are suffering. Tell me what it is and I'll help you!'

'I'll tell you gladly, it'll be a relief,' said Bukhur, 'it's been gnawing at me like a bad illness. You know, grandfather, I've been worrying terribly because we have no children.'

'You shall have them!' said the old man. 'And what else do you wish for? I can fulfil three wishes for you.'

'Children, grandfather,' said Bukhur, 'I really do not need anything else!'

'Boy, think carefully, think carefully! I ask you for the third and the last time. What else do you wish for?' And Bukhur whooped and threw his hat above his head: 'Children and only children, so that the house is full of them!'

Suddenly he stopped, surprised. His hat was in his hand, but the old man was no longer sitting by the road, there was not a living soul around.

'I worry everywhere I go,' said Bukhur to himself, and now I've started losing my mind.'

At home, 100 children were waiting for him.

'How Father Bukhur Fed His Hundred Children',
V. Adascalitei, *Weaving, Weaving Fairy Tales*

'After the wedding, we will stop using birth control and have a child.' What a simple plan. Not this month, we are going to a dance, and I do not want to be worried about one or two glasses. Not the next one, we want to enjoy the last quiet holiday for a long time to come. Not even in September, I will be taking an exam in Spanish and do not want to add to the stress by worrying about morning sickness. In October, yes in October we will get started. But October does not work out, or November, or even December, January, February. Just as previously you had your mind filled with all kinds of tasks and interests, now you can think only about children, children, children, like Bukhur from the fairy tale. Fortunately, today we do not have to rely on accidentally running into a magic old man, but have a range of diagnostic and therapeutic options. But we are going to discuss those in the next chapter. For now, let us look closely at the map.

A Map of the Quest for a Child

I had promised that I would provide you with a reliable walking map. I am not sure whether you expected the kind of map that I have created, but hopefully you will be able to orient yourselves. It will be easy for those with an understanding of programming.

A small oval indicates the beginning and the end of the trail. A small rectangle means some activity (for instance, choosing a therapist, undergoing treatment). Finally, a rhombus is a crossroad, a point at which you have to make a decision. These signs are connected by lines with arrows that show the direction you could go.

Psychologists sometimes divide mental activities into acting, experiencing and knowing. The map follows this division.

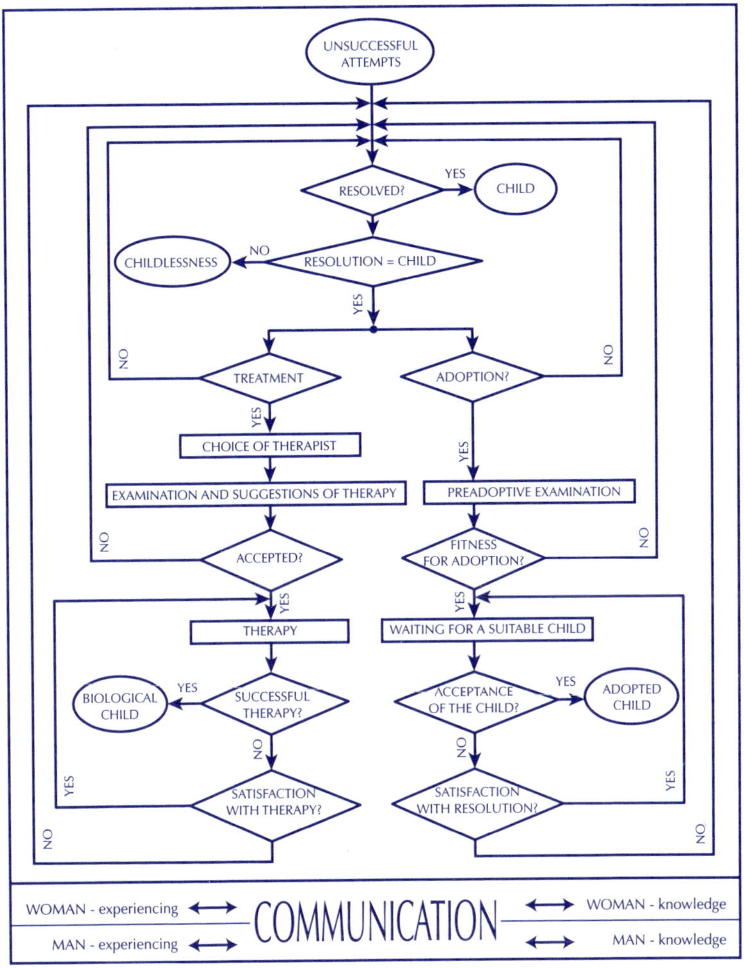

Figure 2.1: A map.

Acting on the quest for a child refers to the respective steps that you may take. Usually, you first establish that you are not succeeding (unsuccessful attempts), then you decide how to resolve the situation, then you engage in the process of resolving it and in the end the solution is achieved and you find yourselves at the end of the quest. If only it could be done as quickly as it is said! A detailed description of the individual steps will be provided in the next chapter.

The seemingly illogical placement of the question whether the situation is resolved immediately after unsuccessful attempts has its reasons. It often happens that after a certain period of unsuccessful treatment a couple chooses adoption as an alternative solution of the situation and enters into the adoption process without interrupting the treatment. It may then happen that, during the adoption process or while waiting for a suitable child, the couple have their own child. They stop the adoption process, they do not wait for the adoption or do not accept the adoptive child (but sometimes they do). The situation is resolved. Of course, the opposite can happen as well when, during treatment, a couple adopt a child and after the adoption they terminate the treatment. To make it possible to resolve such situations in the diagram, I had to place the question about the resolution of the situation before the decisions about the mode of solution.

Everything that happens to us and everything we do, including the quest for a child, creates some feelings in us and influences our experiencing. Of course, this also holds true the other way round—our experiencing more or less influences our decisions and what we do.

But it is not just our feelings that influence our everyday actions. We also decide according to our knowledge about the particular issue. In this case, knowing does not mean an awareness of a dry piece of information but information formed by our own mode of perception, the current situation, our relationship with the source of the information, our emotions. When you try to explain something to a group of people in which each member has a different personality and each is in a different mood, you can be sure that each person will understand what you say differently.

Our personal knowing is formed by a system of our opinions, our prejudices, attitudes, and values. Similar to the relationship between acting and experiencing, the influence between acting and knowing is mutual. Our knowing influences our acting and, vice versa—our acting enriches our knowing.

The diagram does not capture all the alternatives. For example, it would be hard to show the frequent situation when a couple is undergoing several kinds of treatment with various therapists at the same time, often without the therapists' awareness (such as combining hormonal treatment, the Mojzis method, and acupuncture; it is also common to work with several different gynaecologists at the same time). Hopefully, it will not be difficult for you to adapt the map to your own situation.

Apart from certain forms of foster care, it still takes two to gain a biological child. Infertility is a special kind of illness, for it is an illness of a couple. Even when the cause of the illness (the lack of success on the quest for a child) is on the side of only one partner, the whole couple is ill. Even when sometimes only one partner undergoes treatment, he or she is solving a problem of the couple. Each person has a special, individual, different way of experiencing and knowing. Thus, as a couple you have two ways of experiencing, two ways of knowing, but always only one way of acting that is common, on behalf of both of you. It is the age-old situation: you have to decide what furniture to buy, or where to go on your holiday. You did not have the option of buying two sets of furniture and you could not be together if one were to go to the sea and the other to the mountains. You had to look for a common solution.

What Can You Find in the Map?

'Somewhere the journey will end, but the way will stay hidden until you get there' is a line from a song. When you get a bit oriented in the map, you will realise that the quest for a child eventually leads to three possible destinations: your own child, an adopted child, and childlessness. I want to use bold and large letters now to draw attention to the fact that none of these destinations is inferior to the others. The sooner you accept this, the better, because then you will avoid running into a dead-end when, for example, all the available therapeutic methods have failed you or you do not have any more money for another IVF cycle. You will always have an option. However, accepting the option to adopt a child or stay childless is a task for strong people, and it can take a long time to achieve. I will talk about this in the next chapter, and, more importantly, I will share with you the testimonies of people who have lived through it. When I encourage you right at the beginning to consider various options, I do not want to suggest that you should give up the quest for your own biological child early on. The other way round! You must not give up or lose faith; you have to struggle and do your best. For you to have enough strength for a long fight, it is necessary to have several irons in the fire, that is, to think ahead.

You will notice that there are quite a few crossroads in the map. Usually you make the decisions. Therefore, you are not helpless, as it may often seem, but the quest for a child is, to a large degree, in your own hands! The map shows clearly whether you are going in circles (for instance, the first IVF, the second IVF, the ninth, the fifteenth—one client said that she had 19 treatments) and whether you are using all the opportunities to decide. When we realise that we have freely and consciously decided, we feel more in control of the situation. Often when people make a decision, they do not realise that they themselves have made the decision. They feel that they are being weighed down by fate. Then they refuse to take their future into their own hands and expect others to decide for them. And then they start feeling sorry for themselves…

The quest for a child is almost always a journey of two people who have different ways of experiencing and knowing. For optimal decision making and acting, it is necessary to communicate with each other. Even when people do not talk about their problems together, they communicate. But the probability that they will find an optimal solution through such communication is, of course, reduced.

I hope that the previous section has not weighed you down so much that you are thinking about giving up this book-length quest for a child. If you are tired, take a break and relax for a while.

I'll Toss a Coin

> *Once upon a time, there was a father and a mother, and they had a farmhouse, a pretty farmhouse, quite free of debts. They had lived together for ten years, but they did not have any children. When they saw that there was no one to keep running the farm, the mother said, 'Listen father, since we have no children, we could just live easily and fritter away the farmhouse in food and drink so that nothing is left when we die.' 'And so we could, dear mother,' he said, 'you are quite right.'*
>
> 'Two Keys', Josef Štefan Kubín,
> *A Book of Fairy Tales*

After 10 years, the couple from the fairy tale decided that they would enjoy life without children. When and what do real couples plan?

> I've formed no particular plan, perhaps we'll find out in time that we want to adopt a child. We'll see, at the moment it's hard to say. Otherwise there's a whole range of activities, both work related (especially for me) and social ones. (m)
>
> We're thinking of adoption. On the other hand, I am afraid of this step. (f)
>
> We've submitted an application for adoption. We thought about it for a long time, and we consulted it with a female acquaintance who has an adopted child. (f)
>
> I haven't much of an idea. I have not yet reconciled myself to such an option, I don't want to, really. I am considering adoption, but right now I am not able to accept it. (f)
>
> Yes, adoption. We were both for it and planned everything together. (m)
>
> I was planning to become a nurse and later a mother in an SOS children's village—if I can fulfil all the requirements and if I am mentally strong enough. (f)

I didn't have a clear plan. I always had the opportunity to repeat the IVF. Perhaps, in the extreme case, I would want my husband to find a woman with whom he would be able to have children, and I would look for a man with a child. I don't know, I don't have any other ideas. (f)

I had a plan, I wanted adoption, but my husband didn't want it. In this situation, both must want the same, that's why I gave in. A chance would have been a child from a test tube, but at the time when the experimenting had finished and the method was being introduced into practice, I'd passed the age limit for this kind of treatment. (f)

We didn't undergo treatment, we knew that no treatment would have helped. The decision was very spontaneous and unanimous, we adopted a child. (f)

We've remained childless. The solution has come with the passing years. I cannot really call it interruption of treatment. (f)

The couple wanted to place an advertisement in a magazine saying that they were looking for a surrogate mother who would give birth to their baby. (p)

We already have two children of our own. For nine years we have wanted a third; if we aren't successful soon, we'll probably take a child into foster care. (f)

I've not been able to imagine adoption so far, I can't imagine that I would accept somebody else's child. It is still too early, we haven't yet exhausted all the therapeutic and diagnostic methods. But we got some information about adoption in advance. (m)

We're planning adoption, but so far there is still time. (f)

I have no idea. I don't know how many more times I'll have the IVF (she says she has had it 19 times, she is 45 years old [author comment]. (f)

I have applied for adoption, next year it should work out. We were at one, there was nothing to discuss. (f)

I strongly believe in it [treatment], so I am not thinking about other options. I simply believe that we'll have our own children. But if not, I would go for adoption. (f)

I don't even admit to myself the possibility that the treatment might be unsuccessful, I've rejected adoption. (f)

We've applied for adoption, I assume we'll have a child within two years. Unless our own child comes within that time, we'll be happy, I believe, even with an adopted child. I am more anxious about us remaining by ourselves than about adoption. (m)

I've been trying to reconcile myself to it for a rather long time. I won't do anything extraordinary, probably I'll devote more time to my husband. (f)

My husband was clear about his desire for an adopted child much earlier than I was. Basically it could be said that he 'was waiting for me'. I perceived this and it wasn't always pleasant for me, I felt myself to be the one who is slowing things down. (f)

My friend's husband didn't allow adoption. (f)

At times, the woman wants to and the man doesn't. Mostly men are somewhat less able to accept somebody else's child, they often do it because of the wife. (p)
Before the wedding, we went through courses for engaged couples where we also dealt with the question of what we would do if we could not have a child. We agreed on adoption. Now that the problem has really occurred after our wedding, my husband is for adoption and I am not yet, I am worried that I wouldn't be good to the child. (f)
I've refused adoption. (m)
We learned about incurable infertility two years after the wedding, and we did not submit an application for adoption until another six years later. The six years was a period of reconciliation and search, and also of active testing out various options. I'd even want to say that we would have been able to be happy even childless, but we would have had to finally accept it, to discover joy in childlessness, enter in it, and accept it as a gift. And this is the either/or that we had been deciding on. (f)
We've stayed childless. When I was celebrating my 40th birthday, my husband got tipsy and told me: 'I was always waiting for you to bring home a little Gypsy girl.' I was shocked, I would have never imagined that he would be for adoption.(f)
My husband is for adoption, but I do not have the courage so far. (f)
We went though several IVFs, without success. We said no to adoption, we are both quite ambitious, we wouldn't be able to cope with the fact that the child might not be clever. So we completely devote ourselves to work. (m)

When does an involuntarily childless person start considering alternative ways of resolving the situation? The timing can differ greatly. There are people who consider the issue even before they discover that it applies to them ('Before the wedding we went through courses for engaged couples where we also dealt with the question of what we would do if we could not have a child'), people who consider the alternatives after they have learned the diagnosis ('We didn't undergo treatment, we knew that no treatment would have helped'), after a few months or years of unsuccessful treatment ('I've been trying to reconcile myself with it for a rather long time') and people, who do not consider the question even after many years of unsuccessful treatment, when the hope for success is slender ('I have no idea. I don't know how many more times I'll have the IVF,' 'The solution has come with the passing years. I cannot really call it interruption of treatment'). It seems that treatment by assisted reproduction has alleviated the urgency of the issue and postponed its resolution ('It's too early, we haven't yet exhausted all the therapeutic and diagnostic methods,' 'They were looking for a surrogate mother who would give birth to their baby,' 'I always had the opportunity to repeat the IVF').

What are the alternatives? Most people are thinking about some form of foster care ('I am more anxious about us remaining by ourselves than about adoption'), mainly adoption, rarely some other form ('I was planning to become a nurse and later a mother in an SOS village' 'I would look for a man with a child' 'We'll probably take a child into foster care'). Some choose childlessness ('Probably I'll devote more time to my husband' 'I've refused adoption' 'We wouldn't be able to cope with the fact that the child might not be clever').

The choice is usually accompanied by uncertainties and fears ('I am afraid of this step' 'We thought about it for a long time, and we consulted it with a female acquaintance who has an adopted child' 'I am worried that I wouldn't be good to the child' 'A period of reconciliation and search, and also of active testing of the various options'). It is especially difficult because infertility is an illness of a couple, and therefore the alternative must also be agreed upon by both partners. The partners' agreement can be easy ('We were both for it and planned everything together' 'Very spontaneous and unanimous' 'We were at one, there was nothing to discuss'), at times one spouse is more anxious than the other, or is less hesitant ('My husband was clear about his desire for an adopted child much earlier than I. Basically it could be said that he was waiting for me. I perceived this and it wasn't always pleasant for me, I felt myself to be the one who is slowing things down' 'My husband is for adoption, but I do not have the courage so far'). In some couples the partners' ideas for a solution are mutually exclusive, and so the final solution is always childlessness ('I wanted adoption, but my husband didn't want it. In this situation, both must want the same, that's why I gave in' 'I would even go for adoption, but my husband resolutely refuses').

An interesting testimony is the one before the wedding. Before the problem occurs, we may look at it one way (a mutual agreement on the alternative solution), but when we are suddenly personally confronted with it, we may see it differently ('Now that the problem has really occurred after our wedding, my husband is for adoption and I am not yet').

An unfulfilled desire for a child is a very intimate and sensitive matter, and it is very hard to admit to oneself even in one's thoughts that the final solution may perhaps not be the classic happy ending. Moreover, it is a matter that involves a couple, which means that it is extraordinarily demanding in terms of communication—what is difficult for a person to admit to oneself is even more difficult to talk about with another. But, without an open discussion, you will not come to an optimal solution. The following testimony brings this to our attention poignantly: I was always waiting for you to bring home a little Gypsy girl. I was shocked, I would never have imagined that he would be for adoption.

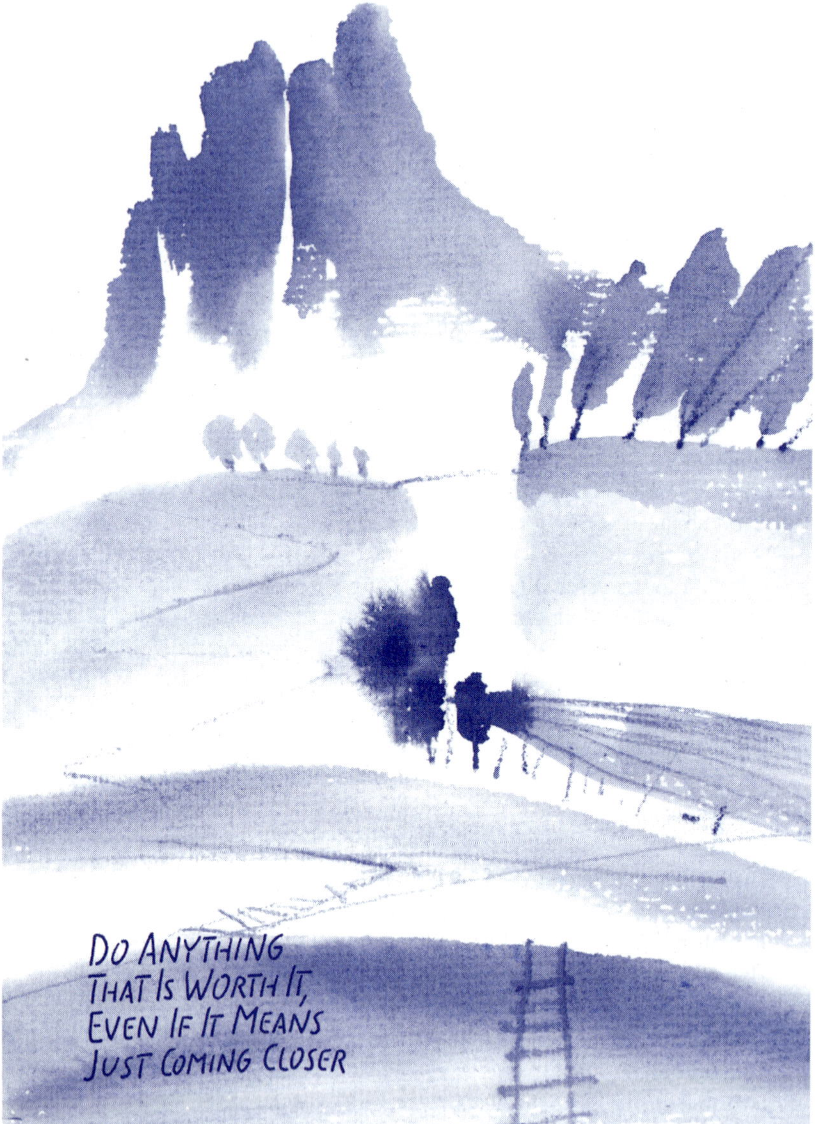
DO ANYTHING
THAT IS WORTH IT,
EVEN IF IT MEANS
JUST COMING CLOSER

Do Anything That is Worth It, Even if It Means Just Coming Closer

The kind king Ashvapahti was advanced in age, as was his wife, but they were still without descendants. He grieved much because of this, so once upon a time he visited a forest hermitage to consult with saints who, due to their repentance, know matters that remain secret and concealed to ordinary mortals. They advised him: Make your personal life more humble and disciplined: dress simply, give up excessive enjoyments, regularly bring sacrifices to gods, repent and fast. Such is godly life. He did so for eighteen years, and then they had 'a daughter'.

'How a Devoted Sahvitri Saved Her Spouse from the God of Death',
V. Miltner, *Legends of Ancient India*

The two small wings of the stork are not here. You have to set out after them yourselves. You will probably not go to visit a saint (where to look for them nowadays, anyway?). Nevertheless, you will talk to various people who you think may know your secrets and you will ask them about how you should solve your problem. I do not want to frighten you by suggesting that you will be given a similar advice to what king Ashvapahti received; nonetheless, you should not expect a walk in the park. As a psychologist, I do not recommend that you give up your fun, unless it is excessive or threatens your mental or physical health. As the title of this chapter says, it is certainly necessary 'to do anything that is worth it' (in your opinion), and to have patience, even though you perhaps will not have to wait 18 years as in the fairy tale.

This chapter describes what one experiences on the quest for a child and outlines the individual concrete steps that one may take. The therapy of involuntary childlessness means the resolution of the situation, and that is why we consider not only therapeutic methods in the common sense of the word, but also include solutions by foster care or by remaining without a child. Essentially, the chapter offers descriptions of various procedures. At the same time, therapy is not just a technical procedure. You will not decide to undergo even the most ingenious, and, according to the statistics, the most effective method, unless you yourselves can believe in it or unless you can trust the person who carries it out. Therefore, besides the procedure itself (including the application criteria), an important part of the therapeutic effect is the therapist (including his or her knowledge, experience, beliefs, and expectations), and the communication between the therapist and the client. We will deal with the role of the therapist and the communication with the client in the chapter 'My Mama Doesn't Know and She Mustn't Know'. The clients themselves will be discussed in the chapter 'Just After I Was Born…'

The Quest for a Biological Child

When you discover that your attempts to extend your family are to no avail, the first step is to try to find out why. Earlier, I said that fertilisation requires a heterosexual partner, the capability of and consent to fertilisation, sperm capable of fertilisation, an egg capable of fertilisation, unobstructed and correctly functioning genital passageways, and suitable conditions for the implantation and development of the egg. Therefore, you will start searching to see whether everything is fine and, of course, you will not search on your own but turn to specialists for help.

Each visit to the doctor means a certain loss of privacy. The conception of children is a very intimate matter, and that is why the examination and treatment of fertility problems is a far greater intrusion into one's privacy than, for example, the treatment of a broken finger.

The diagnosis of fertility problems

> Until now my wife and I have come into contact with physicians very rarely. Maybe the flu about once in five years, nothing else except for my knee surgery after a car accident. (m)

With tonsillitis you go to the GP, for your teeth you go to the dentist. Somewhat more experienced patients may know the orthopaedist who treats the pain in your knee after a football game, from childhood they may remember the 'ear doctor', the shortsighted know about the optometrist, and women regularly go to see the gynaecologist. But whom should you go to with an unfulfilled desire for a child? The first trip is usually to the gynaecologist, but often gynaecologists call on their colleagues from other fields to help, as well. Experts who take part in diagnosing the causes of infertility work in the following fields: gynaecology, andrology, immunology, endocrinology, sexology, urology, genetics, etc. Most often, you get inside the examination circle through the gynaecologist, the GP, the urologist, or the andrologist. The basic examination always includes the methods below.

A detailed medical history. This, despite all the technical possibilities, is one of the most important parts of establishing a correct diagnosis. The history of couples desiring a child should contain detailed information about the illnesses of close relatives, with an emphasis on the genetic impact and fertility problems. You should also discuss the illnesses that each partner has had and the present state of both partners' health, details about the drugs they are taking and about their diet and lifestyle. Also important is information about employment risks, sexual development and use of birth control, as well as about previous pregnancies and the sexual circumstances in the current relationship. Both partners should be present for the history to contribute to accuracy.

> Oligospermia was found in the man, his sperm showed practically no movement. I asked him about alcohol intake, but he answered negatively. A month later, the examination was repeated with the same result. The wife, who was present this time, asked me whether it couldn't be the impact of her husband's hot baths. Every time he goes in the tub, he says 'tssssss'. After another month, this time without the baths, the spermiogram was fine. If the wife had not been present at the [history] interview, the cause of the oligospermia would probably not have been found, and the couple would have had to undergo demanding treatment via the methods of assisted reproduction. (p)

Demands: the examination is not mentally or physically demanding if the physician is good at communicating. For many patients, this is the only pleasant part of the whole treatment.

> The doctor talked with us about all kinds of things and explained everything to us. He was even witty. After eight years of treatment, he was the first one to give us personal attention. (m)

Only after the conclusion of the history does the doctor plan other diagnostic steps. Therefore, do not be surprised that your acquaintances, who are also unable to conceive, may have undergone a different examination process (even though the individual examinations may be the same). It is simply that the conclusions of their histories were different. Now I will try to explain what may be in store for you. I will describe the diagnostic procedures as clearly as possible, always adding a note about their demands on patients and how the patients tend to perceive them.

The spermiological examination. This helps to discover whether there are sperm capable of fertilisation and whether there are enough of them. Nowadays, specialists claim that this should be the first diagnostic step right after the detailed history. The prerequisite for the examination of the ejaculate is a four-day abstinence from ejaculation. The sample should be gained by masturbation, kept in a clean glass and, if possible, immediately taken to the laboratory. What is observed is the overall volume, the number of sperm per millilitre, their motility, shape, capacity for survival, etc. The results oscillate and, even when everything is fine, two–three examinations are required. Sometimes, more detailed and comprehensive spermiological examinations are necessary, for instance microbiological, immunological, etc. Those are performed at specialised clinics. Recently, a home sperm test has become available. You can analyse the basic sperm parameters in the comfort of your home.

Demands: for some men, the clinical environment can cause problems.

> The clinic had a waiting room with exit doors on all sides: the main exit, the door to the examination room, to the lab, and also to the toilet. The collection of the sperm proceeded in such a way that the woman came out of the examination room into the waiting room with a cup, passed the cup to her waiting partner in front of all the waiting people, he went to the toilet, completed the task, then he walked across the waiting room in front of all the waiting people, passed the cup to his wife, and she took it to the examination room. My partner was a very tall man, the room inside was very small, and so every time he tried to begin to fulfil the task, he unwittingly leaned against the flat flushing button in the wall—and flushed—and it was easy to hear this in the whole waiting room. After flushing three times, he understood and came out and, after one look at his red face, I understood, and after that we would go to a beautiful place outside the city where the

collection proceeded wonderfully even in the snow, and we have the most beautiful memories of it. (f)

It is possible for a man to collect the ejaculate at home as long as he brings it within two hours after the ejaculation. The container should be transported in the dark, at a temperature close to body temperature. The laboratory notes that this is a sample that has been brought in, since there is no certainty that the sperm belongs to the man who has brought it in. But for some men, stress can be helpful.

The man (with a stout figure) was unsuccessful in his attempt to collect ejaculate in a clinical environment. I was trying to calm him down, saying that it didn't matter, and explaining to him how to bring the sperm from home. His wife (who was quite small) was present at this exchange and she resolutely refused this possibility. Before the eyes of the other five waiting couples, she pushed her husband back in. The waiting room fell completely silent. After some long, absolutely silent minutes, the man came outside successful, and everybody cheered. Even his wife smiled a bit, I think. (p)

However, for most men this examination is not a problem, as long as the place of collection is at least somewhat dignified. Some men said that various people kept entering the bathroom that was designated for carrying out the procedure and that it was impossible to lock the door. The methods of assisted reproduction have long been used in veterinary medicine and human medicine has taken advantage of this experience. Before it began to be used on a broader scale, physicians worked closely with veterinary professionals, especially in the area of examining the sperm.

In the early 1990s, I was sent for the ejaculate examination. The first surprise was that the examination was performed on the premises of a veterinary school. I was walking past various stables and, with a knowing expression, the female caretakers of the animals pointed out to me where to go. The next surprise was the doctor—a vet. The temporary examination room was the room of the specialist for the insemination of farm animals, decorated with models of animal sperm. Since I am by nature an inquisitive person, and I was not anxious about my problem, the visit with the kind vet was an opportunity for me to discover which animal sperm are similar in structure to the human ones, and which animal is the biggest 'stud'. But I wasn't the only human visitor, and I observed in many of the others that the circumstances of the examination were not that easily accepted. (m)

The basic physical examination. A physical examination of women and men is a common gynaecological or andrological examination of the genitals. The examination is helpful for gaining more information about the couple's history and for optimizing the diagnostic procedure.

Demands: the examination is not pleasant but, as far as I know, it does not cause problems for patients if they are informed about its content in advance.

> I was sent for an examination about which the doctor didn't tell me anything in advance. The specialist told me to take down my trousers and bend over. As I learned later on, he carried out an examination of my prostate *per rectum*. Since I hadn't been informed about the way and the goal of the examination, and since I'd never heard of the examination before, I was shocked, the examination was a nightmare. (m)

Nevertheless, for some people, even the most thorough information provided in advance may not be a guarantee against stress.

> I work as a nurse for a gynaecologist, so I know all the examinations very well. But when I go to my gynaecologist for a regular examination, I am so nervous that I even have to write the date of my last menstruation on my hand because I cannot remember anything at all in the examination room. (f)
>
> In fact there is a lot of information around, but sometimes it may be better not to know everything in such detail because usually you realise that it is even more complicated than you had supposed, and then you perhaps have a tendency to be even more sceptical. (f)

The examination of ovulation. Ovulation can be demonstrated, for example, by blood analysis, uterine mucus analysis and via ultrasound. Women themselves can find out whether ovulation occurs by taking basal temperatures or by using ovulation tests. Some women can recognise ovulation from the quality of the uterine mucus. Ovulation tests are urine tests that show the increase in luteinising hormone shortly before ovulation. These tests are easily available in pharmacies and they are highly reliable. Another test is to use basal body temperature. In the second part of women's menstrual cycle the body temperature rises, mainly caused by the thermogenic effect of the hormone progesterone. The increase in temperature is proof of ovulation and of a functioning corpus luteum, which is reliable proof of the normal activity of the ovaries. The difference between the minimal and the maximal temperature in the course of the cycle is

0.3–0.6°C (32–38°F). The increase occurs 24–48 hours, exceptionally 72–96 hours, after ovulation. One or two days before menstruation, the basal temperature drops again to the levels of the follicular phase. The woman herself takes the basal temperature daily after a peaceful sleep at the same time of the day immediately after waking up, before starting any activities or eating breakfast. The measured temperature is recorded in a calendar. It is possible to assess only the curves that have been obtained from measurements taken in the course of at least three menstrual cycles. The examination of ovulation via basal temperatures is quite a reliable, simple, and harmless. Its disadvantage is that it provides information about an ovulation that has already occurred.

Demands: the examination makes minimal demands on time (5 minutes every day). However, it has a great impact on the psyche, since the woman keeps closely observing herself and focusing even more on her goal to get pregnant. On the other hand, it can bring about a rewarding sense of the woman's own participation in the diagnosis and thus reduce the feeling of helplessness.

> When the patient came for the check-up, she brought me a huge roll of paper on which she had noted down her basal temperatures over the past ten years. For this desperate woman, taking her temperature was the only thing she could do so as not to feel completely helpless. (p)

I am always reminded how difficult it is to communicate matters connected to the diagnosis and treatment of infertility to those who have no personal experience with them. Recently I had a conversation with a colleague about recording ovulation using basal temperatures, and I expressed a strong aversion toward the method. I said that waking up day after day with a thermometer on the bedside table was stressful. He was surprised to hear that; his wife (a mother of two children) has been waking up this way for years and she does not consider it to be a burden in any way. He said the use of this method should be the same for all women, since it indicates the fertile and infertile days. One could agree with this statement on a purely informational level. But a thermometer on the bedside table is a completely different symbol for a woman who is trying to prevent pregnancy and for a woman who is trying to get pregnant. For a fertile woman, it is a symbol of the surplus of her procreative powers, which she is trying to control but, for an involuntarily childless woman, it is a symbol of failure and a constant reminder of the unavailability of the goal of her life.

The examination of the uterine mucus. This examination helps in determining whether the woman has eggs capable of fertilisation and whether sperm can pass through her genital passages. It serves, for instance, to establish the time of ovulation, examine the penetration of sperm, and for microbiological analyses. The aspiration of the mucus is performed using a syringe or the smear is taken from the cervix and from the vaginal fornix using a small cotton brush. A special kind of examination of the cervical mucus occurs the post-coitally; it can also establish whether the sperm are capable of fertilization (the collection is 3–15 hours after sexual intercourse; what is assessed is the amount and quality of the mucus, and the presence of antibodies and fertility problems in the man).

Demands: the examination is not painful and lasts only a few seconds. The disadvantage is that it is usually necessary to repeat the examination. For the post-coital test, the adjustment of the timing of the intercourse and the examination might be demanding.

The examination of the vaginal and the uterine environment. The vagina and the uterus (the womb) form a part of the pathway of the sperm toward the egg and the womb is where the fertilised egg nests and develops. Therefore, as with the environment at the cervix uteri, it is necessary to find out about the conditions in the vagina and the womb. The smear from the vagina is usually collected by a small cotton brush. Then it is sent to a laboratory for examination. Sometimes it is necessary to take a small sample of the tissue in the womb using a small sharp tool; this procedure is called a biopsy.

Sometimes, a curettage is performed, which means removing the complete surface of the uterus. As a diagnostic step, curettage helps in determining the stages of the menstrual cycle and in establishing the quality of the lining of the womb (endometrium) to see whether it is able to retain and nourish an embryo.

Demands: the smear and the biopsy are common outpatient examinations. Curettage is performed under complete anaesthesia; if everything goes well, the woman can go home in the evening (accompanied by another person). Otherwise, she stays over until the next day.

Blood examination. This method gives a detailed overview of the hormonal levels, infections, the presence of antibodies, immunity, genetic equipment, etc. Therefore, it is necessary for investigating the quality of sperm, the quality of eggs, the openness of the genital passageways and the ability to retain and nourish an egg. The blood test is also used to monitor the effect of the prescribed therapy. Demands: most people have had their blood taken, it is nothing new. The procedure is not pleasant, but most people do not mind it. The disadvantage is again the necessity of frequent repetition of the examination because certain indicators (for instance, the hormone level during the cycle) change. Waiting for the laboratory results, sometimes even for several weeks, can be a major mental burden. Possibly the most demanding kind of waiting is waiting for the results of the genetic examination.

Laparoscopy (the keyhole surgery). This enables a direct visual check-up of the abdominal and pelvic organs. In female fertility problems, laparoscopy has a dual purpose: diagnostic and therapeutic. In diagnosis it allows the doctor to determine about the openness and condition of the fallopian tubes, the development and location of the ovaries, uterine abnormalities, endometriosis and perform a check-up of ovulation by proving the corpus luteum, when there is suspicion of extrauterine pregnancy. It is used therapeutically to open obstructed fallopian tubes, correct the dysfunction of certain ovarian abnormalities, and remove endometriosis. The laparoscope is introduced through the abdominal wall, usually through 1–3 cuts through which the tools are introduced into the abdominal cavity, including a light source and a camera connected to a television screen and a video recorder. The surgeon watches the television screen and performs the procedure, using tools that are handled outside the abdominal cavity.

Demands: the intervention is carried out under complete anaesthesia, a one- or two-day hospitalisation is necessary, and the total time required off work is an average of one week. Usually laparoscopy is not painful, and the small scars left by the openings become almost invisible in one week.

Hysteroscopy. This procedure enables a direct observation of the uterine cavity. It examines the openness of the genital passageways of the woman, and the conditions for the embryo's implantation and development. The uterine cavity is widened, most often by the infusion of a gas, the hysteroscope is introduced, the cervix uteri and uterine cavity are observed, and the outlet of the fallopian tubes is located. Hysteroscopy can be used both in diagnosis and in therapy. For example, it can remove a septum within the uterus, or a benign tumour, etc.

Demands: the examination takes 3–5 minutes, it is performed under complete anaesthesia and one- to two-day hospitalisation is necessary. Hysteroscopy is sometimes done together with curettage (the removal of tissue from the vaginal wall), and sometimes with laparoscopy.

Hysterosalpingography. This is an x-ray image of the uterine cavity and the fallopian tubes. It is again helpful in exploring the openness of the woman's genital passageways and the conditions for the embryo's implantation and development. The womb, and sometimes the fallopian tubes, is filled with a contrasting material and x-rayed.

Demands: the examination is not performed under anaesthesia and, for some women, the filling with the contrasting material may be painful; after the examination, one- to two-day hospitalisation is necessary. The contrasting material is gradually absorbed; it is not toxic.

> I had a womb X-ray. When they were administering the contrasting material, it was painful. I complained to the nurse that they should have informed me about that, so that I could have mentally prepared for it. The nurse snapped at me, said I couldn't bear anything. (f)

Sonography. This procedure is better known as an ultrasound. It shows the inner organs via ultrasound on a screen. The wand is placed on the abdomen or the scrotum, or it is used internally in a vaginal or a transrectal (through the rectum) examination. The procedure is used for examining ovulation, the quality of the eggs, the openness of the genital passageways, the condition of the womb, the age and condition of the embryo and, in men, for examining the condition of the testicles and the prostate.

Demands: the examination does not burden the patients, it is not painful and no preparation is needed. The disadvantage is the need to repeat the procedure several times (in women several times during the cycle).

The examination of fertility problems is not as pleasant as a chat in a cafe. Nevertheless, the more methods we have, and the more precise they are, the better.

> Patients are sad when no cause is found. It is much worse for them. That's clear: the known enemy is half the enemy. When they do not know 'why', they lose hope. (p)

Therapies for Fertility Problems

Now you perhaps know why your have been having difficulties, and you are getting ready to undergo treatment. The following section describes what possible therapeutic methods you can undergo on the quest for a child. Of course, it depends on the conclusions of the diagnosis. As I did in the section about diagnostic methods, I again try to simplify things, but those who are interested in more detailed information will need to search further in other sources. Progress in this area is so rapid that the following information and the references to the literature might already be somewhat outdated; please consider them as just a basic guideline. I do not deal with the effectiveness of this or that therapy because that, of course, depends on how suitable it is for a particular person. In addition to the 'conventional' methods, I also include the 'unconventional' methods. I may upset some people by doing so, but many couples seek the unconventional methods of therapy as well and find hope in them. They seek anything that is, in their opinion, worth it. I am convinced that anything that offers hope to someone is worth our attention, although the attention should remain critical and observant. I use the word therapy and not treatment on purpose. The word therapy comes from the Greek *therapeia*, which means to heal or to treat.

1. Medical methods

The most basic and frequent therapeutic method is medical therapy, in which the kind of drug used is determined by the kind of illness. In the treatment of fertility problems, there are three main medical therapies: therapy of infection, therapy of immunological infertility and hormonal therapy.

A. Therapy of infection

The cause of failure to become pregnant can be inflammation of the reproductive organs. In women, discharges or inflammations change the acidity of the vagina and reduce its immunity, and the danger of transfer of the infection to the uterus arises. Inflammation of the cervix, the uterine body or the vagina results in the reduced motility of sperm or in their immobilisation. Inflammation of the fallopian tubes can often cause their irreparable obstruction. Inflammation of the ovaries can cause a hormonal imbalance. In men, infection in the exit channels of the testicles or the epididymis may cause oligospermia (fewer than normal sperm); if the infection is not treated, it can cause obstruction in the exit channels, the result of which can be azoospermia (no sperm at all).

Infection is diagnosed by blood analysis, spermiological examination, and microbiological examination of the vaginal environment, the uterine environment and the uterine mucus. As therapy, antibiotics and vitamins are administered locally and generally.

B. *Therapy of immunological infertility*

Together with the nervous and the endocrine systems, the immune system shares the task of maintaining balance in the inner environment—homeostasis—within the body. Its basic function is the ability to differentiate between harmful and beneficial elements. This ability manifests itself as: a system of defence (it recognises harmful external influences and protects the body against infections), immunity control (it continuously recognises harmful internal influences, i.e., it removes old and altered cells), and auto-tolerance (it recognises one's own tissues and maintains tolerance towards them).

There are three immunological causes of fertility problems:

a. Immune reaction against sperm. In a man, antibodies against one's own sperm can be found in the spermal plasma in cases of injury, inflammation, operation, tumours, etc. The antibodies cause the sperm to form clusters so that they cannot travel all the way toward the egg or they are stopped completely. The antibodies can also harm the acrosome (the sperm's head). Cellular autoimmunity against the tissue of the testicles and against the sperm disrupts, and in severe cases, completely annihilates, the creation of sperm. Sometimes, cellular autoimmunity can also limit the production of hormones in the testicles. For a woman, sperm are considered alien cells. In the case of a certain dysfunction of the immune system, the woman creates antibodies against the sperm (which are found for instance on the cervix uteri); this may cause the sperm to form clusters and lose their aggressive motility, which prevents them from reaching the released egg waiting in the fallopian tube in time.
b. Immune reaction against an egg. Even a woman's own mature egg might not be recognised by the her immune system as her own cell since, at the time of birth, when the immune system makes a certain audit of its own tissues, the eggs are not yet in the stage they reach later in the fertile age of the woman. In certain cases, the immune system then acts against the egg (specifically against its envelope, the so-called zona pellucida), which allows the sperm get to the egg but not inside of it because the zona pellucida is impenetrable for them.
c. Immune reaction against the embryo, specifically against the trophoblast (the cell layer important in early development of the embryo).

Through complex, mutually interacting regulatory mechanisms of the immune, hormonal, and central nervous systems, certain functions of the immune system are inhibited during pregnancy. If this were not the case, pregnancy could not occur since, to the woman's immune system, the embryo is an alien tissue. However, in some cases, sufficient protection of the development of the embryo and the foetus does not occur. Oversensitivity toward the components of sexual cells or their environment can very frequently lead to early miscarriage. It has been stated that 20–30% of repeated miscarriages have an immunological cause. An immunological cause also lies behind some late miscarriages (in the second or the beginning of the third trimester). Autoantibodies (antiphospholipid syndrome) can lead to a thrombotic (blood clotting) process in the veins and arteries that results in reduction of the blood circulation in the placenta. This then causes a disturbance in the nourishment of the foetus and consequently a miscarriage or a preterm birth.

The diagnosis and therapy of immunological causes

The basic examination is the post-coital test, which consists of the aspiration of the mucus from the uterine uvula 6–8 hours after unprotected intercourse. This is a way of finding out whether there are antibodies against sperm. This examination is performed at any assisted reproduction centre. For a special reproductive-immunological examination, it is necessary to collect the woman's blood, sometimes both partners' blood, as well as the sperm. This special examination is currently performed only at selected laboratories. If immunity against sperm is established, condom therapy is recommended (the use of a condom for a certain period to inhibit immunity against sperm), in combination with drugs called corticoids. Sometimes, intrauterine insemination is recommended. Corticoids are administered in cases of immunity against zona pellucida and against the trophoblast. Sometimes IVF, together with immunosuppressive treatment is recommended, which sharply increases the effectiveness of IVF in the indicated cases.

C. Hormonal therapy

Hormonal or endocrine therapy is used mainly in cases of infertility problems caused by hormonal insufficiency, which disturbs the progress of ovulation or the production of sperm. It can be used for hormonal stimulation or for substitution of the missing hormones that are necessary for conception. Some sources estimate that 40% of female fertility problems have a hormonal cause associated with insufficient activity of the ovaries, which are in a close relationship with other hormonal, nervous and immunological stimuli (the reduced activity of the ovaries is then secondary). The ovaries are controlled centrally from the brain. A problem related to functioning of the ovaries can also occur as a result of a dysfunction of the thyroid gland, of reduced activity of the adrenal glands, and of an untreated metabolic illness, such as diabetes.

The diagnosis and therapy of hormonal causes

The levels of hormones are derived from the blood. In women, hormonal levels change during the cycle, therefore it is necessary to repeat the examination several times (usually three times). At the same time, a check-up of the growth of the follicles is performed via ultrasound. Any gynaecologist, urologist, or andrologist with medium-level equipment in their examination room can perform the hormonal examination.

In women, fertilisation drugs can influence the induction of ovulation, or the support of the egg's release. These include, above all, clomiphene and gonadotrophins. Clomiphene is administered mainly to women who have normal concentrations of female hormones, oestrogens, and simple anovulation, and to women with polycystic ovaries. In the normal menstrual cycle, the hypothalamus produces the gonadotrophin releasing hormone (GnRH), which prompts the pituitary gland to release the hormones that control follicle development and ovulation (FSH and LH). The substance is used for initial stimulation of the GnRH from the hypothalamus. Gonadotropines are suitable for women with low oestrogen concentrations and with normal or reduced levels of FSH. They have a stimulating effect on the ovaries and enable the maturation of eggs. They stimulate the growth of the follicles in women who have not achieved pregnancy after therapy by clomiphene. They are also used in treatment through the methods of assisted reproduction in women who have a normally occurring ovulation, to allow a larger number of follicles to mature. Choriogonadotrophin (hCG) causes the release of eggs similarly to LH. It is administered to the woman in a single sitting, usually 24 hours after the last dose of FSH. Some drugs are administered intramuscularly, and sometimes this is even necessary several times a day. If the hormones are administered to induce ovulation (for instance before the collection of eggs for the IVF), they are administered in the first half of the cycle. The efficiency of the hormonal treatment of men with fertility problems is low.

Demands of Medical Therapy

What do patients have to say about therapy of infection, immunological therapy and hormonal therapy?

> I had regular health problems lasting months following each hormonal therapy. (f)
>
> I probably underwent all the possible methods of treatment, starting with hormonal drugs, after which one feels sick. (f)
>
> Under hormonal treatment I started being aggressive, depressed, I had constant feelings of tension and anxiety. I thought it was impossible that infertility would change me so much. I asked the doctor whether it could be a side effect of the drugs and he denied it. I asked for an information leaflet in the pharmacy, and there were all these side effects described in detail. I was relieved that I was not such a lunatic, but I got angry at the doctor because he hadn't told me and needlessly put me under even greater stress and fear for my mental health. (f)
>
> A 25-year-old woman has been trying to conceive for two years. Her husband and she have both passed several basic examinations, without any findings. Although she has strong ethical reservations against the methods of assisted reproduction, she'd decided to undergo therapy soon. We were discussing the possibilities, and we found out that she had not yet undergone the examination of the openness of the fallopian tubes and the immunological examination (not even the post-coital test). When she discovered that she would have to wait for a month for the results of the complex examination at the clinic of reproductive immunology and that, when the tests come out positive, the therapy takes several months, she said that she wouldn't go there, that she would go straight for the IVF, since she was fed up with all the examinations and drugs, and that it had all been for nothing. (p)
>
> My husband looks at the immunological examination quite sceptically, he says that even if some conclusions were reached on the basis of such an examination, it would lead in the same direction anyway—to artificial fertilisation...so it may take a while for me to convince him. (f)

Sometimes the administered drugs have unpleasant side effects, the women describe themselves as vulnerable, irritated, anxious, and their emotions are hard to control and change quickly. After the termination of the drug administration, their condition returns to normal. A complication of this treatment is that it is time-consuming. It is necessary to go for injections and check-ups. Recently the possibility of subcutaneous (under the skin) application of certain drugs has appeared, the advantage of which is a reduction in the time necessary for treatment and hence a reduction in the accompanying stress. However, the disadvantage is a higher price. From the point of view of some of the patients, the big disadvantage is the slow effect of the therapy, where sometimes the result does not become apparent until after several months.

> The biggest enemy of the treatment is the patients' impatience. For them, each day is like a year further away from getting a child, they telephone all the time to see whether they can try to conceive, they don't want to wait for the laboratory results. (p)
> If the effect of the treatment manifests itself only after a long time, most patients lose interest in the treatment, even though the prognosis is optimistic. They do not consider the fact that the lack of treatment can, for example, take its toll later when they reach old age. (p)
> Patients often lose interest in the immunological treatment, it takes too long. They say that when they have the IVF, they get a baby in a month. Which is, of course, not true. (p)

It is not always wise to choose the faster ways. Infertility can be only one of the symptoms of an illness, and not even the most serious one.

> A couple who were getting ready for assisted reproduction because of the man's infertility came to see me. The man was supposed to have a microsurgery procedure, in which his sperm was to be taken from the testicles or the epididymis, if any could be found there, for the *in vitro* fertilisation of the woman's eggs. The couple were in a hurry, they already had an appointment, they didn't want to wait for anything else. They'd heard from friends that the efficiency of assisted reproduction could be increased by the hormonal treatment of the man. They asked me for this treatment. I performed all necessary examinations and I found that the man had testicular cancer. It is even possible that the assisted reproduction might have been successful, but the question is how long the man would have enjoyed his fatherhood. (p)

2. Surgical therapy

If the fertility problem is caused by an anatomical defect in the reproductive system, the problem can often be solved by a surgery. Sometimes the defect is the result of previous infections or inflammations, after which scars and adhesions often remain in the reproductive system. In some cases, surgical operations can resolve the problem completely, but they are often combined with other therapeutic methods.

Diagnosis and therapy of surgery
The cause of the fertility problem can sometimes be found during a basic examination (for example, abnormalities of the cervix), or it can be established by laparoscopy (the keyhole surgery), hysterosalpingography, or sonography. The surgery can be regular macrosurgery, laparoscopy or microsurgery. In men, surgery can remove a varicocele (abnormal enlargement of the veins in the scrotum) and an obstruction of the urethra (the tube semen exits from). Microsurgery, done under general anaesthesia, is often used to gain sperm directly from men's testes when they suffer from obstructive azoospermia. In women, surgery can sometimes remove obstruction of the fallopian tubes, more serious forms of endometriosis, and uterine and cervical abnormalities. Surgical therapy is also necessary in women with polycystic ovaries when, even after hormonal treatment, ovulation cannot be stimulated.

Demands of Surgery

Macrosurgery is performed under general anaesthesia and requires several days of hospitalisation. The post-surgery condition depends on the extent of the surgery and the treated area can remain painful several days or weeks. Laparoscopy requires general anaesthesia and usually one to three days of hospitalisation. There is usually no pain after the surgery. Apart from the above mentioned difficulties (pain, hospitalisation), the disadvantage of surgical therapy is that, even more than with medical treatment, the effect of the surgery is felt only after some time, in certain cases only after several months. Often the biggest enemy of this therapy is the patients' impatience, as when they prefer bypassing the causes to actually curing them, which is not necessarily the best solution; the untreated cause can have other effects than just fertility problems.

In recent years, advances in medicine have significantly reduced the length of hospitalisation, which is, understandably, perceived as a plus, but it also has its drawbacks.

> Before, patients spent more time in the hospital. They had the opportunity to talk to each other and discover that they are in a similar situation. They had someone to talk to and cry with. Many of them initiated long-term friendships, they wrote and called each other and thus supported each other. Today, everything is done quickly, people spend hardly any time in the hospital at all, and in the waiting rooms couples often just pass by other couples. (p)

Therefore, technical progress has increased feelings of isolation and reduced the opportunity for a spontaneous psychosocial support. Not only involuntary childless persons can be affected by sharing infertility experiences:

> After my third spontaneous miscarriage I was waiting in the pre-surgery room before undergoing surgery. I was in the room with a young woman who was waiting for the same surgery but for very different reasons: she was having an abortion. I was beside myself. I envied the woman her pregnancy. I thought how unjust that was. Why should someone who does not want a child get it, and I have been so desperately longing to have a child for years and I cannot get it. I thought it would be nice if the child could just be transferred. I wanted to try to persuade the woman to keep the child. But I knew she would not listen. And then, I don't know why, I started to tell her my story. I told her how much I wanted a baby, how hard my husband and I have been trying, how happy we are for the short time we know it is there and how devastated we are when we always learn from the doctors a few weeks later that the baby is not living any longer. Then I was taken to the surgery. After the surgery I did not see the woman again. But about four months later I was shopping in a supermarket and I saw her there. With a tummy. She also recognised me and she came towards me. She came to thank me. (f)

3. Assisted Reproduction Technologies (ART)

A big breakthrough in the therapy of fertility problems occurred with the introduction of methods of assisted reproduction, which you may be familiar with under the terms of 'artificial fertilisation', 'in vitro fertilisation' or 'test-tube fertilisation'. The first 'test-tube baby' was Louise Brown, born in 1978 in England. Assisted reproduction does not treat the causes of infertility but bypasses them.

The two most common methods are intrauterine insemination (IUI) and in vitro fertilisation/embryo transfer (IVF/ET). I will discuss these methods in more detail below. Other methods include gamete intrafallopian tube transfer (GIFT), which is transfer of the gametes (egg and sperm) into the fallopian tube, and zygote intrafallopian transfer (ZIFT), which is transfer of the already fertilised egg into the fallopian tube. The later two methods are rarely used.

A. *IUI*

Intrauterine insemination is the introduction of specially modified sperm into the womb using a unique tool. This method is usually employed in cases when the couple's infertility is caused by problems on the side of the male partner, when the causes of infertility are immunological, or when there are abnormalities of the cervical mucus. The success of the intervention can be enhanced by hormonal stimulation of the ovaries, which incites the maturation and release of more eggs. It is possible to use the sperm of the woman's partner (called homologous insemination) or the sperm of a donor (called heterologous insemination, used when the man is infertile, or has a genetic dysfunction or is a transmitter).

B. IVF/ET

In vitro fertilisation is conception outside of the body. Therapy through IVF can bypass all the conditions necessary for the birth of a child. Whether this is permissible depends on the ethical and legal norms in a particular area. In vitro fertilisation is most useful when the woman has damaged fallopian tubes, when there is an andrological cause of infertility, or when it is necessary to use donated eggs.

IVF begins by hormonal stimulation that ensures the maturation of several eggs during her menstrual cycle. According to an individual schedule, the woman takes hormonal drugs, usually in injections, for a certain time. The injections are administered by the GP, a nurse, or in some cases, the woman can inject herself. The course of stimulation is observed by ultrasound so that the dose of the drugs can be adjusted, negative side effects reduced, and the precise date of ovulation established. When ovulation occurs (this is approximately 32–36 hours after the last hormone injection), the eggs are collected through the vagina, usually under brief anaesthesia; the collection takes about 10–20 minutes. The sperm is also collected on the same day that the eggs are collected. It is also possible to use frozen or donated sperm.

The eggs and the specially modified sperm are placed in a container and then a period elapses in which some of the eggs may become fertilised. The fertilised eggs (embryos) are then left to mature (called cultivation). Between 2–4 days after fertilisation, the embryos are transferred into the womb. Then the waiting begins.

a. The most recent techniques used in IVF/ET

Micromanipulation techniques are methods in which the egg, the sperm and the embryo are manipulated under the microscope so that the probability of the egg's fertilisation and its nesting in the womb is increased. Today, the most frequently used methods are: intra-cytoplasmic sperm injection (ICSI), when one sperm is artificially introduced into the egg by a microneedle; subzonal insemination (SUZI), which is the introduction of 1–4 sperm under the surface envelope of the egg; and assisted hatching (AH) and zone drilling, in which the probability of the embryo's nesting within the womb is increased by disruption of the envelope of the embryo.

Microsurgical techniques have been used since 1992 in cases of reduced fertility in the man: microsurgical collection of sperm from the epididymis (MESA); microsurgical collection of sperm from the testis (TESA); and, microsurgical collection from the semen-producing ducts (TESE) which, in the ideal situation, also contain free sperm.

Preimplantation genetic diagnosis (PGD) is a technique used to identify genetic defects in embryos created through IVF before transferring them into the uterus. Because only viable embryos are transferred to the uterus for implantation, PGD provides an alternative to modern post-conception diagnostic procedures (for example amniocentesis or chorionic villus sampling), which are frequently followed by termination of the pregnancy if the results are unfavourable. PGD is performed in conjunction with IVF and is offered to fertile and infertile couples. Other supplementary methods include: for several decades, sperm donation has been used in the case of andrological fertility problems; donation of eggs is a method for women who do not develop their own eggs or their own eggs cannot be used, for example because of a genetic problem; donation of embryos, sometimes called pre-implantation adoption, is also possible. For long-term conservation of sperm and embryos in a viable condition, cryoconservation, preservation under deep-freeze conditions, is used. Prolonged cultivation of embryos (72–96 hours) has the advantage of the womb being better prepared to accept the developing foetus and of the ability to better discern the more viable embryos.

b. Risks

The most frequently cited serious complication is the syndrome of hyperstimulation of the ovaries, which can occur after an unusually strong reaction of the hormonal system to the administration of the hormones.

About 5% of women face the risk that the nesting of the embryo after its transfer will occur outside the uterine cavity, for instance in the fallopian tube. The percentage of spontaneous miscarriages is also high, about 20%. Although the rate of occurrence of these miscarriages seems to correspond to the rate of miscarriages in unassisted conception, in this situation they have a greater mental impact because the patients are aware that the egg had been implanted.

The IVF method increases the probability of pregnancy by using more eggs, not just one, which is related to the risk of a multiple pregnancy. An artificially conceived multiple pregnancy, similar to a spontaneously conceived one, entails a greater probability of miscarriage and of reduced birth weight of the infant.

All pregnancies achieved by the IVF method are centrally registered. It is apparent from published sources that the risk of a developmental problem in these children is not any higher than in the general population.

c. *Ethical and legal aspects*

Only a few areas of medicine are related to so many ethical questions as the techniques of assisted reproduction. For all therapeutic procedures, it is necessary to obtain informed consent from the patient, to ensure that the patient is aware of all the circumstances and risks of the therapy.

The oldest problem, the donation of the eggs, sperm or embryos is still unresolved from the ethical and legal viewpoints, as well as from the perspective of the third party. These rules should also take into consideration the ever more frequently mentioned right of the child to know its biological parents.

Perhaps the most serious ethical problems are the result of manipulation of embryos. This is because the success of assisted reproduction is based on gaining and using more than one embryo. The complicated question is their selection and freezing, as well as the destruction of fresh or frozen embryos. In the effort to increase the likelihood of conception, several eggs are introduced into the womb at once. This, of course, leads to a higher probability of multiple pregnancies, which is a risk both for the woman and for the fetuses. To reduce potential health complications, the multiplicity of the pregnancy can be reduced. This surgery is known as reduction of a multiple pregnancy or cardiocentesis. Some specialists suggest that the surgery should be called abortion.

The use of preimplantation genetic diagnosis (PGD) is a very serious aspect. Who should decide which embryos are good and which are not, and according to which criteria? PGD was originally developed for detection of serious genetic diseases. Some of them are bound to sexual chromosomes and thus only girls or boys are at danger. PGD can, of course, also be used for psychosocial reasons: what happens when a couple want only a child of a certain sex? The advances in the development of drugs and technologies have significantly increased the rate of success of IVF. In recent years, it has been possible to collect a small number of eggs and to create one or two embryos for the transfer, called single embryo transfer (SET), without reducing the efficacy of the procedure. This removes the need for problematic reduction of the number of embryos, their freezing, or their eventual destruction.

A widely debated issue consists in surrogate motherhood, where a woman other than the biological mother carries and gives birth to the child. Another ethical question has arisen: using the method of assisted reproduction, it is not technically impossible to make a mother of a woman who is well beyond her fertile age or woman whose husband has died but has frozen embryos or sperm. The ethical and legal questions are discussed in more detail in the chapter 'My Mama Doesn't Know...'

The ways of resolving these issues differ from one country to the next, which is one of the reasons why patients travel to other countries where procedures are permitted that their own country prohibits. The price of treatment is also a factor in this respect.

d. Reimbursement

Treatment of fertility problems is an expensive matter. Each country approaches the subject of covering the costs of treatment differently. In some places, health insurance companies cover a substantial part of the cost of diagnostic and therapeutic procedures, while this coverage is much less in other countries and, in some places, this is not covered by health insurance at all.

Demands of ART

> When we found out after a certain time that it (the IVF procedure) hadn't succeeded, an extraordinary disappointment followed, but in view of the statistics we thought that the second time it would come off. Not even the second attempt was successful, though. I was starting to get angry then. During one cycle there are 4–6 visits plus the procedures themselves, which is also time-consuming. (m)
>
> With all the unsuccessful attempts I just cried myself silly. (f)
>
> The worst was the first unsuccessful attempt for IVF. It was like after an unsuccessful suicide. (f)
>
> For two months, going every other day to a town 50 miles away, and every day to another town 20 miles away for a shot. I had to hand in my resignation at work. I felt like a hunted animal. (f)
>
> The long-term mental burden of the repeatedly unsuccessful attempts. I was off work two months out of six because of the therapy, and the remaining months were spent rushing around from one doctor to the next. (f)

When they told me 14 days after the procedure that 'unfortunately, we are very sorry, come and try it again in a few months,' an immense part of my hope collapsed, the hope that had kept me going so that I could bear it all. Then I decided that I would never undergo it again, and now I am thinking I might try it because the desire for a family is stronger than the fear of repeated failure. (f)

The horrific moments related to the infertility treatment, where the IVF method was the last hope. I ended this suffering on my own. The long-term mental burden of the repeated failed attempts led me to hate the child that I could have. The form and the means of using ART and their dehumanisation offend me strongly. (f)

Always just one week after the transfer I pulled the pregnancy test out of the drawer and then I put it away again for the next day. I feared to use the test and I wanted to prolong my hope. The next day the same thing was repeated until menstruation, so I never used the test. (f)

I had many eggs, even my tummy was under pressure. Then there were 17 embryos, but all of them disintegrated, so there was no transfer. It was dreadful. (f)

The first time I was calm, hoping that the next time it would work, but the fourth time I collapsed and cried. But I reproach myself for being weak. (f)

I fear the next transfer, how will it end again? (f)

A total collapse of the family budget and the occurrence of a vicious circle. Earning money for the fourth and the next trial takes some time. When you need to make money, you cannot be taking sick leave for the therapy, and time passes by and your age goes up, which reduces the probability of successful therapy; when you are undergoing therapy, you are earning less and so on. (f)

The couple couldn't go for the planned IVF because the man was unable to produce ejaculate at the given time. They lived in a place more than two hours away from the centre of assisted reproduction, so he couldn't use the advantage of the 'home environment' and the centre didn't tolerate any longer distance. (p)

I underwent IVF eight times, I probably went through everything that was possible and available. The doctors recommended donation of embryos. I saw the embryos on the screen and believed again that this time it would surely finally come off, but it unfortunately didn't. I have no more strength, and so I'd rather be a loving aunt to my nephews and the children of our friends. (f)

I had a horrible time after the transfer. I knew that I had two beautiful embryos in me, and I was afraid to make an abrupt movement, take a big step or jump a bit so that I wouldn't interfere with the nesting process. (f)

One of my patients always lies down in bed and doesn't move after the transfer, she even lets people bring her food in bed. In this way she spends the

> fourteen days until menstruation. I have explained to her that this is useless, that she cannot influence the implantation of the embryo, that she can go to work and behave as if nothing were happening. But she does the same thing again after the next IVF. And she's a college graduate. (p)
>
> I have undergone many things in my life, I have recovered from several operations. But the worst experience was after the transfer. I knew that I had new lives in my body, and I feel completely helpless, I didn't know what to do to make the lives continue. After the first four IVFs, I stayed in bed all the time for two or three weeks, my husband, mother-in-law, and mum rushed around me, if I made 40 steps a day that's too many. But it was useless anyway. After the last transfer I didn't stay in bed, I haven't got the nerves for it, and anyway it's no good. (f)
>
> After each transfer I kept observing myself all the time to see whether I had any of the pregnancy symptoms of which I'd read thousands of times in books. I also kept going to the bathroom all the time to check whether I was still okay or whether the hope was over. (f)
>
> It worked only in the fourth stimulation cycle (still covered by the medical insurance company). In the seventh transfer. And I (foolishly) hoped that I would become pregnant after the first (!). And in the meantime my friends kept getting pregnant and giving birth and I had nothing. (f)
>
> Only later did I realise how much real physical pain all the procedures cost me. But it is like giving birth, one forgets the pain. And the undergoes it again. (f)

One IVF cycle means about one month of daily visits to the doctor ('For two months every other day to a town 50 miles away, and every day to a town 20 miles away for a shot'). It is not possible to predict how things will work out in terms of time, whether any eggs will be available and when, so it is necessary to come in regularly to see whether the eggs got fertilised, whether embryos are developing, and when it is necessary to come for the transfer. The couple must be prepared to respond quickly to the situation. It is immensely difficult to manage focusing all of one's attention on the treatment for a month, the partners often use up all their time ('I had to hand in my resignation at work. I felt like a hunted animal' 'I was off work two months out of six because of the therapy, and the remaining months were spent rushing around from one doctor to the next'), mental ('The long-term mental burden of the repeatedly failed attempts led me to hate the child that I could have') and sometimes even financial ('A total collapse of the family budget and the occurrence a vicious circle'). The treatment is, especially for the woman, physically demanding ('How much real physical pain all the procedures cost me'). Sometimes patients think that they have come across a half-educated doctor who is still learning the dosages of the hormonal drugs on them. But the reaction to the drugs is really individual and even the most experienced doctor has to first carefully monitor the reaction and then respond to it accordingly.

Therapy by methods of assisted reproduction is special because it is quick, or rather, it offers a quick gain because it can bypass many obstacles to natural fertilisation and it can be successful after just one month. Therefore, this therapy offers a lot of hope ('The IVF method was the last hope' 'The first time I was calm, hoping that the next time it would succeed' 'And I (foolishly) hoped that I would become pregnant after the first (!)'). The hope is enhanced by the fact that patients know about the partial successes of the individual steps. In vitro fertilisation enables the partners to see the obtained eggs and the resulting embryos, the embryos of the children that might be born to them ('Then there were 17 embryos, but all of them disintegrated, so there was no transfer. It was dreadful' 'I saw the embryos on the screen and believed again that this time it would surely finally come off, but it unfortunately didn't').

The time after the transfer is mentally especially demanding ('The worst experience was after the transfer' 'Always just one week after the transfer I pulled the pregnancy test out of the drawer and then I put it away again for the next day. I feared to use the test and I wanted to prolong my hope' 'After each transfer I kept observing myself all the time to see whether I had any of the pregnancy symptoms of which I'd read thousands of times in books. I also kept going to the bathroom all the time to check whether I was still okay or whether the hope was over'). The couple is seemingly only a little step away from success, but they do not have the little step under control ('I know that I have new lives in my body and I feel completely helpless'). For some people, the feeling of helplessness can be so unbearable that they will try anything to contribute by their own effort ('I was afraid to make an abrupt movement, take a big step or jump a bit so that I wouldn't interfere with the process of nesting' 'One of my patients always lies down in bed and doesn't move after the transfer, she even lets people bring her food in bed' 'After the first four IVFs, I stayed in bed all the time for two or three weeks, my husband, mother-in-law, and mum rushed around me, if I made forty steps a day that's too many'). Here is a splendid way how to try to bring the situation under control:

> The fairy tales for the Little One. These fairy tales came to be during the time when we were waiting to see whether the little embryo that I was given in

> the fall of 2003 would get attached and nest in my tummy. I spent the ten days filled with expectation as well as fear by showing the whole world to the Little One: home, work, school, the second home, the landscape behind our house, the cinema, the theatre, the church, travelling by train and by bus, an exhibition, the pub… And to attract the Little One even more, I used Scheherazade's old trick. I promised him that I would tell him a story every evening and I hoped that he would very much want to hear how it continued and so have one more reason to stay alive. I got help with all of this from an old stuffed penguin that we had brought from our honeymoon trip. The penguin slept with us and travelled with us (although it did not go with us into the theatre or the cinema). Besides the Little One and the Penguin, Daddy also got to listen to the stories when he did not go to sleep in the morning. (f)

Usually, the bigger the hopes for the method, the worse the disappointment ('Not even the second attempt was successful. I was starting to get angry then' 'With all the unsuccessful attempts I cried myself silly' 'The worst was the first unsuccessful trial for the IVF. It was like after an unsuccessful suicide' 'the forth time I collapsed and cried' 'When they told me 14 days after the procedure 'unfortunately, we are very sorry, come and try it after a few months again,' an immense part of my hope collapsed, the hope that had kept me going so that I could bear it all'). Women often check the success of the procedure soon after it by the pregnancy test and so may find out that the following menstruation was not a menstruation but an early miscarriage. Many people perceive even an unsuccessful transfer as a miscarriage; they have seen the developing living embryo, the future baby. The next planned attempts instigate fear ('Then I decided that I would never undergo it again and now I am thinking I might try it because the desire for a family is stronger than the fear of repeated failure' 'I fear the next transfer, how will it end again?'). A successful treatment brings up the question of how to tell other people and the child how it was conceived (not normally?), especially when a donor's gametes were used.

The use of the methods of assisted reproduction presents a special kind of difficulty.

> They came out with a very bad spermiogram for my husband. They recommended a donor, which he refused, saying who knows from whom it could have been taken, bad genetics. Only if he knew the donor. (f)
>
> My husband and I don't have to have children at any cost. I certainly wouldn't want my child to be burdened by potential infertility. I respect human life to the extent that I refuse any manipulation with eggs and embryos, or the

injection of sperm. Not only Christians think that a human being has a right to life even before birth. (f)

We were discouraged by the idea that the embryos created from the eggs of an unknown donor and my husband's sperm would be frozen, and in time used for an attempt at fertilisation. I'm thinking now of the strictly ethical aspect of it. My gynaecologist tried to convince me of the harmlessness of this method with the various arguments that I had also found on the internet. We still feel that it is a very serious thing to manipulate the life of unborn people. Unacceptable. (f)

I don't think that IVF is against God's will. In the method, so much depends on chance (for the egg to be maintained, for the embryo to develop, for it to nest) that God must be present. (f)

We refuse artificial fertilisation, we are believers, we don't like manipulation with embryos. (m)

The pain and the desire for a child were stronger than any attempt to rationally submit to certain ethical norms that I would (otherwise) follow. (f)

A young couple, the man with azoospermia. As a possible treatment doctors suggested assisted reproduction with the use of donor cells or by micromanipulation techniques. The couple refused, it is 'against nature'. After two years of various attempts with other therapies, they went to one of the centres and on the second attempt they had twins. (p)

We had one child thanks to the methods of assisted reproduction. We want a second one, but in the meantime we have become believers and artificial fertilisation is now unacceptable for us because of the manipulation. (f)

We weren't happy with the environment and the way of performing the IUI, so the physician suggested to us that we should choose a friend and do it with a syringe at home. We seriously considered the possibility, but in the end we didn't find a friend from whom we would really like to have a baby, and at the same time, we didn't know how we would cope with the situation mentally, with all three of us living in the same village. (m)

A couple came to see me, both partners had fertility problems, neither the egg nor the sperm was healthy. Doctors had suggested they use at least one donor gamete for the treatment. But the partners couldn't agree whose gamete would be substituted. The woman wanted donated sperm, the man wanted a donated egg. We discussed the problem, we talked about the fact that using a donated egg is therapeutically much more demanding than using donated sperm. The man said, 'okay, but the child will call me Uncle.' (p)

After the transfer, three embryos became nested. I decided for reduction of one. But, after some time, another one died on its own. I have a beautiful and healthy child, but also horrible reproaches that I wasted one life, perhaps

I am to blame for both. I despair and sometimes I ask: What would you have been like, my baby? What would you have looked like? (f)

I am waiting for one more hormonal therapy. If that doesn't help, the last option is artificial fertilisation. We are believers, we have a problem with accepting artificial fertilisation. My husband has a bigger problem than I do. But if I don't go for it, I will feel that I haven't done all that I could have. I can't imagine how I could live with that feeling. I've read a lot about the techniques of assisted reproduction, and I believe that it is possible to perform it in a way that doesn't harm anyone. (f)

In the IVF centre, they suggested to us that they could try to fertilise part of the eggs by my husband's sperm and part by donated sperm to see how they develop. For me it is hard to accept, my husband is for it, he has no problem with it. I have trouble reconciling myself with it because we have a case like this in my family, and there is a strange atmosphere around it. I was thinking that it would be necessary to do it in secret, but I would tell somebody about the donor, so that someone knows in case something happens to me and my husband. (f)

Our problem is that the embryos don't develop properly. I suspect that the egg could be to blame, so I am preparing myself for the possibility of using a donated egg. I don't mind it in any way. What I mind is just that the whole procedure will get more complicated again. (f)

We discussed the possibility of donor sperm with my husband and we agreed on the fact that if no other chance were available, we would try it. My husband even said that he definitely would not want to deprive me of motherhood. (f)

The IVF went really well, one of the two embryos became nested, and we still have another six embryos frozen. My husband and I agreed that we would definitely give them all a chance as soon as it is possible. (f)

I have a daughter after an IVF. I haven't got the nerves for another IVF. No one understands what a burden on the psyche it is. Moreover, I had major trouble having my daughter and I am terrified that this time it might be twins. I had five other embryos frozen, though. I'm still paying for the storage, I cannot cope with the thought that someone would just flush them down the toilet. I was thinking of donating them to someone. But I haven't had the courage to decide yet. I am afraid that the people wouldn't be good to the child. After all, it is a piece of myself. (f)

Of course I am afraid and have some doubts. For example because in the history of the relevant couple (the donors of the embryo, author's note) I read about the man's pathological spermiogram, about her problems with the production of oocytes, or maybe because I'll have a giant child since the parents are 201 and 182 cm high and weigh 105 and 93 kilos... That is linked to another complicated question—when and where to tell the child the truth? Tell it at a casual meeting with a doctor that the child is going to

> see about a simple illness and who is going to ask about the ailments of the parents and grandparents? I am convinced that no, it shouldn't be told in this way, but even the child will be asked by doctors again and again what his mother died of... (f)
> The solution to our problem is the donation of an embryo. I am quite afraid that I won't feel a relationship to the child when it isn't mine. But the doctor told me that of course it'll be mine since it'll have my blood. (f)

When donor cells are used, it is necessary to accept that, for at least one of the parents the child will not be biologically his or her own ('Okay, but the child will call me Uncle' 'I am preparing myself for the possibility of using a donated egg. I don't mind it in any way' 'My husband is definitely for it, he has no problem with it' 'That if no other chance were available, we would try it'), some people worry about the genetic input of the donor of the gamete ('We didn't find a friend from whom we would really like to have a baby' 'Saying who knows from whom it could have been, bad genetics. Only if he knew the donor' 'In the history of the couple, I read about the man's pathological spermiogram, about her problems in the production of oocytes, I'll have a giant child since the parents are 201 and 182 cm high and weigh 105 and 93 kilos' 'I am quite afraid that I won't feel a relationship to the child when it isn't mine. But the doctor told me that of course it'll be mine since it'll have my blood'), and, mainly, partners are concerned about the psychosocial effects of the fact that donor cells might be used ('At the same time we didn't know how we would cope with the situation mentally, with all three of us living in the same village' 'We have a case like this in my family, and there is a strange atmosphere around it'). In some countries, donation is anonymous, and doctors usually do not include the information relating to the use of donor cells in documents sent outside the centre. However, it is not always possible to keep this fact a secret, and many couples also consider the right of the child to know its biological parents.

A very complicated situation can arise when more than one embryo is implanted and it is recommended to the couple that this number be reduced ('Horrible reproaches that I wasted one life'). Their long-term efforts have been directed toward the conception of a new life and now that they are successful, they are faced with the question whether they should reject one of them, a procedure which brings a certain risk for the rest as well. Moreover, it is necessary to apply for the operation in writing. It is just as difficult to decide what to do with the extra embryos

('I'm still paying for the storage, I cannot cope with the thought that someone would just flush them down the toilet. I was thinking of donating them to someone. But I haven't had the courage to decide yet. I am afraid that the people wouldn't be good to the child' 'We still have another six embryos frozen. My husband and I agreed that we would definitely give them all a chance as soon as it is possible').

For some people, the techniques of in vitro fertilisation are ethically hard to accept as a solution ('I refuse any manipulation with eggs or embryos' 'We were discouraged by the idea that the embryos created from the eggs of an unknown donor and my husband's sperm would be frozen, and in time used for an attempt at fertilisation' 'It is against nature' 'We are believers, we don't like the manipulation with embryos'). Sometimes one's desire for a child is stronger than one's worldview ('The pain and the desire for a child were stronger than any attempt to rationally submit to certain ethical norms that I would (otherwise) follow,' 'But if I don't go for it, I will feel that I haven't done all that I could have. I can't imagine how I could live with that feeling').

4. Other, uncommon therapies

In some countries, there is infertility physiotherapy called the Mojzis method. This can treat the kind of infertility caused by a disruption of the musculoskeletal system. The therapy consists of very specific exercises of the pelvic floor muscles and a repeated intervention of a trained physiotherapist. Through regular relaxation and strength-building exercises, the weakened muscles will firm up and any blockages may be removed, resulting in a removal of the dysfunction of the spinal column and the irritation of the organs. Due to the complex nature of the excercies, the physiotherapist must be properly trained. For more information: www.mojzis-methods.com.

A further therapy called balneotherapy consists of various medical procedures carried out in a spa under the guidance of a doctor. These spas are not the kind we normally think of, but rather spas where one 'takes the water' of which there are many in central and eastern Europe (for example Karlovy Vary in the Czech Republic or Baden-Baden in Germany). Spas are in nice, natural locations which help with relaxation and the procedures are followed in a set schedule, sometimes for up to a month. For some this constant company and routine is comforting, for others it is a nightmare.

5. Psychotherapy as a causal treatment

We have already discussed that psychological causes of infertility have not yet been reliably confirmed. Therefore, it would be difficult to recommend psychotherapy as a treatment. In my opinion, designating mental issues as the cause of the failure can have two effects: some people may calm down because the cause is now known and there is something to work for, and when the cause is removed, success may arrive. However, if psychotherapy is not successful, the patient can get into a worse mental condition than before. For other people, the possibility that the cause of their infertility is mental makes them nervous. The need to seek out a psychologist is considered by many people to be one's own failure, as an inability to solve one's own problems. Therefore, for certain people, mental causes of infertility only strengthen their belief that the inability to conceive is not an illness but a form of incompetence. Moreover, for some involuntarily childless people, the diagnosis of mental causes can incite feelings of guilt: I cannot have a child and I myself am to blame.

But this is not to say that you should not seek the help of a psychologist. To the contrary. The unfulfilled desire for a child and the troublesome quest for it is a complicated life situation. The fact that a person uses all the available avenues of dealing with the problem is not a sign of incompetence but a sign of competence! The psychologist can help you orient yourself in the demanding life situation, look for the optimal solution, and consider the alternatives. In addition, a psychologist can help you to learn to manage stress, to search for appropriate forms of communication with your partner, family, physician and other people, etc. After all, if you get pregnant while undergoing supportive psychotherapy, then it is only for the good. In the end, it does not matter what exactly has cured you, does it?

Sometimes, I hear that a couple got the following advice: adopt a child, that will calm you down and then you will succeed with your own. I consider this advice inappropriate. No relation has been found between adoption and pregnancy. The fact that you may know a couple like that does not mean that they would not have conceived without the adoption. I even consider the advice harmful! Adoption of a child cannot be a means to an end; this could make both the child and the couple unhappy later. Adoption must be a goal, the resolution of your quest for a child, not just one of its steps. Of course, nothing prevents you from setting out on another quest for another child. Perhaps this time it will be a biological child. Do not be afraid of this scenario, the experience of specialists in adoptive parenting indicates that if you approached adoption in an honest and responsible way, you will be quite capable of handling the relationship to your own child as well as to the adopted one.

6. Acupuncture

According to Chinese doctors, one is healthy only when one's energy (qi) circulates throughout the body without interruption. Acupuncture is an old Chinese method that treats patients through stimulating certain points on the body surface by the pricking of fine needles. It relies on the inner strength of the person. Acupuncture has several modifications, such as laserpuncture, magnetopuncture and others. Alternatives to acupuncture include acupressure, which uses firm pressure instead of needles. As a diagnostic method, acupuncture often uses electrical stimulation or EAV. This consists in measurement of the electrical resistance at certain points and it is said to provide full information about the condition of the organs. Pulse diagnostics is also used.

Not even the critics of alternative medicine have significant objections against acupuncture (except for the erroneous explanations of its principles) and sometimes they acknowledge its therapeutic effect. Even if the effect of acupuncture was just the 'placebo' effect, anything that relieves us of pain for a while improves our mood, improves our appetite, and in the end can objectively improve our health. The treatment carries very little risk when performed by a competent professional.

Demands

Diagnosis via EAV or pulse is not painful or uncomfortable. It can be interesting and pleasant for the patient to discuss other health issues unrelated to the fertility problem with the therapist. In some people, the thought of acupuncture needles can incite the fear of pain, but if done correctly, the sensation should be pleasant and not cause any pain.

7. Homeopathy

Homeopathy functions on the principle that treatment should be 'like for like'. The principle, which was introduced by the German physician Samuel Hahnemann (1755–1843), is based on the idea that in illness very small amounts of substances produce the same symptoms in healthy people when given in larger doses. Homeopathy is meant to enhance one's vital power towards higher activity. The treatment is individual and should be performed in conjunction with a registered professional. The goal is to support the vital power, which is capable of encouraging the defence of the body against illnesses. Critics of homeopathy point to its unscientific principles. As a risk they emphasise that, sometimes the remedies are made from medications in very small amounts which may cause some harmful effects. This is why it is necessary to use caution and a registered homeopath.

Demands

The requirements of homeopathic diagnostics vary; sometimes the process can take several hours. For some patients, the homeopath's interest in topics other than the date of the last menstruation, and the opportunity to talk to a therapist for a longer time can be literally a balm for the soul—a pleasant change from the routine experience of just receiving prescriptions like on a conveyor belt. Homeopathic drugs are usually very small sugar-based tablets and the treatment is not unpleasant. The disadvantage is that homeopathic therapy is a long-term process and homeopaths themselves emphasise this fact; patients often terminate the therapy before the necessary time has passed that the homeopath estimated for the achievement of success.

8. Phytotherapy

> *Once upon a time, there lived an emperor and an empress, both were young, both were beautiful, both had everything they could think of and yet they were not happy. Well, these are the ways of the world, and sometimes not even the emperor's gold can buy everything: the emperor and the empress did not have a baby. There were as many doctors at the palace as there are ants, but the stork kept knocking on the windows of simple houses, as if he were not at all attracted by the gorgeously laid nest, and the empress had eyes full of tears.*
>
> *Until one day a stranger came to see the emperor. It was a man who had come to the empire from afar and he knew spells and magic. He bowed to the ground before the emperor and said, 'I have heard, emperor, that you would like to have a son. If you want to, I will help you to have him. Give a command to brew these powerful herbs and then give the infusion to the empress to drink. Within a year and a day you will have an heir.'*
>
> 'About Prince Dafin, Faithful Afin and Beautiful Kyralina',
> V. Adascălitei, *Weaving, Weaving Fairy Tales*

Phytotherapy is one of the world's oldest therapies. This is not any different in the treatment of fertility problems. When one looks around in the drugstore, pharmacy or health food store, one will surely find several teas that advertise that they adjust the menstrual cycle and improve various 'male' difficulties. Usually, the powerful herbs used for women's illnesses are yarrow, lady's mantle, the bloom of marigold, and the bloom of deadnettle. In addition to teas, many herbalists recommend baths. Teas are differentiated into healing teas and herbal teas. According the UK Medicines and Healthcare products Regulatory Agency, herbal medicines licensed in the UK have a PL (product licence) number on the label. Traditional herbal medicines registered in the UK have a THR (traditional herbal registration) number on the label. Opponents point out the risk of the use of unapproved mixtures and the possibility of undesirable interactions with drugs or other teas.

Demands

The search for the recommended herbs and the preparation of teas and infusions can be time consuming. Moreover, some ingredients can be expensive. In contrast to drugs, though, teas can have a pleasant smell and taste. The making and drinking of teas can be relaxing and can reduce the feeling of helplessness. Many people, largely women, say that phytotherapy is a method that helps them influence their own situation.

9. The application of hands

The word healer most often conjures up the image of a person who heals by applying his or her hands directly to the body or closely above the body surface. This is called therapy through magnetism, bioenergy, biocurrents, bioplasm, etc. For many people the mention of this treatment produces an indulgent smile, but our response to the human touch (however we explain it) is deeply embedded in us. Nurses often call this 'therapeutic touch' and some forms of physiotherapy and psychotherapy use this method. Nowadays, when diagnosis is performed mainly by machines, the physician often does not even touch the patient leading some to view the physician as cold and some patients may miss the human touch. In some people, touch can have a relaxing effect and can relieve anxieties. Opponents of this method point at its non-scientific principles. I can see a risk in a potentially unethical behaviour of some practitioners who may abuse the opportunity for tactile contact.

I conceived very soon after undergoing treatment at the healer. My gynaecologist was very surprised because he said I had a reversed womb. This diagnosis agreed completely with the diagnosis of the healer who had diagnosed it even before the gynaecologist. (f)

After seven years of a childless marriage, during which we wanted a child, I happened to meet a healer who heard me out and recommended to wait with the x-ray and the tubular clearance. After the first therapy, within two months, I could officially announce to my husband that we were expecting a baby. In February, we had a healthy girl. (f)

When I do IUI, I stroke the patient's tummy. They relax, they are not under such stress. (p)

I used to go to a healer but it didn't help me. They may not have the results they claim to have. (f)

My wife is significantly helped by the therapy; after the treatment she has more energy, which the healer has passed on to her. (f)

I had various gynaecological problems and for a long time I was on hormonal treatment, but now, since I've been going to see healers, I have no problems and don't take anything. (f)

At the healer's, it is relaxing, they have time to talk to people. (f)

The therapeutic session has a calming effect. The healer cannot harm, the psyche is positively influenced by the session and the therapy. (f)

A colleague had a shock at the healer. To make a diagnosis he pushed his finger in her vagina, and then during the treatment he touched her breasts and the lower tummy. (f)

Demands

For some people the application of hands has a relaxing or even stimulating effect ('My wife is significantly helped by the therapy, after the treatment she has more energy which the healer has passed on her') and in some cases the symptoms disappear. The mode of some of the healers' communication with clients favourably impresses many people. Some consider the application of hands to be a therapy that leads to success. Others consider it ineffective, but usually they are not too disappointed, because they simultaneously underwent other therapeutic procedures.

10. Astrology

The royal husband and wife, Laius and Jocasta, were childless. They wished to have children with all their hearts. To be sure that they were not going to wait in vain, Laius went to the oracle. But the prophecy was not joyful. It said: 'Do not have a destructive wish against gods and do not ask to have a son.

> *If it is born, he will kill you later on and he will take his own mother as a wife. And all your kin will wade in blood.'*
>
> 'Oedipus', R. Mertlik, *Ancient Greek Myths and Legends*

A special kind of therapy is derived from astrology. It deals with one condition of conception only—the right timing of sexual intercourse. The suitable and unsuitable periods for conceiving a child are determined with the help of astrological calculations.

> We were considering going to an astrologist, my cousin recommended it to us; she went there, and paid quite a lot of money for the calculation. But she wasn't successful. It probably doesn't work (what if I have tonsillitis on the calculated day). (f)
>
> A friend had a calculation done by an astrologist. He designated several suitable days. The friend got pregnant, the astrologist even forecasted correctly that she would have a girl. (f)
>
> After many unsuccessful IVFs, I had a calculation done. I decided to plan the next IVF on the calculated suitable day. After talking with the gynaecologist in the centre of assisted reproduction, we planned a three-month hormonal treatment to shorten the menstrual cycle so that the ovulation and fertilisation in the test tube could occur on the calculated day. (f)
>
> A patient came to us with a request to plan the IVF according to an astrological calculation. Moreover, the astrologist said that the transfer had to be done by a blonde female doctor. We accommodated her, we even found a blonde female doctor. We consider the mental side of the therapy very important and we try to use the inner mental powers of the patient. But, unfortunately, the procedure still was not successful. (p)
>
> We had an astrological calculation performed, we went all the way to a town 250 miles away for this. Together with the doctor, we then tried to plan the artificial fertilisation for the recommended date. It wasn't precisely to the day, so I don't know if the embryo didn't nest because of the imprecise date or because it is all nonsense. (f)

Demands

For the diagnosis, the complete date of the woman's birth, including the hour, and place of birth are needed by the person doing the calculation. It is possible (and common) to do it by mail. You will also get the calculation with the suitable days for the conception of your child by mail. From the viewpoint of a psychologist, I see two theoretical possibilities for the influence of this method on the patient. Knowing the date when one should surely conceive according to the stars can be either stimulating or stressful.

The Quest for an Adopted Child

So they put aprons around their necks, to pretend to have royal robes with a train, and they put on ribbons, and then walked beautifully around in it. Then the Kitty and Doggy sat down on little chairs and pretended to drink coffee. But Doggy sighed and said: 'Today, my queen, I won't drink any coffee because I am sad.'

'And why are you sad, my king?' asked Kitty.

'I am the king of the golden land and the silver land and the diamond land behind the nine-fold mountain ranges, behind the ten-fold rivers, and behind the blue, yellow, and green seas, but we have no daughter, no royal princess, and kings should have princess daughters, and that's why I'm sad.'

'I will advise you, my king,' said Kitty, 'I know about one royal princess. She is far away in the white land, far behind the black land, so I will go there by car and I will buy the daughter for us.'

And now Kitty took a box, as if it were a little suitcase and pretended to go by car and left. Doggy remained sitting royally and pretended to drink coffee, and he kept saying that he was looking forward to the princess, to the little daughter.

Kitty put a doll in the box and blew the horn: 'Tutututu!' and arrived. 'Here I am Doggy, I have brought the little daughter, the princess, I had to pay 100 Crowns for her.'

'I am not a Doggy, I am a king,' said Doggy, 'You know it, and you are the queen.' Then he took the doll in his arms and cradled her, and rejoiced very much that now they had a little daughter, a royal princess.

'We must raise her well,' he said, 'you know, my queen, such a royal princess must be raised well. We will have her trained in everything, even in playing the piano and cooking.'

'How They Played Theatre and What Happened on St. Nicholas Day',
Josef Capek, *Yarns about Doggy and Kitty*

The royal husband and wife did not have a little princess daughter, so they acquired her from the fairyland. The same is done by non-royal husbands and wives, when they desire a princess. For many people their desire is fulfilled by the adoption of a child. However, you will not simply pay for a child like the Kitty.

Adoptive parenting from a legal viewpoint

The best known and the most common form of adoptive parenting for childless couples is adoption. In adoption, couples or single people accept an orphaned child as their own and have the same rights and responsibilities toward her or him as if they were the child's biological parents. In a great many countries, this is defined in that the mutual rights and responsibilities between the adopted child and the biological family disappear as a result of the adoption. The adoption is decided by the courts and, in most countries, the proceedings must be preceded by a period of several months, during which the interested party takes care of the child at their own expense.

It is possible for a married couple, the spouse of the child's parent, or a single person to adopt a child. Adoption by a single person is possible in some countries only if it can be concluded that the adoption will fulfil its social role. In the case of adoption by couples, it is likely that, if one of the spouses does not agree with the adoption, the court would not approve such an adoption. There should be a suitable age gap between the adopted child and the adoptive parents. Another option consists in international adoption, which is regulated by the Convention on Protection of Children and Co-operation in respect of Intercountry Adoption accepted by the Hague Conference on Private International Law on May 29th, 1993. This form of adoptive parenting is a viable solution when an adoptive family cannot be found in the child's country of origin.

Foster care constitutes another way of providing substitute parenting. This option is used especially by couples who have their own children or by involuntarily childless couples, who have already adopted their first child and then accept a child into foster care as a sibling for the first adopted child, because they do not want to wait a long time for another adoption. The main difference between adoption and foster care is that a foster parent is not the child's legal representative, contact between the biological parents and the child is not entirely excluded, and the biological parents have the right to decide on the most important issues (unless the biological parents' parental responsibility has been removed from them).

Where do orphaned children come from?

Today the system of adoptive parenting only rarely addresses cases of actually orphaned children, whose parent or parents have died. A large majority of these children are socially orphaned and already have a mother and a father or at least one of them. However, these parents cannot, will not, or are unable to take care of their children.

Children can be entrusted to the new families from various children's homes or other institutions. From there, the children are placed into adoptive parenting either based on an agreement of the biological parents or the legal representatives, or without the parents' agreement, on the basis of lack of parental interest or legal removal of the parents' responsibility. Children can also be entrusted directly from the biological family, when that family creates an agreement with the adoptive family. In some countries, especially outside of Europe, this type of adoption, called private adoption, is very common. This has its advantages, but also its risks.

A young student became pregnant and, because she was not able to look after the child, she decided on adoption. According to her rights, she chose the adoptive family. After six weeks, the child was entrusted to that family. But the student started having doubts about the correctness of her decision and went to visit the adoptive family. The door was opened by the adoptive mother with the child in her arms. The student was thinking about taking back her decision. The adoptive mother understandably defended herself as she had already bonded with the child. It took several months to find a solution and the negotiations were difficult. In the end the student did not change her decision and the child remained in adoption. But this was a mentally demanding situation for both women that required prolonged psychotherapy. (p)

We had a possibility of direct adoption. A woman already had three children and she didn't want the fourth one that she was expecting. We seriously considered it. We were even prepared to meet their financial demands. But after a week we learned that the woman's husband said that if it were a boy, he would probably keep it. So we began to have doubts. When they had second thoughts before the birth, what all might they want to change and do later? (f)

It was an experience that I certainly do not like to remember. The adoption was organised by a young woman who succeeded in gaining for herself the child we were supposed to get. (f)

How to give a child for adoption

Usually adoption requires the agreement of the child's legal representatives, which means, as a rule, the biological parents, unless the parents' responsibility or their competence for legal action has been legally removed from them. In many countries, the law for the protection of the mother post-partum is in effect. Only after the end of this time (usually about six weeks) is her agreement with the child's adoption valid. However, it often happens that the biological mother does not present herself for this decisive legal action and the child is therefore not legally free. Then it is necessary to wait for another legal procedure, the court's proclamation of what is called qualified lack of interest. In other words, if the parents of a minor sheltered in a private home or in an institution have revealed a manifest lack of interest in the child, seriously compromising the proper bonds of affection during the several months prior to the submission of a petition to the court requesting the entrustment of the child for future adoption.

What is in store for a person who decides for adoptive parenting?

It is impossible to describe the formal procedure for the adoption of an orphaned child with precision for readers around the world, as custom and laws vary from one region to the next. Thus, the description should be taken as a basic guideline.

A person who has decided to adopt an orphaned child needs to submit an application for the adoption of a child into adoptive parenting to the state authority or to an organisation authorised by the state to perform these tasks. The completed application should be accompanied by other documents, for example confirming the person's nationality, state of health, economic circumstances, etc.

After the submission of the required documents to the relevant department, a social investigation in the home of the applicant/applicants usually follows. This is usually performed by a social worker who checks whether the child will have suitable living conditions. This report becomes part of the application. Other documents will be added to this file, depending on local customs. For example:

- the applicants' criminal records
- a written agreement that the adoption agency is authorised to make any further background checks
- that there has been no change in the decisive facts stated in the documentation in the file
- a statement confirming whether or not the applicants are interested in adoption from abroad
- a statement of the adoption agency expressing their position toward the application for mediation of adoption or foster care.

The documentation about the applicants is then forwarded by the district authority of social and legal protection of children to the higher regional office. The applicants are then invited for a psychological assessment. The goal of this assessment is to enquire into the suitability of the applicants from the viewpoint of their personal qualities, their motivation, their prerequisites for raising children, and to ascertain that there exists sufficient marital harmony to ensure a stable environment for the child(ren). The psychologists gain this information by consulting the application and added documents, by carrying out interviews focused on family and personal affairs, by talking with the applicants about issues related to adoptive parenting, and by examining the applicant. After processing the results, they invite the applicants for a supplementary interview. The investigation has two phases: investigation of the suitability for the position of adoptive parents or foster parents, and investigation of the appropriateness for a certain child. The investigation includes physical factors (health, appearance), developmental factors (age, personality; mental health issues, especially those caused by the applicants' infertility, are not a contraindication for adoption or foster care), social factors (marriage, the applicants' other children, extended family), and situational factors (material and social circumstances of the applicants). Then the psychologists prepare a report with the recommendation to either reject or accept the applicants.

Before the adoption of the child, the applicants take a preparatory parenting course. The course has various forms, from several-hour discussions to weekends, but the content is always the same. The applicants are familiarised with common problems related to adoption and with the possible solutions to these problems, for example with the question when, how or if at all to tell the child that he or she was adopted.

When the report is finished and the applicants have been recommended, the time of waiting for a child begins. This differs according to region and according to the kind of child the applicants are requesting.

How does the selection of applicants proceed? A board, made up of experts from various professions, such as psychologists, paediatricians, sometimes social workers from infants' homes and children's homes, and social workers from the district where the relevant applicants live, meets regularly to assess individual cases of orphaned children and, on the basis of a comprehensive evaluation of the applications, they recommend an appropriate family for each child. The applicants are proposed according to their suitability for the offered children and according to a waiting list. Sometimes it happens that the applicants submit the application before they intend to adopt a child, for example, they want to continue fertility therapy for some time. They have submitted the application in advance, so that they can ensure that they will not stay childless. This procedure is common in many countries, but it is necessary to inform the responsible officials about it.

The adoption of a child into the family

They took off the royal robes, Kitty put a scarf around her head and Doggy put on a piece of an old rag. Then they rang the bell and again it was theatre time.

'Now I am no longer a king and Kitty is not a queen,' announced Doggy to the children, 'we have become poor.'

'And you are a poor cottage man and I am a poor cottage woman. What shall I cook, my dear husband, when we don't even have bread? And what shall we do with our daughter when we cannot feed her?'

'You know what,' said Doggy, 'We must take her to the forest, perhaps someone will take her home.'

They took the doll and pretended to lead her to the forest and they were play-weeping. 'We cannot take her to the forest, a wolf might get her,' said Doggy, 'If we meet some good people, we'll sell her to them, they may need a little daughter.'

They led the doll toward the bed where the children were sitting. 'Now you must play theatre with us,' said Kitty to Jim and Vera, 'Now you need a little daughter and you'll buy her from us.'

'Here are some people, Doggy called out when they arrived with the doll at the bed, and to Vera and Jim: 'Hey, kind man, hey, kind woman, do you need a little daughter?'

'We might need one,' said Vera, 'we were just looking for one.

'And what can your daughter do?' asked Jim.

'Well, she can do everything,' said Doggy. 'She can cook and clean and do laundry and she can even do summersaults.'

'We might really need that girl,' said the children. 'And what else can she do? asked Vera.

'Many things,' said Kitty. 'She can sleep and eat, jump and sit, and she can even climb the wall if you help her.'

'And when she falls down, she doesn't even cry,' said Doggy.

'We were looking for a daughter exactly like her' said the children. 'And how much is she?'

'Nothing,' said Doggy. 'We will give her to you for free, if you love her.'

'How They Played Theatre and What Happened on St. Nicholas Day',
Josef Capek, *Yarns about Doggy and Kitty*

The selected applicants are invited to take over care of the child by the social worker of the respective regional authority or municipality. Similarly to Vera and Jim, the applicants receive all the available information about the offered child: about its physical and mental condition, about the child's family and the related social and legal aspects. The applicants may learn, for instance, that the family are poor cottage people who have given the child up for adoption because they cannot feed it, but that it was important to them that the new parents love the child. The amount of information also depends on the age of the child. They may learn that the baby can sleep, eat, or that the toddler does not cry when he or she falls. And if the applicants agreed to accept a handicapped child, they might learn that they cannot expect summersaults, but jumping will be fine. The applicants have an opportunity to consider their present situation and openly express their views and feelings. They should not be afraid to admit that they feel that a particular child is not suitable for them.

No one knows when a child suitable for the specific applicants will become available. Therefore, the couple can have only an idea about when they might get a child. That is why they are not allowed to take the child home immediately. This depends on the situation, the child's age, the preparedness of the child and the parents, etc. This deferment is meant to give the applicants time to prepare themselves and their home after they have received the invitation to take over care of the child, so that they do not act under emotional pressure, and so that the child can prepare for departure for a new environment. But the future parents visit the child in the infants' home or in the children's home. They also talk with the physicians, psychologists, social workers, and educators in the home who know the child intimately. The direct assessment of these experts of whether the applicants and the child are well suited to each other is also taken into consideration.

After the taking over care of the child, in some countries there follows a lengthy (up to several months) pre-adoption or pre-foster care period, in which the applicants try to get used to living with the child. They are invited to take the child to a paediatrician or a psychologist for a check-up to see how the child is doing and developing. During this period, it is possible to take the child away from the applicants or the applicants themselves can return the child. If the applicants have serious reasons for returning the child, they can be offered another child after the reasons cease to exist.

Pre-adoption care is followed by court proceedings to confirm the adoption or the foster care.

Adoptive parenting from a psychological viewpoint

What is necessary for the creation of a healthy adoptive family? Here are some suggestions from The Whole Adoption Book[4]:

'Parents show the characteristics of a healthy, functioning family. Parents fully agree with the adoption. Parents express their own conflicting emotions (that means they behave authentically, they can even express disagreement or anger, for instance, but in a cultivated way). Parents have the ability to wait for the feeling of parental fulfilment that results from the child's gratefulness and bonding, and they do not yield to refusal. Parents can feel joy in even small steps toward improvement. Parents are determined to maintain the family relation in hard moments. Parents respect themselves. Parents do not hesitate to seek out professional help or the support of others when needed. Parents respect differences. Parents build up a family with a strong value structure, based on personal conviction that is expressed on the outside and that is respected by their social environment.'

Adoption is not only the couple's affair; it involves the extended family and the close social circles. You must prepare, not only yourselves, but also all the other members of the adoptive environment. Not only do you become adoptive parents but your own parents become adoptive grandparents, your sister an adoptive aunt, etc. They must also be prepared for the adoption. It is necessary for you to acquaint them with your decision to adopt a child and to gain their support, to provide them with enough information so that they understand where their place is, and to discuss with them the aspect of the influence on the other children in the household. For your social environment (friends, neighbours, teachers at school, physicians) to successfully cope with the situation, it is necessary to speak about adoption in positive terms), to provide information selectively, and to prepare oneself for dealing with and forgiving indiscriminate and insensitive remarks.

Are you taken aback and do you have the impression that you will never achieve this sort of perfection? And do you feel it is unfair that some parents do not fulfil even a single criterion, whereas you meet at least one or two, and they have plenty of their own children while you have to humbly request a single one, and strive for perfection? This is what all responsible couples feel, but in the end, they manage to deal with all of these things and become good adoptive parents. Of course, they do not comply completely with all of the above criteria—perfection exists only in books. But books can help you with many questions in your preparation for adoptive parenting. You can do a great deal yourselves if you start learning about the issue. Give yourselves time, so that your resolutions can mature, do not leave it to the last moment when you can be mentally exhausted. You can submit the application for adoption right away; it does not bind you in any way. The clerks are usually familiar with the situation of people suffering from fertility problems and understand it, and it is possible to tell them: we are submitting an application but we want to continue with treatment for some time. I have already rejected the idea that adoption could be a form of psychotherapy leading to conception. However, many couples enter the adoption investigation without interrupting treatment and have not given up hope for their own biological child. Of course they ask the question: what if the treatment is successful? Will we be able to manage the adopted and the biological child together? I know a family that adopted a girl. Several years after the adoption, the woman became pregnant. I talked to her right after she had the ultrasound where it was possible to tell the sex of the expected child, and she said, 'It'll be a girl again.' Notice, she did not say *also*, but *again*!

Demands

What are the experiences of the people who have undergone the process?

> The social worker tried to convince us to change our mind about adoption because, as teachers, we have enough children at school. (f)
>
> My wife went to the appropriate office to collect the forms, and she was told that if we submit them the same week, we have a chance perhaps in the next five years, and if not, then the next chance to submit the application will be in one year, and, moreover, the criteria of screening will be changed. When I read through the forms, I was overwhelmed by anger. The forms clearly [were outdated], and it followed from the forms that, from the moment I submit the application, my apartment becomes a continuous laboratory where any woman who works at the office has the right to look into my privacy and explain to me what the correct values are. (m)
>
> The men are sometimes offended that they should be screened so many times. (p)

The first (as well as the subsequent) meetings with the psychologist from the counselling office was dreadful. Undisguised assessment (and disapproval) of our expectations of the child, the manner of dealing with us from the position of the superior and powerful. We had the feeling that, after a few sentences, she'd placed us in a certain slot, and it was impossible to get out of that niche. A feeling of helplessness and humiliation. (f)

Is the psychological assessment really so decisive? And are the sometimes unscrupulous interventions of the social workers necessary? The longer you wait, the less prepared you are, because you 'fall asleep'. How long can you bear the pressure, when you do not know the day or the hour? (f)

To my question about when we may expect to get a child, the psychologist responded that he didn't know, it could be next month or in four years. I am desperate, I do not know when. We know that people wait at least four years, that's why we have submitted the request now. We plan to continue therapy for another two years. But what if they give us a child next month? And when we refuse it at the moment, will they remove us from the waiting list? (f)

We tried everything, maybe 10 artificial fertilisations at various places throughout the country. It wasn't working, so we submitted an application for adoption. But we had to fill out a questionnaire with questions like: Describe your character qualities. I wrote down 'I am a crook and a liar' because I was irritated that I should assess myself in this way. And then another question: What age children do you want to adopt? So I wrote down: 'From zero to infinity.' And the next line: What profession should your child have? Such nonsense. So I wrote down: 'An astronaut'. Of course they took offence. And then my wife and I had an appointment for a personal interview on the basis of the filled out questionnaire. By coincidence the date of the meeting [was during a] break in the shooting of a film. We were just in the middle of a scene where I was going as St. Nicholas to visit a friend at the hospital. I wasn't allowed to take off the makeup because they would have been unable to put the makeup on the same way again, and therefore I was unable to take off the St. Nicholas costume, which would have damaged the mask. When my wife and I (as St. Nicholas) entered the counselling room, the present clerk scolded me, and said that she would recommend the adoption to my wife if she divorced me. I was outraged and I wrote her a letter. A harsh one, I must say. What does the screening itself involve? You must undergo many tests, medical, psychological, sociological examinations. An investigator will come to your home to see whether it is big enough, where you keep the clean clothes, where the dirty ones. (m, a famous actor)

It was immensely complicated and humiliating; various investigations, how we live, check-ups. We were supposed to participate in a psychodrama with people who wanted to adopt children. I considered that useless. Now I am

> glad that we have a nice and kind son. We are a relaxed family, and I imagine that we could adopt another one. After the experience with the pre-adoptive investigations, though, I am not sure I would be able to go through it again. (m)
> It certainly doesn't have an optimistic effect on me to always come to the office and watch the clerk fish out our application from the bottom of the folder, verify that everything still holds as we stated many months ago, and return it to the bottom of the folder again. (m)

I do not want to terrify you with these testimonies. You need to take into consideration that usually it is the people who perceived the situation negatively that tend to express their views. Those who experienced the situation in a relaxed state of mind usually do not comment on it. But I want to prepare you for the fact that the investigative process for the suitability for adoption is unfamiliar territory, the applicants are under stress to see whether they pass and perceive everything in stronger terms. And even if the majority of the people who work in adoptive parenting are pleasant, there are always some—as in any area—who are insensitive or unprofessional and who can hurt you. Adopting a child is a time-consuming matter and it is mentally demanding.

The whole adoption process is underwritten by uncertainty and doubts as to whether this is the optimal solution. Couples who set out on the quest for an adopted child miss the feeling of privacy and of being in control. They must go through unpleasant investigations by strange people, from social workers to court clerks. They have a (justifiable) feeling that they must be careful about what and how they say to whom, so that a seemingly unimportant remark would not threaten the process of adoption.

When the process of investigations for adoption is closed, the real uncertainty arrives. Each phone call can be the notice that you can have a child.

> When I hung up the phone after talking with the clerk, I had a moment of fear, wondering about how I would announce to my boss that, starting tomorrow, I will be on maternity leave for several years. But that is how it is with adoption; for a long time nothing happens and then you have a child from day to day. (f)

Fear as to how you will manage the first contact with the child sets in. There is also the anxiety that, at the last minute, someone could designate you as unsuitable applicants.

You may have arrived at the decision, gone through the adoptive investigations, done everything possible for the creation of a good adoptive family, the waiting time has passed, a suitable child has been found, and you are getting ready to take the child home. You are looking forward to hugging the child. But you should be prepared that things will not go so smoothly. If you have any children in the extended family, you know how it is. Some children easily establish contact, even with strange people, others are wary even with people from their own family. You have experienced the situation when the eager grandmother comes to visit the grandchild, brings many sweets and toys, and then leaves in tears because the child refused to talk to her and did not give her a good-bye kiss. Not even a baby will necessarily immediately cuddle up to you. In older children, the length of time required for accepting the adoptive parents, some people call it courtship, varies. The time necessary for the adoptive parents to say: yes, this is the right child for me, I want to look after this child, can also vary from case to case. Simply, sometimes the adoptive parents and the child are immediate friends, sometimes the bonding takes time. Difficulties in building up a relationship, in getting to know each other and getting accustomed to each other are also familiar to parents and children who share a biological bond, but that is rarely discussed. It seems inappropriate to admit that a mother was not filled with a feeling of motherly love right after the birth but had to build a relationship with her child (the same is true for fathers). The following observations come from parents who did not have fertility problems.

> It took me a long time to create a relationship with and emotionally bond with my first child. Things got sorted out after my departure from the marriage. I definitely was not overwhelmed by a wave of motherly love, it was more a feeling of compassion for the helplessness of the infant; I developed a relationship to my children gradually. (f)
>
> No parental instinct exists. At least not in me. I wanted a child because I was curious what it would be like to have my own child. The reason why I looked after the baby up to a state of complete mental exhaustion was a feeling of responsibility. It is not possible to speak about maternal love in me until the child was about one year old, when the child would come on its own to cuddle up to me, to show me or tell me something. Parenting is about communication, not about instincts. (f)

Therefore, if the chosen child does not rush into your arms, do not despair; do not judge the child or yourselves—give it time. You are stranger to the child, and even if you come with your heart in your hand, the child may not be so sure of it. Do not forget that the child has already been abandoned by adults at least once, and that it is not easy to give up the certainties and relationships that he or she had found in the children's home.

> A couple was called to take over a pair of school-age sisters. Both the man and the woman liked the girls and they were looking forward to having them. But the girls liked the children's home and they didn't want to go to a strange environment, they even refused to talk with the potential parents. The couple didn't give up, every weekend they commuted many kilometres to the children's home and spent time with the little group of children to which both the sisters belonged. After a while the group of children got used to the couple and, after making arrangements with the administration of the home, the couple began to organise various activities for them: once they took the whole group for ice cream, another time to the fair, another to the cinema, etc. So it went weekend after weekend for several months. In the meantime, one of the sisters decided that she would go to the adoptive family, but the other didn't want to, then the other wanted to and the first didn't. Only after many months did the potential parents gain the trust of both the sisters and could start a family. The period of courtship was long, the financial, temporal, and mental strain was enormous, but it was worth it, today it is a good and happy family. (p)

Some well-known writer said in an interview that, at the time when it seemed that she and her husband could not have their own children and decided to adopt two Gypsy boys, she had romantic ideas about adoption.

> Those film ideas when the children throw themselves into your arms and you are happy and content in a moment. (f)

The next obstacle emerges immediately after the child's arrival, during the three-month pre-adoptive care: the question of the parental responsibility towards the newest member of the family. When do adoptive parents really become parents? On the day of the child's arrival? Physically yes, legally no. The child continues to stay in the legal care of the legal guardian.

During the pre-adoptive care, the parents and the child can see various specialists or the paediatrician in the institution where the child has come from. They also have to accept check-up visits from social workers. The reason is clear: to find out whether the child is doing well. For the parents, though, it again means a loss of privacy, a feeling that they are being assessed all the time, and permanent anxiety. In the case of children younger than one year of age, this anxiety does not go away with the end of the pre-adoptive care; the so-called permanent adoption is possible only after one year of age.

What can you do to be able to cope with this mental load? Above all, you need to know about it in advance and count on it. Perhaps you will be better able to handle the process if you imagine yourselves in the role of those who are responsible for the screening of suitable candidates for the orphaned child. Such a child has been disappointed once before by parents, and those who are now responsible for the child are doing everything they can to prevent this from happening again and to compensate the child as much as possible. What do you think? Would you not be just as or even more careful as a social worker and a psychologist? I also strongly recommend that you do not hesitate to seek out specialists with your questions, uncertainties, and doubts. If you are afraid that acknowledging your uncertainties to those who have the power to decide your case would complicate the adoptive investigations, turn to one of the non governmental organisations.

The Quest for Childlessness

According to demographics[5], between 15–30% of the world stays childless. Childlessness will increase gradually in almost all industrialised countries. Among women born in the 20th century, low childlessness levels associated with the generations born in the 1940s and having children in the 1960s and early 1970s appear to be more unusual than the more recent increase in lifetime childlessness. I assume that this number includes both voluntarily and involuntarily childless people.

Some of the involuntary childless men and women often end the treatment not because it is easy for them to accept childlessness, but because they have exhausted their mental strength, they have run out of financial resources, or they have passed the age when it is possible to conceive. People who remain childless do it either out of their own decision when they end the treatment and do not consider adoption a suitable solution, or when they have fought for biological parenthood so long that they are now past the age that would have allowed them to adopt the kind of child they would like. The section on 'The Quest for a Biological Child' is long. The section on 'The Quest for an Adopted Child' is shorter. And this section on 'The Quest for Childlessness' is even shorter. But the length of the description does not correspond with the length of the actual route that may lead to this destination. The quest for a biological child can be considerably shorter than the quest for childlessness, since the quest for childlessness usually follows a long time spent on the quest for a biological child. The description is short only because this route has no clearly defined steps; it depends on each individual person.

Perhaps the quest for childlessness is the kind of quest most concerned with the words at the end of the chapter title, the words 'if it means just coming closer'. Come closer to yourself and to your partner, and search for an answer to the question about what a fully lived life means when it for various reasons cannot be a life with a child. And fill your life accordingly. A life without a child is just as meaningful, it is up to you to make it so.

THE PATH IS DISAPPEARING,
WITH EVERY STEP
MY HEART IS ACHING

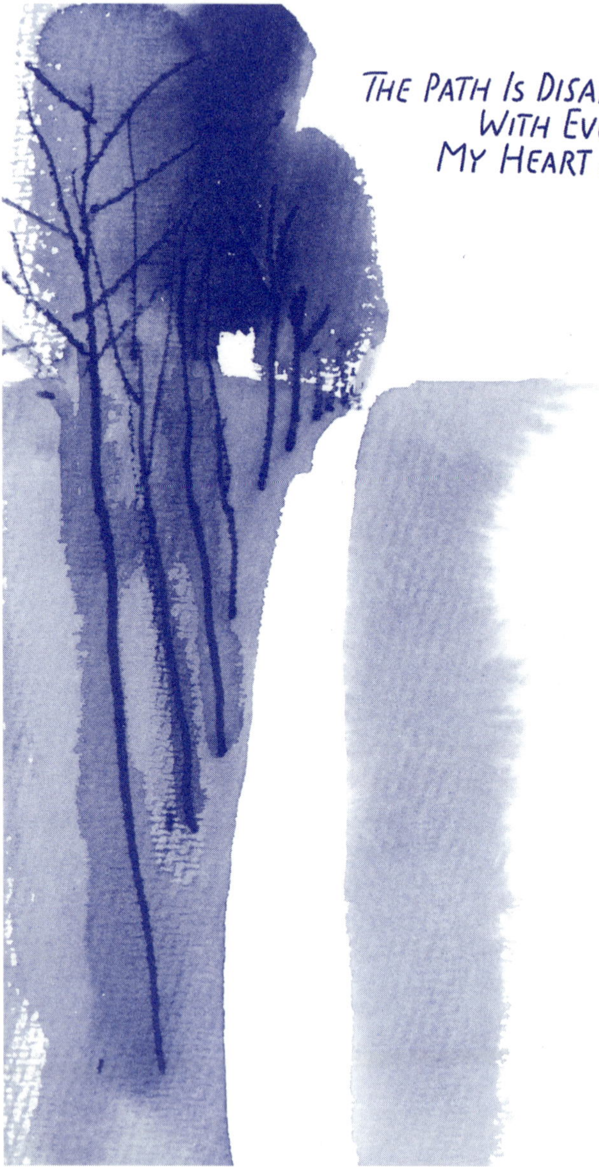

The Path is Disappearing, with Every Step My Heart is Aching

Human beings are not like machines; they have their dreams, hopes, and desires. When the journey is demanding, they can grow tired, their feet hurt, the luggage weighs them down, and the destination remains beyond the horizon—humans suffer. But, when the trip is going well, the sun is shining, and the destination is within reach, humans rejoice.

All that we go through influences us, effects our experiencing, and vice versa. Therefore, just as it is helpful to become oriented in what you are doing or could be doing on the quest for a child, it is useful to get your bearings in regards to what you and your partner are or could be experiencing. When you can recognise and name your feelings, you can get them somewhat under control, you can better cope with them, and you have a better chance to convey and explain them to your partner. This way, your partner will also be able to form a better picture and get a better overview of the situation and thus cope with it better. It will be easier for you both to search together for an optimal solution. It is often said: know your enemy.

Involuntarily childless people often tell me, 'I am not probably normal any more, I think about it all the time and cannot reconcile myself to it.' When I ask how they determine what is and is not normal in their situation, they do not actually know. Most often they do not have contact with anyone else dealing with a similar problem, so that they cannot compare their feelings and find out whether they have gone crazy or not. In the following chapter, you will read the testimonies of those who have undergone the quest for a child or who are still on it. Take advantage of the fact that they have tried to name their feelings. With the help of these testimonies, try to identify your own feelings, experience them, and accept them. They are yours; do not be ashamed of them. That is an important starting point for you to come to terms with them and learn how to handle them.

Before I start to differentiate between testimonies about women and about men, I would like to share an insight that can concern women as well as men.

> A number of our friends have a similar fate. The basic feeling is the feeling of being taken aback: something that they considered matter-of-course is not possible to plan in the same way as their studies, the acquisition of an apartment or their own professional growth. Then times of a feverish search for help from anywhere alternate with times of resignation and helplessness. Today people are not very patient, and when things do not go according to their plans, they panic. (f)

Human life is a sequence of bigger and smaller certainties. The certainty that one will have a child when one wants to is the type of certainty that most people put in the category of the most certain certainties. The failure of a bigger certainty surprises one more than when something that one did not count on too much fails (for example, when one does not win the lottery). The response is determined by the position of the certainty on one's value ladder, by one's personal predispositions and current mental state, and by outside circumstances.

How Do Women Respond?

> *There was a man whose name was Elkanah...and he had two wives; the name of one was Hannah, and the name of the other Peninnah. And Peninnah had children but Hannah had no children. Year after year Elkanah went from his town to worship and sacrifice to the Lord at Shiloh... Whenever the day came for Elkanah to sacrifice, he would give portions of the meat to his wife Peninnah and to all her sons and daughters. But to Hannah he gave a double portion because he loved her, and the Lord had closed her womb... And because the Lord had closed her womb, her rival kept provoking her in order to irritate her. This went on year after year... her rival provoked her till she wept and would not eat. Elkanah would say to Hannah, why are you weeping? Why don't you eat? Why are you downhearted? Don't I mean more to you than ten sons? In bitterness Hannah wept much and prayed... And she made a vow, saying, If you will only look upon my misery and give me a son, then I will give him to you for all the days of his life. Hannah was praying in her heart, and her lips were moving but her voice was not heard. Eli thought she was drunk... 'Not so, my lord,'*

Hannah replied, 'I am a woman who is deeply troubled. I have not been drinking wine or beer; I was pouring out my soul to the Lord. Do not take your servant for a wicked woman; I have been praying here out of my great anguish and grief.'

1 Samuel 1: 1–16

A biblical woman speaks about grief and resentment. What do non-biblical women experience?

My wife probably suffers from depression because of it, she longs for a baby very much and because of that she has lost joy in other things. Before, she was afraid she would not know what to do at home alone. (m)
I've been handling it well because I believe that it will turn out well. Without faith, one could not cope with anything. (f)
I was sad about it, after about seven months I was quite unhappy, we both desired a child. (f)
Periods of hope alternate with periods of suffering, fear. (f)
On the outside, it seems that I am coping well, but I'm quite sensitive about the topic of children. When someone says something to me in that sense, it can make me mad. (f)
I'm taking it hard, especially when I am somewhere among children and realise that I am already 30. (f)
Sometimes I'm handling the situation well, at other times it's hard. The biggest hurdle is the constant awareness of the inability to conceive. (f)
I'm handling the situation well. Thanks to my husband, adoption of a child, interests, hobbies and work, I am not currently thinking about the fact that I haven't got my own child. (f)
It isn't easy. One goes through many disappointments and hardships. One gets to feel at home at the doctors', every month one waits for what's going to happen, waves of hope and depression come and go. (f)
Under the influence of the gynaecologists, I perceived the problem rather clearly: either now or never. I felt inferior, of little value, which the doctors reinforced with their statements about my age, statistical probabilities, etc. (f)
Before each menstruation, I was nervous, and when it came, I always cried. With each new drug my hopes increased, and then disappointment came. I even argued with my husband out of nervousness. When I saw babies in prams or when a friend of mine conceived, a wave of sadness and of blaming myself came over me. (f)
It was hard for me to cope with the repeated disappointments, but I didn't want to resign myself to such a cruel fate, I really fought hard. (f)
At the age of 23, I didn't fully realise the impact of the fact that I would not be able to conceive. I only started dealing with the problem two years later with my husband. (f)

I didn't want to boast anywhere of the fact that I had no child, it was unpleasant for me to speak about it, especially when I met my schoolmates. I avoided my colleagues' discussions about children and grandchildren. (f)

When people in my presence talked about children, I automatically switched off. Even more, I felt alone, 'out of the picture', it wasn't my topic. Women talked about their children—it didn't concern me, but I pretended I was listening. Often I even tried to listen and be honestly interested but I felt out of the scene. I was living through utter loneliness. (f)

Despite all the denials and rationalisations, my anger and resentment against God was growing. Against God who knew what I was experiencing, who knew of my pain, emptiness, loneliness, and who kept calmly looking at it. The first time I told him that I hated him it was in front of several close people. (f)

I've never stopped feeling a certain emptiness, seeing pregnant women has never stopped hurting me, from time to time I again have to struggle with self-pity. (f)

Even though neither my husband nor I will ever stop hoping, I am slowly getting used to the idea that I'll probably never have my own child. The dreadful moments connected with the infertility treatment where the IVF method was the last hope. I ended the suffering myself. The long-term mental load of the repeated unsuccessful attempts, which made me hate the child I cannot have. I haven't done anything wrong, I simply cannot have my own child. Am I any worse than those who can have their child? (f)

When they told me 14 days after the surgery, 'We're sorry. Come try it again in a few months time,' an immense part of my hope collapsed again, the hope that had kept me going so that I could stand it all. Then I told myself that I would never undergo this again, and now I am thinking again that I might try it because the desire for a family is stronger than the fear of repeated failure. (f)

My sister cannot conceive, she is getting ready for artificial fertilisation and is terribly ashamed of it. (f)

My friend is unhappy because her husband doesn't agree with adoption. She is a teacher at a kindergarten. She says that makes it even worse because she realises all the time that she has no children of her own, she cannot avoid these thoughts. (f)

I'm handling it well since I already have two children. We've been trying to have a third one for nine years, and nothing has happened so far. (f)

It was getting on my nerves, I was blaming my husband, I always cried during menstruation. Now I would like a second one but I am afraid that things would not go well again, that I'd be unbearable, that we'd be heading for a divorce. (f)

The miscarriage got me down totally, and I'd gone through a lot. Then I was unable to conceive for two months, and I thought that was the end of the world. (f)

I couldn't have children and I've had trouble coping with it my whole life. A few months ago my husband died, and now I am totally alone. (f)

I was desperate, even 25 years later I still think about it with dread. (f)

I didn't cope with it well, especially the miscarriages. (f)

Always when I go to visit my little niece, I am sorry that I haven't got my own. I leave for home earlier than I planned, and cry the whole way. I also cry with each menstruation. I know in advance it's coming, and my husband just asks 'Is it?'... I talk about the situation only with my husband, talking with others frustrates me. (f)

It's getting on my nerves. Once my menstruation was eight days delayed, and when it came, I collapsed. For several days, I cried and cried from morning to evening, and my husband didn't know what to do with me. Now I can't enjoy anything. My sister is getting ready to get pregnant again, and I am afraid about how I will take it, if I won't be envious of her—even though I would be happy for her. (f)

I coped well with the first miscarriage, I told myself that every other woman has had a miscarriage. The second one was really hard, when the heart did not beat in the ultrasound and the placenta was peeling off... The third and the fourth ones were dreadful. I can't come to terms with it, even though I keep telling myself it's better than having cancer. At first, I was envious of my friends who became pregnant, and I couldn't bear to see a mother with a pram. Now I've got this under control. When I am waiting at the gynaecologist's and see a pregnant woman, I sympathise with her and tell myself, what if this poor pregnant woman ends up the same way as I did, what nightmares might be in store for her. (f)

I don't give up, I believe it'll turn out well. (f)

I probably won't even try again [3 miscarriages, author's note], I couldn't handle the 9 months, I haven't got the nerves for it. I can't deal with the frequent presence of my step-son, and my husband's interest in him. (f)

I am ashamed to buy the drugs necessary for the IVF, a friend buys them for me in a neighbouring town. (f)

I feel isolated, sometimes it's getting on my nerves. The last two years, I've been completely down, it's too much, and I can't cope with it. I am afraid of late motherhood, that I'd be an anxious mother. (f)

I am afraid of another pregnancy, I can't imagine that I'd be, for instance, in the eighth month. (f)

I think am not normal any more. I broke into tears even in company where not a word was spoken about the problem. (f)

When a woman wants a child, and doesn't have it, she wants it even more. (m)

I comfort myself with the thought that I am able to conceive, and so it is going to turn out well next time. (f)

For me, the world has collapsed. (f)

I gradually started to lose meaning in my life. My desire for a child tied me up so much that, even though I was always full of [other] interests, I couldn't concentrate on anything. (f)

I am worried about it but I am not in a bad mental condition. (f)

I'm still hoping that I'll get lucky and have a child. From my experience, I know that most of my fellow patients got pregnant only after the fourth or fifth attempt at IVF. (f)

I was devastated by the extrauterine pregnancy and the loss of an ovary. I am afraid of another transfer. (f)

More and more, the feeling of emptiness and pointlessness are getting to me. Many of my friends have their families, and that's why my husband and I are quite isolated. (f)

After four IVF failures and one miscarriage, I was desperate. (f)

I know well what it is to feel pointlessness and hopelessness. (f)

My wife can't cope with it, she is depressed, she is an anxious type. (m)

My wife has fixated on her nephew, she is spoiling him terribly. (m)

My wife worries needlessly; the application for adoption keeps her head above water. (m)

I can't come to terms with it; I am unable to relax. (f)

It's terrible for me just to keep waiting, I can't do that. I must be doing something for it all the time. (f)

Our own repeated disappointments, and the fact that I can't fulfil the heartfelt wishes of my close relatives. A feeling of impoverishment that the meaning of life is unfulfilled. A pity that there is no one to whom we could pass down the good in us, as our parents passed it down to us. (f)

I am always afraid of whether I'll be able to sleep at night at all. After the worst miscarriage, I felt so bad that I could not sleep at night, and in the morning I would be thanking God for the fact that I'd survived the night. (f)

My own parents were involuntarily childless for eight years and, for the second child, they waited another eight years. At that time childlessness wasn't as frequent as it is now, they themselves felt like outsiders, especially my mother felt it as her unworthiness, imperfection, she didn't feel as a fully valuable woman or human being. She felt unfulfilled, unable to give the love that she had within her, and the wish to have a child became almost an obsession with her. (f)

When I first learned that I could not have children in a normal way, I took it as a big injustice. Countless times, I've asked myself why it had to be me. (f)

We're getting ready for the second attempt at IVF in a short time. And I dread that it won't come off. Before, I thought that I was so strong, that I could stand almost anything, but now I feel completely the opposite. My sister has an eight-year-old girl who is mentally retarded. It happened during the birth, but I still ask myself, what if it happens to me too. I feel as if I don't know

> exactly what I want. On the one hand, I really wish to have a child and, on the other hand, I am scared of it all. It may be normal, but I rather think it is not normal. I am afraid that people would take me for a mad woman if I confessed my feelings to someone. It is simply utter isolation from people, even from the closest ones. (f)
>
> On the other hand, I mind seeing prams and pregnant women more and more. I also prefer avoiding my friends who have young children. I am probably a typical example of how a woman experiences these troubles. Probably I will have to go through all the suffering from the beginning to the end...there is no other way in life. At the moment, having a child is simply an unattainable idea...something like a rare natural phenomenon. (f)

Women are usually sad about their failures on the quest for a child. Psychologists would say that the failures bring about a depressive tuning in the women, even though to various degrees ('I was desperate, even 25 years later I think about it with dread' 'The last two years I've been completely down, it's too much, and I can't cope with it' 'My wife probably has depression from it' 'I had trouble coping with it my whole life' 'My wife can't cope with it, she is down, she is an anxious type' 'It's getting on my nerves' 'I can't come to terms with it, even though I keep telling myself it's better than having cancer' 'It isn't easy. One goes through many disappointments and hardships' 'It worries me but I am not in a bad mental condition' 'On the outside it may seem that I've been handling it well' 'I was even cheerful and optimistic' 'I've been handling it well'). Women experience feelings of helplessness ('It's terrible for me just to keep waiting'), fear of the future ('I am afraid of another transfer' 'I am afraid of late motherhood, that I'd be an anxious mother' 'I am afraid of another pregnancy, I can't imagine that I'd be for instance in the eighth month' 'On the other hand, I'm scared of it all'), and self-pity ('From time to time I struggle again with self-pity'), some women feel anger ('When someone tells me something in that sense, it can make me mad' 'I was even argued with my husband out of nervousness' 'I was blaming my husband' 'my anger and resentment against God were growing'), or injustice ('I took it as a big injustice. Countless times I've asked myself why it had to be me'). The women who already have a child, whether an adopted one or their own, cope with the situation better, but this is not a general rule ('Now I would like a second one but I am afraid that things wouldn't go well again, that I'd be unbearable').

The situation is full of losses. The main loss is the loss of a child, which is only rarely expressed in words ('At the moment, having a child is simply an unattainable idea...something like a rare natural phenomenon'). This loss is subconscious, usually experienced with the arrival of menstruation ('Once my menstruation was delayed 8 days, and when it came, I collapsed. For several days I cried and cried from morning to evening, and my husband didn't know what to do with me' 'Before each menstruation I was nervous, and when it appeared I cried' 'It was hard for me to deal with the repeated disappointments'), as a response to miscarriage ('I coped well with the first miscarriage, I told myself that every other woman has had a miscarriage. I couldn't cope with the second one when the heart did not beat at the ultrasound, and the placenta was peeling off. The third and the fourth ones were dreadful' 'After four IVF failures and one miscarriage I was desperate' 'The miscarriage got me down totally' 'I couldn't cope with it, especially the miscarriages' 'After the worst miscarriage I was feeling so bad that I could not sleep at night and in the morning I would be thanking God for the fact that I'd survived the night'), in contact with pregnant women or with children ('Always, when I go to visit my little niece, I am sorry that I haven't got my own. I leave for home earlier than I planned, and cry the whole way' 'My sister is getting ready to get pregnant again, and I am afraid of how I will take it, whether I won't be envious of her—even though I would be happy for her, too' 'I'm not coping with it well, especially when I am somewhere among children' 'She is a teacher at a kindergarten. She says that makes it even worse because she realises all the time that she has no children of her own, she cannot avoid these thoughts' 'When I looked at babies in prams and when a friend of mine conceived, a wave of sadness and of blaming myself would come' 'At the beginning I was envious of friends who became pregnant, and I couldn't bear to see a mother with a pram. Now I've got this under control. When I am waiting at the gynaecologist's and see a pregnant woman, I sympathise with her and tell myself, what if the poor pregnant woman ends up the same way I did' 'Seeing pregnant women has never stopped hurting me' 'I mind more and more seeing prams and pregnant women. I also prefer to avoid my friends who have young children'), but also when talking about children ('I avoided my colleagues' discussions about children and grandchildren' 'I talk about the situation only with my husband, talking with others frustrates me' 'I'm quite sensitive about the topic of children').

It seems that what affects a woman most is that she does not have a child. One of the first toys that a little girl gets is a doll. This is then usually supplemented with little beds, furniture, clothes, dishes etc. From early childhood, women prepare themselves (or are being prepared?) for a maternal role. A majority of women do not at all take into consideration that a child might not be a part (and often even the main or only goal and meaning) of their life. Women experience their fertility, their hope and loss, not only mentally, but—unlike men—also physically. Menstruation, let alone miscarriage, is not something that one can just not think about and notice, something that is possible to ignore. Moreover, menstruation always comes again. It is therefore a regular monthly source of feelings of sadness, disappointment, despair, a source that cannot be removed. But menstruation can also bring hope:

> A women's cycle has the advantage that when the bad days are over, a new month of hope begins again. (f)

Other stress factors are children, toys, pregnant women, advertisements with children; they are everywhere, and it is impossible to avoid them.

I would like to return to miscarriage because, for many people, it is a traumatic experience. Our culture has no rituals to help us cope with miscarriage (which is curious, since we live in a culture partly shaped by Judeo-Christian values, according to which life begins with conception), it does not give the partners a chance to weep over the loss of a child, to mourn over it. We do not even have an acceptable expression that would identify the unborn child: we use the medical terms embryo or fetus that do not express the emotional value of the unborn child for a person whose parenthood has not been fulfilled. Our social environment often does not accept the pain of the loss, and people offer cheap consolations such as, 'it's normal, every other woman has miscarried', 'be glad, nature knows what it's doing', or 'next time it will turn out well.'

> I have to admit that the hardest part was the response of other people, especially of my father and brother who didn't mention it in a single word, probably so that they wouldn't hurt me, but I was really hurt by that and felt very sad about it, and I'm still sad about it today. My husbands' parents' response was completely different, they told me how sorry they were, and I must say I was so grateful that they acknowledged it. We went through the loss of the child together with my husband, even if I sometimes feel that I forget that it was not a loss of my baby, but of our baby, equally painful for him as for me. I must remind myself of this all the time, so that I do not concentrate in my sadness just on myself. Also my mom was an immense support for me. (f)

In the American newspaper, *The Washington Post*, there is a column called 'Dear Abby'. In response to a reader's question about how to react to a colleague's miscarriage, 'Abby' replies that it is important to acknowledge the loss, and she recommends that flowers and a card expressing sadness be sent. Perhaps you will find this too much, but is it better to pretend that nothing happened?

Japanese Buddhists have a temple, Zozo-ji, devoted to Bodhisattva Jizo who looks after miscarried fetuses[6]. It is possible to bring him sacrifices—gifts for one's unborn child. The ritual is called mizuko kuyo (the Japanese word for the fetus is mizuko), which can be translated as 'a water child'. By saying this, I do not want to send you off to Japan to see Jizo, I only want to show that other cultures do respect mourning for a miscarried child. If a child represents an important value in your life, you definitely have the right to weep over it if you have lost it. There is indeed a difference in losing a five-day-old embryo and a five-year-old child, but this does not mean that miscarriage is not a reason for mourning.

> My brother died in childhood, so I have some idea how terrible it is to lose a baby. Perhaps it might sound cruel from me, but when a child dies, you have memories, you have photos, you have someone to cry for. We can't have a child so we don't even have the memories and the photos, we simply have no one to cry for. It seems we have no reason to cry, and that probably makes it even worse. (m)

Hopefully, it will not be too hard (perhaps with the help of a psychologist or a priest) to find one's own ritual to express the loss and cope with it. It can be expected that the experience of miscarriage is going to concern a growing number of women. More women will postpone motherhood until they are older (when the probability of miscarriage is greater), parenthood will more often be planned and wanted and, thanks to better and more widely available diagnostic techniques, it is possible to confirm pregnancy at home in the very early stages. One looks forward to a planned and wanted child, and from the moment one finds that the child exists, the child is considered an equal member of the family.

> We have three fertilized eggs and I should go for the transfer on Friday. My husband says that, until Friday, the child is away at camp. (f)

This perception is enhanced by the (sometimes-exaggerated) research results from the area of intrauterine development. An unsuccessful embryo transfer could be counted as a miscarriage situation, too: a life that came to be, but unfortunately did not continue. In one very good centre of assisted reproduction, there was a notice board in the waiting room that clearly explains the process of in vitro fertilisation to patients. The individual steps are titled: the first day of your baby (the day the egg is fertilised), the second day of your baby, the third day of your baby, and so on. It may be the case that this text, which is surely well meant, is also, due to its suggestiveness, iatrogenic (harm caused by a physician) in its effect.

It is interesting how few women mention the demands of the treatment ('The dreadful moments connected to the infertility treatment' 'I couldn't handle the 9 months, I haven't got the nerve for it' 'How much real physical pain all the performances cost me. But it is like with giving birth, one forgets the pain. And undergoes it again'). Probably the demands are, in comparison with the fact that one wants a child but does not have it, less important.

Sometimes a loss of hope occurs ('An immense part of my hope collapsed again'), but not always and with everybody ('The desire for a family is stronger than the fear of repeated failure' 'I comfort myself with the thought that I am able to conceive, and so it is going to turn out well next time' 'I'm hoping all the time that I'll be lucky and will have a child' 'The application for adoption keeps her head above water'). Some people lose their sense of meaning in life ('For me, the world has collapsed' 'I gradually started to lose the meaning of my life' 'The feeling of emptiness and pointlessness' 'I thought that was the end of the world' 'I know well how pointlessness feels'), their interest in other things ('Now I can't enjoy anything' 'My desire for a child tied up me so much that, even though I was always full of interests, I couldn't concentrate on anything').

Some women are ashamed that they do not have a child, they have feelings of inferiority ('I felt inferior, without full value' 'I am ashamed to buy the drugs' 'She is really ashamed for it' 'I didn't want to boast anywhere of the fact that I have no child'), or guilt ('I can't fulfil the heartfelt wishes of my close relatives'). It is interesting that, for women, there is usually no important distinction in the experiencing of the situation when the causes of infertility are on their side and when they are on the side of their partner. It even happens that a woman protects her husband from the consequences of the unfavourable diagnosis and from other people (and sometimes even from himself), and puts herself in the role of the disabled one (in this situation this means the incompetent one). I have come across this myself, and I have found such cases in some literature sources, too. This can happen for two reasons. The first reason is that the woman feels that, in the eyes of most people, the worse stigma is male infertility, and hence she chooses the lesser evil for the couple. The second reason may be that the woman carries a heavier burden as far as a descendant is concerned: in addition to conception, she must ensure the development and birth of the child. Therefore, it is she who was supposed to bring the child into the world and has not done so, regardless of the cause.

Many women feel lack of understanding in their surroundings, they feel isolated from their contemporaries ('Many of my friends have their families, and that's why my husband and I are quite isolated' 'I feel isolated' 'but I felt out of the scene. I was living through utter loneliness' 'An utter isolation from people, even the closest ones), it is difficult for them to find a common conversational topic ('I talk about the situation only with my husband, talking with others frustrates me' 'I avoided my colleagues' discussions about children and grandchildren' 'It was unpleasant for me to speak about it, especially when I met my schoolmates' 'When they talked about children, I automatically 'switched off.' Even more—I felt myself alone, "out of the picture", it wasn't my topic').

Often women reproach themselves that they are not coping with the situation ('Before I thought I was so strong, that I can bear and stand almost anything, but now I feel the complete opposite'), and they fear for their mental health ('Perhaps it is normal, but I rather think it is not normal. I am afraid people will take me for a lunatic').

I have talked with many unhappy women and I would like to point out that these feelings and states of mind are not manifestations of mental weakness. They are a normal response of a normal healthy woman in a demanding life situation.

What is the worst part for a woman?

The worst period was after the miscarriage. (f)
The worst part is that I wish to have a child and I want to know why we haven't got it so far. (f)
The stress of miscarriage. (f)
The feeling of loneliness, of an unfulfilled meaning of life. (f)
I keep missing something in my life. The worst is when my friends have children, and I feel overwhelmed by sadness. (f)
Being with children and then the subsequent loneliness at home. (f)
Emptiness. (f)

The worst is finding out every month that, once again, nothing. Then the results of constant examinations that do not show anything specific, and also other people. The families of friends where there are children without a problem, constant queries at work, pregnant women. (f)

Before adoption, I was sad when I saw a mother with a pram. (f)

The dreadful talk of the gynaecologists. I think they inflated the problems needlessly and made them appear critical, which also made my attitude critical. Then the monthly menstruation. (f)

Probably the constant feelings of helplessness. The alternation of hope and disappointment. The feeling that it may never work out, that not all people have children, there are many childless couples, and perhaps we belong among them. There was a lot that was going on in my mind, that I was thinking about again and again. (f)

The response of my surroundings (sometimes). (f)

The waiting for lab results, whether I was pregnant or not. Then, whether it was a normal or extrauterine pregnancy. The waking up after the surgery and realising that again it did not turn out, and one must start over. And the first unsuccessful attempt at IVF. That was like after a failed suicide. (f)

The waiting for adoption, the uncertainty, and what the situation will be like then, whether the child will be fine and healthy. (f)

The waiting, everything takes too long. It is demanding in terms of time, money, nerves, taking time off work. (f)

In the miscarrying women, the worst time is the period from the conception to the time when they are out of the woods (25th week), or after miscarriage. They cry about this, and then it is better. In women who cannot conceive, the waiting for a diagnosis is worst. (p)

The worst is the 'good' advice of other people. (f)

The fact that physicians don't pay attention to me because I already have two children. (f)

The self-complacency of the doctors. (f)

It was worst after the last miscarriage (in the 13th week). I told myself then that rather than this again, I'd prefer to remain without a child. I gave up on the treatment. When I conceived unexpectedly, I didn't admit to myself until the 20th week that I was pregnant, I felt dread that I would start being happy, and it would end up badly. It was also terrible when, after the miscarriages, I stayed in the same room with women who'd had abortions. (f)

My mother-in-law's pressure and each menstruation. (f)

It's bad all around. I was set up for motherhood, and it hasn't come. Probably the worst are mothers with tummies and prams. (f)

The biggest stress is when I am pregnant and I have ultrasound, what they will say (I've miscarried 4 times). When they say that the baby has grown by two millimetres, I grow by two meters. When they say the heart is not beating and the baby is not developing, it is the end. (f)

Is everything bad also good for something?

Certainly. It has given me more humbleness and inner maturity. I know now what it is like when someone is awaiting a child and the child isn't coming. (f)

Reinforcement of marriage. I can completely rely on my husband. (f)

The quest for a child has brought me to a different assessment of life values. (f)

I think it has strengthened our marriage, I talk a lot about everything with my husband. (f)

I've discovered that I can completely rely on my husband. We have a nice relationship. (f)

I know that, as far as dealing with problems is concerned, even those that might still come, there are two of us. (f)

I am not alone with it. (f)

I am trying to convince myself that everything bad is also good for something, that I can go on a holiday, live a life without major limitations, feel younger than my friends who have 12-year-old children. (f)

I am trying to be more open towards the problems of other people, to not just see myself. Our home is a meeting place for many people. If we had a child, this surely wouldn't be possible…and not the least advantage is the better financial situation of our household. The cementing of marriage. (f)

I know that I can rely on my partner, and that he would not leave me because of my 'illness'. (f)

I do not consider having children as simply a matter of course. It has also been important for me to realise that I cannot not force my husband into something. I was then probably better able to cope with the drawbacks of motherhood. (f)

Certainly! I do not believe that, eight years ago, I would have been able to enjoy motherhood in this way. I am definitely more patient, I am better able to differentiate between the more and the less important problems, I can take certain things with a healthy attitude, I try not to rush around, and I especially devote myself to my little daughters. Basically, we enjoyed eight beautiful, free years. (f)

Probably I have more regard for my baby, for the fact that I have it. I am experiencing motherhood better than if I were 18 and the child arrived unwanted. (f)

I have much more patience. (f)

Perhaps only the fact that we're not going to experience the pain our children experience, since we don't have any. But we aren't going to feel their joy and happiness either. (f)

Yes, we're older, we deal with various problems more calmly, we are financially and materially secure, we could concentrate just on the child. (f)

Each problem that a person solves, including this one, brings some personal growth. (f)

I've fully enjoyed the prayed-for motherhood. (f)

> Reinforcement of marriage. (f)
> A happy marriage. (f)
> My marriage works. (f)
> We have had a happy marriage for a number of years even without children. (f)
> The six years of our struggle for a child were long, but during that time we met so many good people who completely voluntarily help infertile couples, so that in retrospect it seems to me that it just flew by. I wouldn't want to repeat it, but I am grateful that we could get to know all those who helped us. (f)

The biggest gain for a woman is the reinforcement of the partner relationship ('Reinforcement of marriage. I can completely rely on my husband' 'I think it has strengthened our marriage, we talk a lot about everything with my husband' 'I can completely rely on my husband' 'I've discovered that I can completely rely on my husband. We have a nice relationship' 'I know that as far as dealing with problems is concerned, even those that might still come, there are two of us' 'I am not alone with it' 'A happy marriage' 'My marriage works' 'I know that I can rely on my partner, and that he would not leave me because of my 'illness'').

In the women who had to wait for a child, the quest for it has brought a more intensive experience of motherhood ('I do not believe that, 8 years ago, I would have enjoyed motherhood in this way' 'I was then probably better able to cope with the drawbacks of motherhood' 'Probably I have more regard for my baby, for the fact that I have it. I can experience motherhood better than if I were 18, and the child arrived unwanted' 'I've enjoyed the prayed-for motherhood').

Many women observe personal growth ('Personal growth' 'More humbleness and inner maturity'), above all patience, calm, and realisation of life's priorities ('I am definitely more patient, I am better able to differentiate between the more and the less important problems, I can take certain things with a healthy attitude, I try not to rush and I devote myself more to my little daughters' 'Patience' 'Yes, we're older, we solve various problems more calmly' 'A different assessment of life's values' 'I do not consider having children as simply a matter of course'), and more empathy ('I know what it is like when someone is waiting and the child isn't coming' 'I am trying to be more open towards the problems of other people, to see not just myself' 'The realisation that I cannot force my husband into something'). It is also possible to meet kind people on the quest for a child ('I am grateful that we could get to know all those who helped us').

A life without a child brings a certain freedom ('Basically we enjoyed 8 beautiful, free years'), especially in terms of time and personal space ('I can go on a holiday, live a life without major limitations, feel younger than my friends who have 12-year-old children' 'Our home is a meeting place for many people. If we had a child, this surely wouldn't be possible'), financially ('We are financially and materially secure' 'The better financial situation of our household'), and to a certain degree, emotionally ('We're not going to experience the pain our children would experience, since we don't have any').

. . . How Do Men Respond?

> *Once upon a time there was a farmer. He had enough money and fields and, though he was respected and well off, something was missing in his happiness: he and his wife did not have children. Many times, when he went with other farmers to a market in town, the others taunted him and asked him why it was he who did not have children. Once he got utterly annoyed. He came home, hit the table and he shouted with rage: 'I want a child, even if it were a hedgehog.'*
>
> 'Hans-Hedgehog', *Grimms' Fairy Tales*

The fairy tale may have encouraged the impression that we are going to talk about enraged men. But draw your conclusions only after you have read the testimonies.

> I am sad that I haven't got my own child. (m)
>
> He doesn't talk about it, and he isn't very enthusiastic about various examinations. He never speaks about it himself, the discussion is always prompted by me. Nonetheless, he longs for children very much. (f)
>
> He was sorry about it, but he was trying to support me mentally, and he has even reconciled himself with the idea that we won't have children. (f)
>
> He feels very much for me, he always goes with me to all the medical examinations. He is my support. He never reproaches me with anything. (f)
>
> He was trying to keep the problems with a child secret. He is very nervous about it, he couldn't cope with it very well. (f)
>
> My husband has been handling the problem much better than me. He doesn't keep an eye on any bodily changes and, moreover, he is very busy at work. But he is a big mental support for me. (f)
>
> He's been handling the situation well. Without inhibitions, he has undergone all the various examinations with me. In the future, he would like to have his own child, but I think that he would get reconciled with the fact that unfortunately we may not be successful. (f)

My partner is quite young, and on the outside very strong and calm. He was surely worried about the situation, but he didn't show it much. Also, his desire for a child wasn't yet as strong as mine. He's helped me a lot. (f)

He was probably worried about it, but he didn't show it. He was trying to distract me from the problem mainly by sports activities. (f)

He didn't show anything, he supported me. (f)

He reconciled himself to the fact that I couldn't have children, and we mutually complemented and supported each other. (f)

He didn't show it, but he wasn't coping with it well (azoospermia). (f)

At first he reacted by denying the problem and by showing a great reserve toward me, then he calmed down and maintained the position of the support in the background. (f)

For a successful entrepreneur, this was a bitter defeat in life. (f)

I don't feel like writing about it much (about my experience with the treatment) because I'm already getting angry again. (m)

Men want children less than women, mostly they want them because of their wives. (p)

My husband never liked children much. When we planned how many children we were going to have, he wanted one and I wanted five. Now we are trying to have a second child for the third year; we have a five-year-old boy called Tom. It is not successful and I am gradually becoming reconciled to this. I have work that I enjoy and this helps me. However, my husband is worse off. He longs terribly for a baby, practically nothing makes him happy any more, he just keeps on asking me if I got it or not. (f)

My husband is coping with it far worse than I am, he keeps asking whether it has come off yet. (f)

Nothing that terrible happened. I'm searching for information about what next. (m)

My husband yelled at the woman doctor who told him that the spermiogram was 'nothing much'. Next time she told him it had the parameters for a donated one. He likes children a lot, he is very good with them, he's been the first one to suggest adoption. He supports me. (f)

My husband has trouble coping with it, much more than I do. (f)

He copes with it well, but he doesn't understand at all what I'm living through. But he is a big support, he always strokes me and gives me a hug. But he doesn't feel like doing it much any more, he takes it hard when I complain. (f)

It took me a year to get my husband to have an examination, he kept refusing stubbornly, saying that he wouldn't go. (f)

My husband sometimes yells at home, who am I building the house for, only dogs will be left after us. (f)

I am coping with it well, I am looking into the future. (m)

A friend of mine couldn't conceive, and they found out that her husband was completely infertile. He has been mean to her since. He has refused the use of donor sperm. When my friend goes for an examination, he tells her that he hopes that something is found in her as well, so that it is fair. (f)

It seems he doesn't care much to have a child because he has one already. (f)

Nothing matters to him, not even the payment of IVF. (f)

He enjoys his work, he is an athlete, he can distract himself by sport. He copes with it well. (f)

He yelled at the woman doctor when she told him he had a bad spermiogram. (f)

He didn't handle the diagnosis well at all, but he was brave during the treatment. (f)

My first husband couldn't bear it, the second one knew about the problem. He's never mentioned a word about wanting a child, it's more as if he were quite happy that he has me for himself. (f)

He found fulfilment in his job, which he enjoyed. He was completely satisfied with the relationship and he didn't feel an intense need to have a child. It was him who first came up with the idea of adoption. (f)

He was devastated when they told him about it. (f)

When they found a worsened spermiogram in me, I told myself it was for the better when we both had to cope with it. (m)

I am not stressed. I believe that it will turn out well and, if not, there'll still be some sunny days. (m)

I do not doubt that it will turn out well. My graphologist told me. (m)

I wouldn't mind not having a child, I've become a bit lazy, I have my work and interests. (m)

I do not like the type of company where people speak only about children (m)

He didn't want to have a spermiogram, it was hard to get him to go there. When the diagnosis arrived (azoospermia), it was a shock. (f)

I could not get him to have a spermiogram, he had an appointment several times and he didn't show up, so I had to smooth it over. He went after half a year. (f)

The healer's statement that he has plenty of energy, that the results of the spermiogram are nonsense, and that he will have loads of children keep him going. He certainly isn't giving up. (f)

I have always had the impression that he stands somewhere to the side, that he isn't going along with me, or that he is afraid—yes that's perhaps it—that he is afraid of my pain. (f)

The worst is to look at my wife and see her suffer from it. And my mom's remarks that she would like to have a grandchild are also unpleasant. (m)

We found a good spermiogram in one man. He got terribly angry and scolded us that we had a mess in the lab, that we substituted the samples because he'd had a bad spermiogram twice. Even though he upset me, I didn't ask

> him to leave, but told him that the substitution of a sample is impossible, that he can see for himself. I asked him to come for another examination when he would spend the whole time with his sample in the lab. He came, sat in the lab, had his sample before his eyes all the time. The lab assistant processed his sample before him and showed him the living sperms under the microscope. It was fine. The man was happy, apologetic, and hugged the lab assistants. (p)
>
> My wife has gone through four miscarriages. Over the years, she always remembers all the four times she's lost a baby, and says: so today it's been eight years since the first one, today it's been two years since the fourth one… I had a hard time coping with the miscarriages too, but today I would not be able to put together not only the days and months, but not even the years…when it happened. (m)
>
> Only many years later, when we'd given up on the attempts, did my husband start talking about how he suffered from the situation and how much he longed for a child. I worked among women, and always when my husband and I were leaving for a holiday, my colleagues were wishing me success so that we would bring back a baby. My husband didn't experience that, among men they don't speak about these things. (f)
>
> When my wife became pregnant after eight years of attempts, they sent her to have a genetic examination of the fetus water. After that she miscarried. The next two years were the worst in my life. I am a tough guy, but even now when I see a moving film, I start crying. (m)
>
> My husband is a physician. A superb physician. But when it comes to his illnesses, he falls apart and doesn't try to solve anything. It was the same with the treatment of infertility. First, after the miscarriages, when the cause was found in me, he encouraged me, searched for information, went everywhere along with me. But then it was discovered that there were problems in him too. After that, he didn't talk to me, he avoided the conversation, he didn't make an effort, didn't want to go anywhere. (f)

If you put the testimonies about the female and the male ways of experiencing this complicated situation next to each other, you will discover a very interesting thing. In the testimonies about women, it is not obvious what the cause of the couple's infertility is. They are concerned above all with the fact that the child is missing. However, in the testimonies about men, it is often clear from the context of the telling when the cause is in the man.

The discovery of reduced fertility is a heavy blow for a man ('He couldn't cope with the diagnosis' 'He was devastated' 'When the diagnosis arrived (azoospermia), it was a shock' 'He is very nervous about it, he couldn't cope with it very well' 'He didn't show it, but he wasn't coping with it well (azoospermia)' 'For a successful entrepreneur, this was a bitter defeat in life'). Sometimes he responds by denying the problem and trying to keep it a secret, other times by resigning himself to his fate ('The results of the spermiogram are nonsense, and that he will have loads of children' 'He was trying to keep the problems with a child secret' 'He avoided discussion, he didn't make effort, he didn't want to go anywhere'), by anger ('He yelled at the doctor when she told him he had a bad spermiogram' 'He hopes that something is found in her as well, so that it is fair'), or by feeling guilty ('He is afraid—yes that's perhaps it—that he is afraid of my pain').

A positive response is an exception ('When they found a worsened spermiogram in me, I told myself it was for the better when we both had to cope with it') and it is evidently a victory of the man's love toward his wife over potential loss of self-value. A paradoxical case is an angry response to favourable diagnosis ('They found a good spermiogram in one man. He got terribly angry, and scolded them'), but when we think about it, this is not a reaction to the diagnosis but to its unexpectedness. The man had probably reconciled himself to his reduced fertility to a certain degree and the change took him aback. So his response can be explained better by his great sensitivity to the topic. This sensitivity is expressed also in his response to the favourable diagnosis ('He was happy and hugged the lab assistants').

We can only try to guess whether it is worse for a man to face the result of an unfavourable diagnosis (I cannot have a child), that is the loss of a child, or to face the cause of this diagnosis (I am infertile), i.e. the potential loss of one's self-esteem, the loss of control over the situation. Another factor could be a feeling of guilt towards the woman ('He is afraid—yes that's perhaps it—that he is afraid of my pain').

Why is it such a sensitive issue for men? Fertility, virility, and potency are close relatives in people's common understanding of things. If a man is infertile, according to traditional thinking, it is because he is impotent (in a broader sense, absolutely incapable of anything). The subject of the perception of male infertility is mentioned in a film. The couple is returning from an examination in which infertility was found on the man's side. The man is in shock, probably also drunk. He assumes that the doctor sent him to the examination on purpose, so that he would emabarass him before other people: So that people can point at me: look, a capon!

The testimonies seem to suggest that men do not experience the loss of a child as intensely as women, even though here, too, both poles are represented ('He copes with it well' 'He reconciled himself to it' 'He says that nothing horrible happens' 'My husband handles the problem much better than myself' 'He was sorry about it' 'He would be unable to put together, not only the days and months, but even the years when it happened' 'He does not like the type of company where people speak only about children' 'He copes with it much worse' 'How he suffered from the situation, and how much he longed for the child' 'He longs terribly for a baby, practically nothing makes him happy any more' 'She miscarried. The next two years were the worst in my life'). Specifically, men experience sadness ('I am sad') and rage ('My husband sometimes yells at home, who am I building the house for').

The question is, why? It can be because a child is not as exclusively important for a man on his scale of life's values as it is for a woman ('He was fulfilling himself at work, which he enjoyed. He was completely satisfied with the relationship and he didn't feel an intense need to have a child' 'He's never mentioned in a word that he would want a child, as if he were quite happy that he has me for himself' 'I wouldn't mind staying without a child, I am a bit lazy, I have work and interests'). Surely an important factor is that men do not express emotion as easily as women ('He never speaks about it himself' 'Only many years later did my husband start talking about it' 'Perhaps he was worried about it, but he didn't show it' 'He didn't show anything') and fatherhood is not as frequent a topic of their discussion ('Among men, they don't speak about it'). This would indicate that the lesser intensity of their experiencing of the loss of a child is only seeming. This is further confirmed by the fact that it has been difficult for me to find a man who would be willing to talk about it—mostly not because they would not be interested in the topic, but because they do not like discussing it. Notice that the majority of the testimonies about male experiencing of the complications on the quest for a child are by women. An important role is played the fact that—as expressly indicated by one testimony—a man does not observe any bodily changes. A woman experiences the hope and the loss even at the bodily level, for her, unlike for a man, there is no escape from it.

It is also well known that very little attention has so far been devoted to the emotional factors of fatherhood. Motherhood is constantly emphasised, but interest in fatherhood lags behind. When I speak somewhere about the psychological problem of being involuntarily childless, I am always asked: What is the woman's response? What about her unfulfilled motherhood? And I say: and what is the man's response? What about his unfulfilled fatherhood? I usually embarrass my interviewers. But it is clear that better times are coming. In one magazine, I discovered an article titled The New-Style Virility that was devoted to the ideal of a man. According to the article, in the near future, the ideal will become a handsome, pleasant guy, well-secured, with a big dose of self-esteem, and, moreover, with a baby in his arms. I cannot help voicing the ironic remark that I would be glad if the baby could remain in his arms longer than for posing for the picture.

The man is concerned only with conception; the woman must also ensure the development and the birth of the child, and so each partner's participation in the treatment is different as well. Sometimes, it is difficult to get the man to participate physically ('He didn't want to undergo the spermiogram, there were problems to get him to go there' 'I could not get him to have the spermiogram, he had an appointment several times, and he didn't show up, so I had to smooth it over. He went after half a year'). One possible reason may be that he does not want the child hard enough, i.e. the motivation is not strong enough. The second possibility is that he either does not doubt his fertility or, to the contrary, he is not sure and is not interested in the official confirmation of the diagnosis. Or perhaps he has heard something about the way of collecting the sperm and he finds it undignified. The next possibility is that men very often dislike going to see a doctor ('When it comes to his illnesses, he fails. He…didn't make an effort, he didn't want to go anywhere') Do you see that a big role on the quest for a child is played by the motivation, the attitudes, and the prejudices of each partner? Many therapists consider the man's refusal to participate in the therapeutic procedure to be an exception, and from the fact that only some women mention such a refusal one can conclude that most men do not have any difficulties in accepting their share in the quest for a child ('Without inhibitions, he has undergone all possible examinations with me').

The man is mostly aware of the demands of the treatment and tries to alleviate the suffering, whose bulk lies on the woman ('He always goes with me for all the medical examinations. He is my support' 'He's helped me a lot' 'He was trying to distract me from the problem' 'He supported me'). His specific activity may have the form of encouragement ('Definitely he isn't giving up' 'He believes that it will end well' 'He looks toward the future') or search for solutions ('He reconciled himself to the fact that we couldn't have children' 'He's been the first one to suggest adoption' 'He's searching for information about what next'). If his activities run against obstacles, the man can experience the feeling of losing control over the situation and the feeling of the resulting anger ('I don't feel like writing everything (about my experience with the treatment) because I'm getting angry again' 'He yells at home, who am I building the house for').

Not even the lack of understanding from other people is a major problem for most men. Sometimes they dislike the topic of the conversation ('I do not like the type of company where people speak only about children'), but this does not seem to happen too often ('Among men, they don't speak about it').

In the UK, there is a website specifically for men. Its authors say: 'Any professional involved in fertility counselling and/or treatment will tell you that it is the women that tend to ask the questions and drive the process forward. This in itself often adds to the infertile man's feeling of insecurity and identity crisis which drives him further from the place he need's to be. Whilst many efforts have and are being made to address the uniquely "male" issues affecting choices of treatment, gender communication and counselling, the reality remains that men are largely "unreached". The aim of MENSFE is to determine whether creative use of interactive tools now widely used on the Internet may be a means of offering support and even therapy.'[7] (You can visit the website at http://mensfe.net)

What is the worst part for a man?

To look on helplessly as my wife suffers. (m)
The worst is to see how my wife suffers. (m)

Is everything bad also good for something?

One has learned something about a problem that formerly wasn't a concern at all. (m)
It has reinforced our marriage, I respect my wife all the more. (m)
I have a nice relationship with my wife, we have more time for each other. (m)

As in women, reinforcement of the partners' relationship and personal growth dominate as positive aspects in a negative situation.

What is the impact on the partner's relationship?

Now Laban had two daughters; the name of the older was Leah, and the name of the younger was Rachel. Leah had weak eyes, but Rachel was...beautiful. Jacob was in love with Rachel and said, 'I'll work for you seven years in return for your younger daughter Rachel.' ...Then Jacob said to Laban, 'Give me my wife. My time is completed.' ...But Leah was not loved, so her womb was opened, but Rachel was barren. Leah became pregnant and gave birth to a

> *son... She conceived again and she gave birth to a son... When Rachel saw that she was not bearing Jacob any children, she became jealous of her sister. So she said to Jacob, 'Give me children, or I'll die!'...Jacob became angry with her and said, 'Am I in the place of God, who has kept you from having children?' Then she said, 'Here is Bilhah, my maidservant. Sleep with her so that she can bear children for me and that through her I too can build a family.'*
>
> Gen 29: 16–30, 30: 1–3

The quest for a child is a quest of two people, two different people. The woman perceives it one way, the man another way. What is the impact on the partners' relationship?

I have a feeling that the problem strengthens my relationship with my partner. He definitely gives me hope, otherwise I would not be able to undergo the endless and exhausting examinations. (f)

Also important for me is the realisation that one cannot force my husband into something. (f)

The results of my husband's examination came to my gynaecologist. She told me they were bad. I decided not to tell my husband about it and leave it as my fault, since I have endometriosis anyway. He learned about it anyway, when we had artificial fertilisation, the doctor told him about it. (f)

A friend couldn't conceive, and they found that her husband is completely infertile. He has been mean to her since. He has refused the use of donor sperm. When my friend goes to have an examination, he tells her he hopes that something is found in her as well, so that it is fair. (f)

When they found a worsened spermiogram in me, I told myself it was for the better when we both had to cope with it. (m)

What's great about my husband is that he has agreed to adoption. The only thing that keeps me going is a great husband who understands me and supports me. But he didn't stand up for me when his step-mother humiliated me. Also, he doesn't participate in the treatment directly, he didn't go with me for the IVF transfer. Also, he can't fully understand my desire for a child. (f)

If the treatment is successful, I would take my child and leave my husband because I wouldn't need him for anything then. (f)

He is a big support, he always strokes me and gives me a hug. But he doesn't feel like doing it much any more, he takes it hard when I complain. (f)

He supports me, but when it doesn't come off, he is angry for a day, the next day he is already relaxed, he says it doesn't matter, next time it will come off. I'd need to cry before him and talk it out, I keep telling him I need him to hug me. He won't do it, he is angry with me. He hates it when I cry, he says only weaklings cry. (f)

My husband has supported me against his parents. (f)

The results of my husband's examination came by mail to our home. The letter wasn't registered, so I opened the envelope. The diagnosis was azoospermia, followed by the suggestion to use a donor's sperm or adoption. I wanted to hide the letter immediately so that my husband wouldn't see it, but he unfortunately appeared in the door at that very moment. He was in shock. To calm him down, I told him that for me, he is the best guy in the world anyway, and that it is more important for me to be with him than to have children. (f)

My husband couldn't mentally cope with the fact, and the marriage broke down. (f)

My first husband couldn't bear it, my second husband knew about the problem. He's never mentioned a word about wanting a child. (f)

We've remained childless. When we had a party for my fortieth birthday, my husband got tipsy, and told me: I always kept waiting for you to bring a little Gypsy girl home. I was shocked, I would never have imagined that he would be for adoption. (f)

I am 40, and after a 20 year, and, from my viewpoint, a very happy marriage, I've found myself alone. I was very attached to my husband and I did everything only for him. My pain and my blame was that I could not have children. I underwent a long treatment, but without results. My husband claimed he didn't mind it at all, that it was actually pleasant that I gave him all my care and love. He started changing last year. My good husband turned into someone different. I didn't understand anything, and I lost the last remains of my self-esteem. Then I learned that my husband had a relationship with a 30-year-old colleague, a divorced mother of two young children. My husband moved to live with his lover. Then he handed in a divorce petition, and as the main reason he stated my infertility. I had to reconcile myself to it, even if it still hurts, but I don't know what to do with myself. I'm afraid of people, I have no confidence, the divorce and the disgrace lie on me like a stigma. I dread that I will stay alone forever and, mainly, I don't understand why it had to happen. (f)

We've been trying to conceive a child for eight years, and I must say that I am glad I have precisely this husband. He fights along with me, and I respect him a lot for it. Nonetheless, I feel as if there were something between us. We talk about it all the time, but one can see that, for him, the talks are unpleasant. I would need to talk more, to consider together various possibilities, it is as if he were running away from it. I actually don't know what he's experiencing. The other day, he surprised me immensely. We were at the psychological examination of the applicants for adoption, and the psychologist explained to us that we could have a child in a month or in four years. My husband said it would be perfect if it were in a month. I hadn't expected it. He was all hope, and he talked about the problems related to adoption. He knew more than I did! He is concerned about it, but he doesn't talk to me about it. (f)

> Perhaps, as an extreme case, I would like my husband to take another woman with whom he would be able to have children, and I would look for a man with a child. (f)
>
> We got married with the understanding that such is life, and that we would live only for each other. (f)
>
> A woman called me, and asked for contact information for the clinics performing special spermiological examinations. Then she broke into tears, and said that her husband had a bad spermiogram and refused to undergo any further examinations or treatment. She said he even refused to talk about the problem. But I am 100 per cent sure that her husband had called me a few weeks ago and had asked for the same information. His interest was palpable, he even called twice, first at the arranged time and then half a day later because initially I could not find the contacts. He carefully noted down everything and it was obvious that he was well informed in the problem and that he had much interest in solving the situation. But apparently he didn't say anything to his wife (nor did I reveal his activities). (p)
>
> Fortunately, I have a good husband who undergoes everything with me. He keeps calming me down so that I do not suffer. (f)
>
> Then it was discovered that there were problems also in him. After that he didn't talk to me, he avoided discussion, he didn't make any effort, didn't want to go anywhere. When your husband doesn't talk to you at home, you prefer to go to the pub with friends. And a problem is in the making. We like each other a lot, so we've coped with the crisis. But it was close. (f)

I have only a few testimonies about a negative impact of the common quest for a child on the partners' relationship. Sometimes one of the partners cannot cope with the demanding situation and abandons the other. The abandoned partner can be either the woman ('My husband couldn't mentally cope with the fact, and the marriage broke down' 'My first husband couldn't bear it') or the man ('If the treatment was successful, I would take my child and leave my husband because I wouldn't need him for anything then' 'Perhaps, as an extreme case, I would like my husband to take another woman with whom he would be able to have children, and I would look for a man with a child'). But notice the preceding sentence, which shows that the breakdown of the marriage is one of the possible reasonable solutions of the given situation, not the consequence of uncontrolled emotions.

Problems with the conception of a child, the unfulfilled desire for it, and the demanding examinations and treatment present the couple with a difficult situation ('You prefer going to the pub with friends. And a problem is in the making.'). The breakdown of marriage due to the infertility of one of the partners is a disputable thing. It is hard to prove that the marriage would not have broken down if there not been fertility problems (what if the child was born with no problem, but was disabled?), and it is just as hard to know whether the infertility is not a substitute problem, easier to defend before oneself and before society. The longer section about the departure of the husband to the lover with children immediately suggests the question whether the husband did not leave for a younger woman rather than for her children.

The testimonies in the two preceding sections about the experiencing of women and men indicate that, if the quest for a child brings anything positive, it is the deepening of the relationship between the partners. What characterizes the reinforcement of the relationship? Above all it is the discovery that one may count on the partner's support in bad times ('He definitely gives me hope, otherwise I would be unable to undergo the endless and exhausting examinations' 'The great husband who understands me and supports me' 'He always strokes me, and gives me a hug' 'My husband has supported me against his parents' 'I told him that for me, he is the best guy in the world anyway, and that it is more important for me to be with him, than having children' 'He fights along with me'), and the resulting deeper knowledge of the other partner ('The realisation that one should not force my husband to do something').

The partners are willing to share the burden of treatment and the mental consequences, either in the positive sense ('When they found a worsened spermiogram in me, I told myself it was for the better when we both had to cope with it' 'Not to tell my husband about it, and keep it to myself' 'To hide the letter (azoospermia, the author's note) immediately, so that my husband doesn't see it'), or, sometimes, in the negative sense ('He hopes that something is found in her as well, so that it is fair'), which does not show much support for the partner.

Even when women positively evaluate the influence of the quest on the marriage, they often talk about the limits of the partner's emotional support ('But he didn't stand up for me when his step-mother humiliated me. Also he doesn't participate in the treatment directly, he didn't go with me for the IVF transfer. Also, he can't fully understand my desire for a child' 'But he doesn't feel like doing it much, he takes it hard when I complain' 'I'd need to cry before him, and talk it out, I'm telling him I need it him to hug me. He won't do it' 'That he stands somewhere outside, that he isn't going along with me, or that he is afraid—yes that's perhaps it—that he is afraid of my pain'), admitting that they miss talking together and that the partner makes light of the situation. This is, of course, nothing new. It is agreed among psychotherapists[i] that women need to share experiences, to express feelings, to talk about them, and to find an attentive listener. Women convey their worries, difficulties, joys, and injuries. Most often, they do not need to be advised by the man, but they need to be listened to, sympathised with, understood, and consoled. Male superficial commentaries and advice such as 'let your hair down, it's all just nonsense,' are not usually well received.

> I am most worried about our relationship. My wife cries at home and, recently, it has been just too much for me. I try to help her somehow, but that only tends to make it worse. A week ago, I ordered a week-long relaxation stay in a spa, but she refused to go. (m)
>
> All our contemporaries have children, but we have none. We are believers and, in the church, it is common to have children early in life, they look at us as if we were strange. I have no one to visit and talk to. Sometimes, my nerves give way and I cry at home. My husband tries to help me, and keeps thinking of some activities so that I think about something else. We have been abroad on vacation many times, but it is boring to travel alone. Now he has ordered a weekend relaxation stay in a spa, but the idea of lying somewhere in a bath filled with mud and relaxing was horrible for me, so I refused to go. And we argued terribly. I would be completely happy if my husband would just let me cry myself out in his arms and then I would be all right. (f)

Every problem that occurs in a partnership is very demanding in terms of communication ('That I feel as if there were 'something' between us'). Women need to express their feelings and share them with their partners; men, to the contrary, express their feelings related to parenthood only sparsely and unwillingly ('He is angry with me. He hates it when I cry, he says only weaklings cry' 'It is as if he were running away from it. I actually don't know what he's experiencing' 'She said he even refused to talk about the problem' 'Since then he refused to talk about it with me, he avoided discussion, he didn't make any efforts, he didn't want to go anywhere'). Sometimes men express their feelings and views more easily under some special circumstances ('My husband got tipsy, and told me' 'We were at the psychological examination of the applicants for adoption, and…my husband said it would be perfect if it were in a month. I hadn't expected it. He was all hope').

It is necessary to find a certain compromise. The woman accepts the fact that the man is less talkative in this direction, and that it is demanding for him to share strong emotions. Even for Jacob thousands of years ago, it was difficult to cope with the emotional outpouring of his wife: And she said to Jacob, 'Give me children or else I die!' And Jacob's anger was kindled against Rachel... The man, in turn, realizes that the woman needs to feel that she is not alone in her suffering, that she has someone next to her who is looking for the solution of the situation along with her, similarly to Rachel who wanted Jacob to somehow deal with her sadness.

Talking about the problem is nonetheless very important for the solution. When people do not convey to each other their perceptions of the situation and do not discuss their ideas about possible solutions ('He is concerned about it, but he doesn't talk to me about it' 'It was obvious that he oriented himself well in the problem, and that he had much interest in solving the situation'), they may not find an optimal solution ('I was always waiting when you were going to bring a little Gypsy girl home... I was shocked, I would never have imagined that he would be for adoption').

Be Fruitful and Multiply and Replenish the Earth

Genesis 1: 28

An important part of partnership communication is making love. It is not only part of communication, but it is also one of the steps on the quest for a child. However, spontaneous communication and communication as part of completing a task do not necessarily get along well together. As you know, when you *must* do something, it is not always the same as wanting to do it.

> We're trying to abstain (a little) before ovulation, so that there is a greater chance during the fertile days. (m)
> We aren't influenced by it in any way. (f)
> Yes, the daily measuring of temperature and the stress that I haven't become pregnant again have partly degraded joyful sex to work duty. (f)
> Partly. It is influenced by the repeated examinations, the IVF, gynaecological inflammations (formerly without problems). (f)
> We can't achieve pregnancy naturally (azoospermia), so we aren't influenced by it. (f)
> Sometimes I have a feeling that I'm losing appetite, and that I'm overcome by tiredness. (f)
> At the beginning the task to become pregnant influenced us, but it no longer does. (f)
> Of course it did, because our sexual life was determined by the fertile and infertile days, whether we felt like it or not. And you keep thinking about what to do to make it work out. (f)

Completely. The first three months—despite birth control—my partner didn't make love to me at all, then we gradually renewed our love life again. But the healthy spontaneity was often missing. (f)
Minimally. (f)
We weren't influenced by it in any way because my husband wasn't that interested in having a child. (f)
Yes! I didn't enjoy it at all. We made love only so that I would become pregnant. (f)
No, because I couldn't become pregnant anyway. (f)
We each lived in a different city, so we didn't see each other very often. It may seem strange but, for us, IVF was one big rendezvous. (f)
No, but I was strongly bothered by the attempts on command: now the drugs should be working, we must give it a try. (f)
In the fertile days, my wife isn't spontaneous, she is too concentrated on becoming pregnant, then she lies with cushions under her buttocks so that the sperm wouldn't flow out. (m)
During stimulation, her tummy ached a lot when she was ovulating, so the intercourse was very careful and purely pragmatic. (m)
She is meticulous about counting the fertile days, and when it is supposed to come, it doesn't work. Other times, when nothing is at stake, the love-making is wonderful. In the fertile days, I have a feeling that it hurts her more than she enjoys it. (m)
Married sex isn't as passionate and exciting as lovers' sex, I have fixated myself on the thought of becoming pregnant too much. (m)
A married couple I know used to entertain their friends by the stories about how they were trying to get themselves an heir. In addition to carefully following all the physicians' instructions, they also followed whatever someone advised them in good faith as a 'sure thing'. Once someone provided her with the information that a man's fertility increases tremendously after he's had a fright. The moment—it was around three in the morning—when he was woken up by a deafening crash and she was standing above him holding two pan lids, he packed up his shaving things and went to sleep in his office for three days. The method did not get tested that time. (f)

The attempts at becoming pregnant, examinations, and the treatment of fertility problems reduce spontaneity ('Completely. The first 3 months—despite the contraceptives—my partner didn't make love to me at all, then we gradually renewed our love life again. But the 'healthy spontaneity' was often missing' 'In the fertile days, my wife isn't very spontaneous, she is concentrating too much on becoming pregnant' 'Not as passionate and exciting as lover's sex' 'She is meticulous in counting the fertile days, and when it is supposed to come, it doesn't work. Other times, when nothing is at stake, the love-making is wonderful' 'Sometimes I have a feeling that

I'm losing appetite, and that I'm overcome by tiredness' 'I was strongly bothered by the trials on command'). A love relationship turns into a pragmatic one ('The intercourse was very careful and purely pragmatic' 'They have degraded a joyful sex to work duty' 'I didn't enjoy it at all. We made love only so that I could become pregnant').

The right time is determined ('She is meticulous in counting the fertile days' 'determined by fertile and infertile days' 'Now the drugs should be working') and the most effective way of achieving pregnancy is sought ('Then she lies with the cushions under her buttocks, so that the sperm doesn't flow out' 'One thinks all the time what one should do, so that it is successful'). The process is also influenced by the treatment ('The repeated examinations, IVF, gynaecological inflammations' 'At the time of stimulation, her tummy ached a lot after ovulation, so intercourse was very careful' 'The drugs should be working' 'The everyday measuring of temperature'). Even love-making in infertile days is influenced ('We're trying to abstain (a little) before ovulation, so that there is a greater chance during the fertile days'). At first, the joy of love-making can be spoiled by the fear of pregnancy, because you are trying to use the most ingenious techniques of how to prevent the arrival of a child. Then, when the time comes and you want the child, the joy of love-making can be spoiled precisely by the fact that you must be making love, moreover at the predetermined time. And again, you can be thinking up the most ingenious techniques ('That the man's fertility increases incredibly after a fright. The moment—it was around three in the morning—when he was woken up by a deafening crash'), this time so that you would favour the baby's arrival.

Under certain circumstances, the love relationship is not influenced. This is in the case when it is impossible to achieve pregnancy naturally ('We can't achieve a pregnancy by the natural way, so we aren't influenced by it' 'No, because I couldn't become pregnant anyway') or when one of the partners is not engaged in the quest for a child ('We weren't influenced by it in any way because my husband wasn't much interested in the child'). I can imagine that the husband is not influenced when he does not plan for the child. But, unfortunately, it is not clear whether the wife is also not influenced or whether she does not, after all, monitor the fertile and infertile days for herself. It also seems that love-making is not influenced by the planning of the child after a longer time spent on the quest for it ('At the beginning, the task to become pregnant influenced us, but it no longer does').

The situation when IVF is practically the only opportunity for meeting the partner is special ('For us, IVF was always one great rendez-vous').

What is it like in families where they already have children?

> When I didn't get my period, I got a terrible fright, I thought I had cancer, I already saw my children as orphans. A few weeks later, I got up the courage and decided to go to the gynaecologist, and there I was told I was pregnant. It didn't occur to me at all, since I didn't know when I could have possibly become pregnant. Then I remembered that there was something a few months ago. When I told Peter, he claimed it couldn't be his. (f)
>
> We have two girls. The younger one falls asleep only when one of us is in bed with her, at night she sleeps badly, talks and cries in sleep, and she immediately wakes up when the parent distances leaves the bed. That's why we chose a separated sleeping arrangement, each of us sleeps with one daughter in a different room, and we take turns with the younger one. Each Sunday I place my daughters in front of the television and switch on the cartoons. It is the only way to create a suitable moment for my husband and myself. At the same time, we must keep an eye on the clock, so that we don't run over time, and we must listen with one ear to make sure the door isn't opening, and one of the daughters doesn't want to tell us she wants to go on the potty. (f)

Well, you might say, the children will grow up soon, and everything will be as it used to be earlier. It may, but it may not. One marital therapist[8] says that marital sexuality is not a spontaneous phenomenon because, in the course of a marriage, the frequency of situations when both partners want it with the same intensity begins to decrease relentlessly. If we left marital sexuality to spontaneity, then mutual desire would disappear completely because in marriage there are not the right conditions for spontaneous, voluntary, and active sexuality. It is not possible to keep gaining and tempting for three years, let alone thirty. The following joke also shows that, in marriage, the situation differs from the days of dating:

> *Scientists are said to have discovered the food that decreases the female appetite for sex by 90%. It is called a wedding cake.*

The therapist suggests that marital sexuality be put in the category of marital duties, and relegate it to two powerful biological forces: stereotype and regularity. He even recommends that a special day be reserved for it, for example Tuesdays. The Tuesday quite simply solves the burning problem of who should start, how one should start, and if it gets started at all. It was found in a study of peaceful, 30-year marriages that they usually had a fixed day. Perhaps, if they had not, they could have ended up the following way:

> *Do you know why married people are fatter than single people?*
> *The single ones come home, peek in the fridge, and go to bed. The married ones come home, peek in the bed, and go to the fridge.*

It is therefore necessary to see the situation in context. In many phases of the partnership, love-making has a determined time and manner. When you have young children, the time may be when a certain cartoon is on, and the manner is that you watch the clock and listen for the door. Later you introduce the love-making day and, in retirement, you may need Viagra, and you choose the manner of love-making which considers fragile hearts or weakened muscles. During the quest for a child, the time centres around fertile days and the methods that are most effective for becoming pregnant. However, many people submit to the media's fiction that the depth of a relationship is determined by the ability to achieve orgasm. It is necessary to realise that life is full of bigger and smaller limitations, and the depth of a relationship is determined, above all, by the ability to cope with the problems that are brought about by daily life. What do you think: is the relationship better between the partners who say, 'We're trying to abstain (a little) before ovulation, so that there is greater chance during the fertile days, or between the partners whose love relationship is not influenced because 'my husband wasn't much interested in having a child'?

> We are trying hard to have a child and it is quite demanding. My partner is away on business trips most of the time and it is really difficult to organise everything so that he will be home on the right days. If only the international bosses knew what determines the work schedule of the manager of the regional branch! One day he had to return from a trip to a town 150 miles away. He arrived late at night and was very tired after the long day of meetings and the long car trip home. He was not capable of any action, so we said he should first get some sleep and we would try in the morning. At daybreak I woke him up and we tried again. My partner had not had enough sleep and he was not doing very well. I wasn't doing that great myself. Even though I had maximum good will, at one point I caught myself staring into the corner and thinking that I should sweep out the cobwebs. We were also aware of our time limit, his driver was going to be waiting for him in half an hour. Finally we succeeded and he was able to leave with peace of mind. We laughed about it a lot. It was early morning, it was too early for me to go

to work, so I stayed in bed thinking, and in the end I thought to myself that I was probably experiencing the most wonderful sex in my life. (f)

How do Poets Respond?

The song 'The Two Small Wings Are Not Here' always echoes in my ears when I am thinking about the unfulfilled desire for a child. I debated whether I should use this song for this book, since it does not speak about parenthood unfulfilled but about parenthood rejected. After a long consideration, I have decided to include it here.

'The Two Small Wings Are Not Here'
(GIMBEL/FOX/BOROVEC)

Chorus
Walk through the house, see all the corners
You will find shade and only shade
The two small wings are not here
They almost arrived but are no longer
No one knows where they may be wandering
The nest is empty
Quiet the lap.

1.
Who saw a tender woman
Walking to the square in the morning
She went to return the winning
To lock the gate toward happiness
The thing seemed to be common
And now it seems a sin.

2.
A doctor just wrote a brief
Official report
The first mention of someone
And the last
You are no longer a mother
And the bird no longer sings.

3.
Mothers walk from the nursery in the evening
Around playgrounds and street corners

Into white sheets
They tuck two white wings
And the woman draws with her finger
Strange letters.
...

I am not a specialist in abortions, I do not know the feelings of people who have rejected parenthood. But I often hear about the apartments and houses in which the children's rooms are prepared, tidy all the time. If it were not for the first stanza in the song, it would be a good description of the feelings connected with the unfulfilled desire for a child. There is everything: the empty house, the doctor's report about the child that was here at least for a moment, the mothers with prams, even the unwritten letters with the unspoken sentences.

PLAY SOFTLY, MAPLE VIOLIN,
LULL MY BABY TO SLEEP

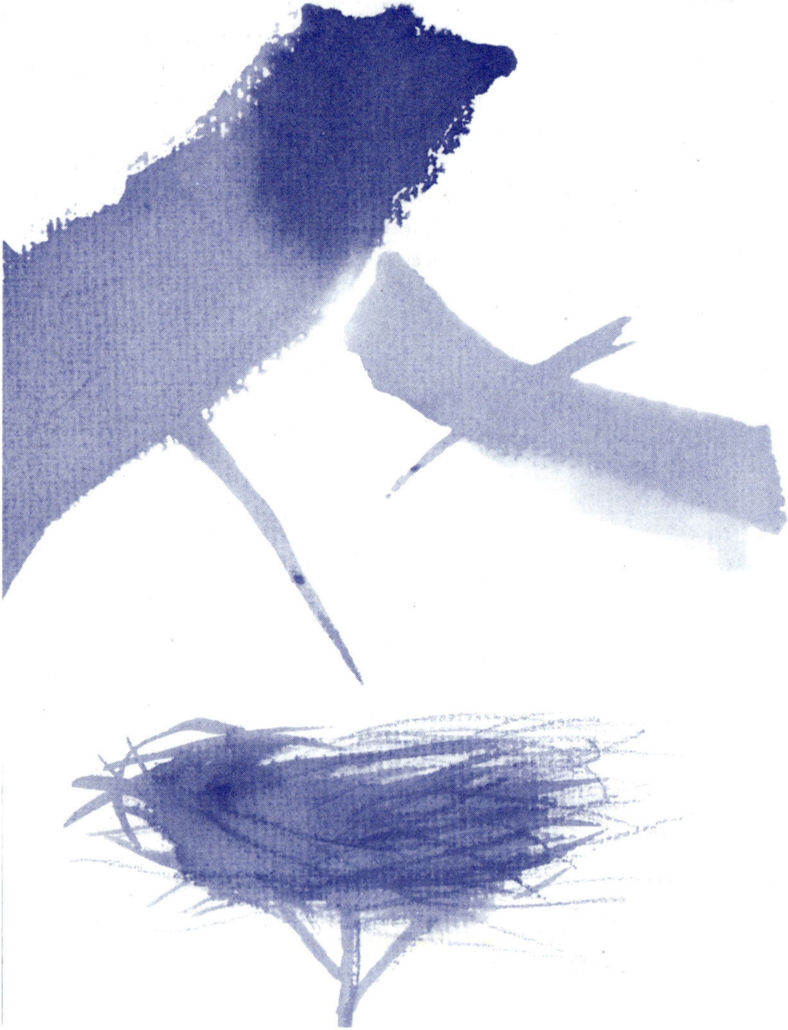

Play Softly, Maple Violin, Lull My Baby to Sleep

There was a king and a queen and they did not have children. The king suffered a lot because of this. The queen pleaded with the Lord to hear her and give them at least a single descendant so that the monarchy would not fall into foreign hands after their death. Finally, the queen had a child, but the women who were around her took it quickly away, to save her from taking a fright. It was a little son, and he had a bear's skin. The queen wanted to see him, the women kept trying to talk her out of it, but she commanded that they show him to her even if he did not resemble a human being. They brought a little shaggy bear, and she took him to her heart.

'The Bear Prince', J. Horák, *The Magic Bag*

The transition into parenthood is a breakthrough transition. Other transitions in life are not so sudden, they occur gradually, but the birth of a child is not a step-by-step process; the baby that was originally not here, is simply around. Parents often are in shock after the birth of their first child. In all the pictures and photos, the babies are always smiling or sleeping. Books about baby care usually mention that babies cry, but a person unfamiliar with the situation may get the impression that babies just beep from time to time, and after they are changed, fed or cradled in one's arms, the crying is over. Many parents are then taken aback by a screaming and resisting baby for whom nothing seems to help. The mother from the title song is begging the violin to lull her baby to sleep at least for a while, and the song continues, 'close your little eyes, so that your Mummy can cook.' I myself lived through my son's infancy on biscuits and yoghurt because the violin did not lull my baby to sleep and I did not even manage to do more urgent things, let alone cooking.

Psychologists have designed a set of criteria to measure the depth of psychosocial burden. According to this measure, the birth of the first child belongs to the category 'heavy burden'. How is parenthood experienced by those whose quest for a child, whether their own or adopted, has been fraught with obstacles?

...the Baby is Biological

Perhaps this chapter should have been divided into four parts: the child is biological for both parents, the child is biological for one parent, the child is not biological because donors' gametes were used and the child was born to a surrogate mother. However, in this book we will consider as biological the child that was born following treatment of fertility disorders.

How do those who have waited for parenthood for a long time perceive it?

> A total change, but pleasant. I wasn't imagining the child in any concrete way, I had more illusions about motherhood, but I soon lost them (not in any painful way). The worst about the first motherhood was the loss of my independence, and to a large degree unlearn planning everything by myself. I was quite devastated that I was unable to do work that objectively takes 30 minutes in three days. With the passage of time, and with the next child, I've stopped planning almost at all, and if I do, then I don't especially dwell on the plans, which is very liberating. (f)
>
> At the beginning, my son cried a lot, and I was worried whether he was alright. The time of lack of sleep and tiredness came. But I'm happy that it's succeeded, that we have David. It's better day by day, and I'm training myself for the life of a mother, and I have a feeling of fulfilment. (f)
>
> Things are livelier. (f)
>
> One cannot even imagine it! When I saw them the first time (the twins from IVF), I cried continuously for two days. My face was swollen, my eyes were red, but I was terribly happy. The girls are one year old now, it's been the fastest school year in my life, in which I've folded x nappies, washed their little butts x times, fed their little mouths x times, and produced x litres of milk. But it has been beautiful! (f)
>
> It's like a miracle. (f)
>
> A complete change. I had twins when I was 30 years old. At that age, one is more careful, moreover all in hope after all the years, so I was trying to do everything perfectly as the books recommended. I was going around with a mask on for half a year. I was breast-feeding for nine months. I am happy that I have the children, I cannot imagine my life without children, but I also can't imagine that I'll be a grandmother, and the crazy carousel will be in store for me again. (f)

When I became pregnant after several miscarriages and decisions to stay without children, I pretended that I wasn't pregnant. I went to see the doctor only after three months. We were very busy at work, I went on business to the Netherlands, I went time and again to Prague. I behaved all the time as if I weren't pregnant, I was afraid that if I admitted it to myself, I would miscarry, and would be dejected. I admitted to myself that I was pregnant only in the 25th week. But still, I did everything as if I weren't pregnant. I was feeling in the best shape, I didn't have any problems at all, and I never looked better. Everything has changed, I haven't much time to enjoy it all yet because we're very busy but we're very happy. At the beginning, until I taught myself the mothering skills, it occurred to me in moments of stress whether I would be a good mother at all, whether nature didn't know very well what it was doing when it was denying me a child. (f)

The keeping up and not losing one's hope is worthwhile. What can be more beautiful than when a two-year-old little child tells you, 'Mom, I love you!' (f)

It is worth it. (f)

One of our patients, a teacher, 40 years old, who had been in treatment for many years, couldn't become pregnant. Then she gave up on treatment and ended it. After some time, she came to the surgery, fat, saying that she has a strange diarrhoea, her tummy and back ache. The doctor discovered that she was giving birth. She didn't know it herself for the whole nine months, she connected the fattening and the omission of menstruation with menopause. She knew from hormonal therapy sessions that the body responds in various ways. The gynaecologist immediately provided for a transfer to the hospital, where she gave birth to a child that weighed five kilos. She was very surprised, but she is looking after the child well, and is happy. (p)

For some women, the attempts to become pregnant become a life program, their single goal in life. When they then become pregnant, they have big mental problems, because they have lost the sense of their lives. They can't cope with the situation, that they are alone at home, and their husband doesn't look after them. They don't look forward to the baby; they weren't interested in the baby, but in achieving pregnancy. (p)

When I announced to my husband that I was finally pregnant, he was terribly happy, but at the same time he became nervous. He didn't let me do anything basically for the whole nine months, he phoned me several times a day from work, he went to all the examinations with me, he looked after what I ate, and how much I ate. The nervousness left him only after the child was three months old. It was very nice of him. (f)

When the treatment has been successful and the woman becomes pregnant, there can still follow a demanding period for her and her partner, full of anxieties and fear for the future, especially if the couple have experienced a miscarriage before ('I was afraid that if I admitted it to myself,

I would miscarry, and would be dejected. I admitted to myself that I was pregnant only in the 25th week' 'He became nervous. He didn't let me do anything basically for the whole nine months'). This fear can even lead to denial of the situation ('I pretended that I wasn't pregnant…I behaved all the time as if I weren't pregnant' 'She didn't discover it herself for the whole nine months, she connected the fattening and the omission of menstruation with menopause'). At the same time, physically the pregnancy can be entirely without any problems ('I was feeling in the best shape, I didn't have any problems at all, and I never looked better').

Physicians still consider a woman who has become pregnant after treatment or who has had an unsuccessful pregnancy before as a case of pregnant sterility. No wonder, the goal has not yet been achieved.

For some, the achievement of pregnancy signifies losing the object that has filled their life with meaning ('They have big mental problems, because they have lost the sense of their lives'). This is a phenomenon known in other areas of medicine as well. Most physicians have some patients whose life plan is not a life without illness but a life spent being ill and undergoing treatment. When they are pronounced cured and healthy, they lose the benefits of being ill: the attention and consideration of the partner and other people, the reason to pity themselves, etc. In the treatment of fertility problems, this can be even more complicated in that this illness is not considered an illness but an incapacity. When pregnancy is achieved, it is proof that the couple are not incompetent, that the woman is a true woman since she has become pregnant and that the man is a true man since he has made his wife pregnant—that proof and nothing more may have been their main goal.

The transition into parenthood is generally experienced as pleasant by the partners ('A total change, but pleasant' 'I'm happy that it's succeeded, that we have David. It's better day by day' 'Terribly happy' 'It's like a miracle' 'I am happy that I have the children' 'They are very happy,' 'The keeping up and not losing one's hope is worthwhile' 'It's worth it' 'She is happy'). The new situation poses demanding tasks ('The worst about the first motherhood was the loss of my independence, and to a large degree unlearn planning everything by myself. I was quite devastated that I was unable to do work that objectively takes 30 minutes in three days' 'At the beginning my son cried a lot, and I was worried whether he was alright. The time of lack of sleep and tiredness came' 'I've folded x nappies, washed their little butts x times, fed their little mouths x times, and produced x litres of milk' 'The crazy carousel' 'We're terribly busy') which are nonetheless manageable ('With the passage of time, and with the next child I've stopped planning almost at all, and if I do, then I don't especially dwell on the plans, which is very liberating' 'It's better day by day, and I'm training myself for the life of a mother, and I have a feeling of fulfilment' 'But it was beautiful!').

At times when the tasks seem unmanageable, the parents may be wondering why they cannot cope. Either they have high standards for themselves as parents ('I had twins when I was thirty years old. At that age one is more careful, moreover all in hope after all the years, so I was trying to do everything perfectly as the books recommended'), or they doubt themselves as parents ('At the beginning, until I taught myself the mothering skills, it occurred to me in the moments of stress whether I would be a good mother at all, whether nature didn't know better what it was doing when it was denying me a child'). Why do parents wonder about themselves in this way? The reason is probably again rooted in the perception of infertility as an incapacity. The difficulties with handling new tasks, which, under normal circumstances, one can ascribe to new, unfamiliar situations, are sometimes connected by formerly infertile parents to the causes of infertility ('Whether nature didn't know better what it was doing when it was denying me a child') or to the consequences of the treatment, for example to their mental exhaustion. Today people are no longer so ashamed about getting pregnant through assisted reproduction.

> Our acquaintances had twins after IVF, and they boast everywhere that their children cost them as much as a good car. (f)

But many still perceive assisted reproduction as an unnatural way of conception and they try to conceal this fact from others. Nevertheless, it is clear that, when the parents have decided to keep the method of achieving the pregnancy secret from the child or from family and friends, then the centre of assisted reproduction will not be a place for afternoon walks and the doctor will not be a friend of the family. Early studies of families with children conceived through the test tube method showed that most parents do not tell their children about the circumstances of their conception, but times change...

After reading the previous paragraph, you will probably understand that it is not easy to conduct research into the topic of the perception of parenthood after the use of a donor's sperm, eggs, or both. The parents have had enough of the interventions of institutions and other external entities into their quest for a child, and now they want to live a normal family life, without anyone's interventions, including those of curious researchers. The conclusions of several international studies of parenthood after heterological insemination (using donor's sperm) are encouraging. The authors[9] claim that, according to their experience, the children conceived in this way are loved more than some children who were conceived naturally, but who were not planned, many of whom grow up without love. The following thoughts are said to occur in many letters written by men or by both partners to their psychologists: that their sense of the meaning of life underwent an essential change after the birth of the longed-for child; that they wish for other couples to experience the same happiness; that the husband has realised that he is a father and has connected biological and psychological fatherhood; that relatives and friends have often found out that the child resembles the parents; and that the partners want another child. Studies of parenthood after the use of donor's sperm and eggs show the same results[i]. If you need to boost your self-confidence as new parents by more results of additional studies, I have encouraging news: most studies indicate good coping with parenthood in successfully treated couples. To assure you that similar uncertainties and exhaustion with parenthood are experienced even by those who did not have the slightest problem with achieving pregnancy, I would like to share with you the following two testimonies. They are also accompanied by the testimony of a paediatrician who deals with parents who have undergone treatment of fertility problems:

> The change was pronounced, mainly in the sense that the day gained a completely different order decided by someone other than myself. The difference between the weekday and the weekend completely disappeared, it wasn't possible to stay in bed late or lounge around on the weekend. As a parent, I needed someone to tell me…that this change would happen, that this would stress me, and that it is normal, and that it stresses others as well. Perhaps I would have handled the situation better with the consciousness that other mothers are in the same boat. (f)
>
> When my second daughter was born, I was completely exhausted. When I accidentally had some free time, I wandered around the apartment and I wasn't able to do anything, although I kept doing something all the time. But it was to no effect. For example, as a toddler, my daughter went to the door and started crying that she wanted to go out. So that I would survive, I dressed her and I went with her to McDonald's. I bought a Coke and French fries for her and a coffee for myself, and she played in the heap of balls and for a while she was quiet. It cost an awful lot of money but there was no other way. There were even times when I wanted to die, really, I am serious. I was simply so exhausted that I kept telling myself if only I could

fall asleep...for ever. Both the girls go to school now, but I am still pulling myself out of it. Even last year I kept giving visitors their coffee directly into their hands, so that it didn't stand on the table, the children didn't tip it over and didn't scald themselves. It is difficult to pull oneself out of it. (f)
I have the best experiences with older mothers and fathers. They have lived through something, they know what they want, they are glad for parenthood. They cope better and in a calmer way with problems, because they have some life experience. They cooperate better, they are able to distinguish between the more important and less important things. That they are sometimes more afraid when the child is sick is understandable exactly because they know what they value. (p)

...the Baby is Adopted

The child does not have your genes nor have you given birth to it. But the child of the parents from the previous chapter might not have their genes either.

The arrival of a child changes one's life. One's life has a goal. At the beginning (the first half a year) I was stressed out from the care of an adopted child, I didn't know whether I would be able to cope with it. I was thinking whether the reason was that I was incompetent, or that I didn't understand the child well when it was not my own. The gynaecologist told me that it was understandable because I had not experienced pregnancy, so that I wasn't set up for parenthood hormonally. Now I quite trust myself as a mother, and we are considering another child. (f)
We haven't our own child. It definitely is a change—definitely for the better. We have something to live for, life has filled itself somehow. Everything turns around the child, but it is beautiful. One has lots of fun with children, at least with the little ones. Neither I nor my husband could imagine it in a better way. (f)
We have had an (adopted) child for two months. A big change, a complete change of the daily regime. It is demanding but beautiful, we are glad that it's succeeded finally, we do not regret it. (f)
After seven years of a childless marriage, my husband and I decided to adopt a child. After a surprisingly quick processing of the application for adoption, they called us one day to say that they had a girl for us. I was indescribably happy, as when they tell you at the gynaecologist that you are pregnant. She wasn't afraid of me or my husband, but she didn't show much interest either. After she got tired, she laid her head on my shoulder for a moment, and that was the moment when I told myself it would all end up well. Even today, I can't avoid the feeling that I make one mistake after another, but I know that we've accepted each other. I don't know what it's like to have

a biological child, but I can't imagine that I would like him or her better than Theresa. (f)

Adoptive parenting, as I experience it today, simply isn't and can't be the same as biological parenthood. We were different, and in a certain sense we have stayed so—in many problems and in many feelings. (f)

Virtually from the beginning of our living together, I realised that something very special occurred which I started calling a miracle without hesitation. The little powerless nothing started growing on me more and more, day by day. A space opened up inside of me that I hadn't known existed at all. I surprisingly discovered that I am a mother, that I feel that I am a mother, although I didn't carry the child nor did I give birth to it. It was clear to me that I found what I was searching for. (f)

We've been left alone to resolve the problems associated with the handling of adoptive parenting, the organisation dealing with adoption hasn't bothered to help us. (f)

I don't know how we'll tell our daughter about it, I am afraid of this. (f)

I wasn't entirely sure about the adoption, so about 80% of me wanted it above all because of my wife. I didn't expect that it would be so great. I study all the books about children, I keep talking with the little girl, playing with her, and cradling her up in my arms. I'm looking forward to the time when we'll go to the circus, and we'll teach her skiing. I am happy with her. (m)

I can't get used to the child, I'm avoiding contact with him. I'm considering returning him within the three-month pre-adoptive care period, but I am afraid of what people would say. My husband wants to keep the child, and he told me that nature knew what it was doing when it made me infertile. (f)

The idea that someone would be coming to oversee you, and inspect your privacy isn't pleasant, but it is bearable in our case. In fact, we still live that way. I've taught myself completely automatic behaviour. In the morning, first of all, to have the girls looking like a magazine picture, the beds made, etc. (f)

Nowadays, even I think that we're a normal family, with normal problems. (f)

Sometimes I realise that I haven't yet entirely coped with the situation. That it is hard for me to admit that I've never had my daughter in my tummy, and I've never nursed her as other mothers did. I realise that I should reconcile myself to reality, so that I could pass this down to the girls completely naturally, but unfortunately… (f)

I've never stopped feeling emptiness, looking at pregnant women has never stopped hurting me, from time to time I still have to fight with self-pity. (f)

Definitely, what's missing is something like follow-up care for emerging families. One can say that the consequences of the former deprivation are a problem. Or after my colleagues told me what can be expected from adolescent adoptive children, including stealing from one's family. One would need to turn to an expert competent in this area. (m)

It is true that you need to count on almost everything. Our children haven't gone through adolescence yet, but from the meetings with other adoptive

> parents we know that we must be prepared for everything possible. Biological parenting simply is not the same as adoptive parenting, and I cannot but try to cope with these things inwardly before my children become interested in them. I never know when they will want to see their biological parents... The social worker was really conscientious in passing on all the available information during the adoption. But there are other burdens, for instance the genetic disposition for certain illnesses, and there are other secrets that our children have in play that my husband and I have no clue about. Of course, I feel happy with the children, and we enjoy being together at the moment, but I must be aware all the time that all the days are not over yet. (f)
>
> The nights when I kept watch over the little sick person, those were the times when something started to happen between us. But it is necessary to reconcile oneself to the fact that things will not proceed quickly. (f)
>
> An unusual experience awaits parents with the arrival of the second child. All of a sudden, I saw that the strange child was hitting mine! It wasn't a normal sibling conflict as I view their nudging nowadays. Simply the first one had been with us for a while, since it was a baby and I felt: it is mine! So the new kid should not hit it! I wasn't able to foresee that I would be in such a situation. (f)
>
> I must confess that it took me a while until I was able to say calmly that our daughter goes to a school for disabled children. That is something that can be quite hard, especially for families where they assign a lot of importance to education. (f)

The arrival of an adopted child is also perceived as pleasant by most parents ('Neither I nor my husband could imagine it in a better way' 'It is demanding but beautiful, we are glad that it's succeeded finally, we do not regret it' 'I don't know what it's like to have a biological child, but I can't imagine that I would like him or her better than Theresa' 'I didn't expect that it would be so great' 'One has a goal in life' 'I was indescribably happy, as when they tell you at the gynaecologist that you are pregnant' 'It was clear to me that I found what I was searching for'). But, for some, the situation brings a heavy burden and is hard to manage ('I can't get used to the child, I'm avoiding contact with him. I'm considering returning him within the three-month pre-adoptive care period').

Similar as for the biological family, the new situation also brings new tasks for the adoptive family ('Everything revolves around the child' 'A complete change of the daily regime. It is demanding' 'Even today I can't avoid the feeling that I make one mistake after another' 'The problems with the handling of adoptive parenting' 'I've taught myself completely automatic behaviour. In the morning, first of all, to have the girls looking like a magazine picture, the beds made, etc.'), which some parents find manageable ('It would all end up well' 'Now I quite trust myself as a mother, we are considering another child'), but others have trouble coping with ('I'm considering returning him'). The adoptive parents can feel isolated and abandoned in their situation ('We've been left alone to resolve the problems with the handling of adoptive parenting, the organisation dealing with adoption hasn't bothered to help us' 'One would need to turn to an expert competent in this area').

Adoptive parents, perhaps even more so than biological parents, can believe that their difficulties in coping with the task can follow from certain causes ('My husband told me that nature knew what it was doing when it made me infertile') or from the consequences of their infertility. Apart from the possible mental effect of long-term unsuccessful treatment (but no testimony has directly mentioned this possibility), the consequences of infertility may also include the biological aspect, that is the lack of biological relation with the child ('Adoptive parenting, as I experience it today, simply isn't and can't be the same as biological parenthood. We were different, and, in a certain sense, have remained so—in many problems and in many feelings, the problems with the handling of the adoptive parenting' 'Biological parenting simply is not the same as adoptive parenting, and I cannot but try to cope with these things inwardly before my children become interested in them').

Among the unique problems that adoptive parents have to deal with are unfulfilled biological parenthood ('It is hard for me to admit that I've never had my daughter in my tummy, and I've never nursed her' 'I've never stopped feeling emptiness, looking at pregnant women has never stopped hurting me, from time to time I still have to fight with self-pity'), temporary loss of privacy ('Someone would be coming to oversee you, and inspect your privacy'), accepting the adopted child ('I couldn't imagine that it would once be our child' 'I wasn't entirely sure about the adoption' 'I'm avoiding contact with the child' 'I didn't understand the child well when it was not my own' 'The nights when I kept watch over the little sick person, those were the moments when something began to happen between us'), accepting the child's differences, be it a difference in the colour of skin or a health disability ('It took me a while until I was able to say calmly that our daughter goes to a school for disabled children'), and sometimes even accepting another adoptive child ('All of a sudden I saw that the strange child was hitting mine! It wasn't a normal sibling conflict as I view their nudging nowadays. Simply the first one had been with us for a certain time, moreover since it was a baby and I felt: it is mine! So the new kid should not hit it!'). A special task lies in conveying of the fact of adoption to the child ('How we'll tell our daughter about it' 'So that

I could pass it down to the girls completely naturally' 'I never know when they will want to see their biological parents, and however difficult it will be for us, I don't wonder').

One psychologist and a respected specialist in adoptive parenting[10], differentiates between biological and psychological parenthood. He points at the excessive celebration of biological parenthood, the exaggeration of the so-called voice of the blood, and the traditional literary description of step-mothers and step-fathers as evil. But does any biologically conditioned voice of the blood exist?

> Thank God they have name tags there! I went to the newborn children's department to look at my just-born child. I couldn't find it! There were about six children, so I was looking at them and searching for my own. But I couldn't find it, even though I saw it after the birth, and held it in my arms. Then I noticed that they had name tags above the beds, so I found it according to the tag. That was good luck, I would be ashamed to ask the nurse. It is a disgrace not to recognise one's own child. (f)
>
> I can't speak about an onrush of motherly love, but I was glad that this baby was my baby, I found it the most beautiful of all I'd seen, but I can't say that I would recognise it if they'd given me a different one from the one I'd given birth to. I didn't see the child immediately after the birth, so sometimes I have the feeling that whoever they'd given me, I took home with me, but they'd chosen well. (f)

It has been proven that the essence of an emotional relationship between children and their families is not that someone feeds the children and plays with them, but that someone gives them support and assurance in their learning about the unknown world. Studies confirm that '...suitably chosen adoptive and foster mothers as well as fathers show better relationships with the adopted child and manifest better prerequisites for raising the child than many biological parents'[11]. Paediatricians[12] add that the areas of parenthood that are decisive from the adult viewpoint—the biological dimension (the parents conceived and gave birth to the child) and the legal dimension (the parents have been given legal responsibility)—are not important to the child. For the child, the psychosocial dimension is decisive: that the parents behave as a mother or father should. In the ideal case, all the three dimensions are linked and integrated.

Adoptive parenting is always different from biological parenting and it brings a number of questions regarding the relationship to the adopted child for which it may be difficult to find answers. But that does not mean that life with an adopted child is not happy. I have heard several times that while the biological child has grown under the parent's heart, the adopted one has grown in the parent's heart.

Biological parenthood of an infertile parent is perhaps more demanding than that of a fertile parent. I think adoptive parenthood is definitely more demanding than a biological one. I personally think that an important influence is the fact that the infertile parents must look for answers to questions that under normal circumstances would not have occurred to them. When you find yourselves in a difficult moment and believe that these tasks are too demanding for you, realise that you are well equipped for the fulfilment of these especially demanding tasks: the quest for a child has strengthened your marriage and given you the opportunity to mature. These are very important prerequisites for good parenthood and very good reasons to trust yourselves.

JUST YOU
AND ME

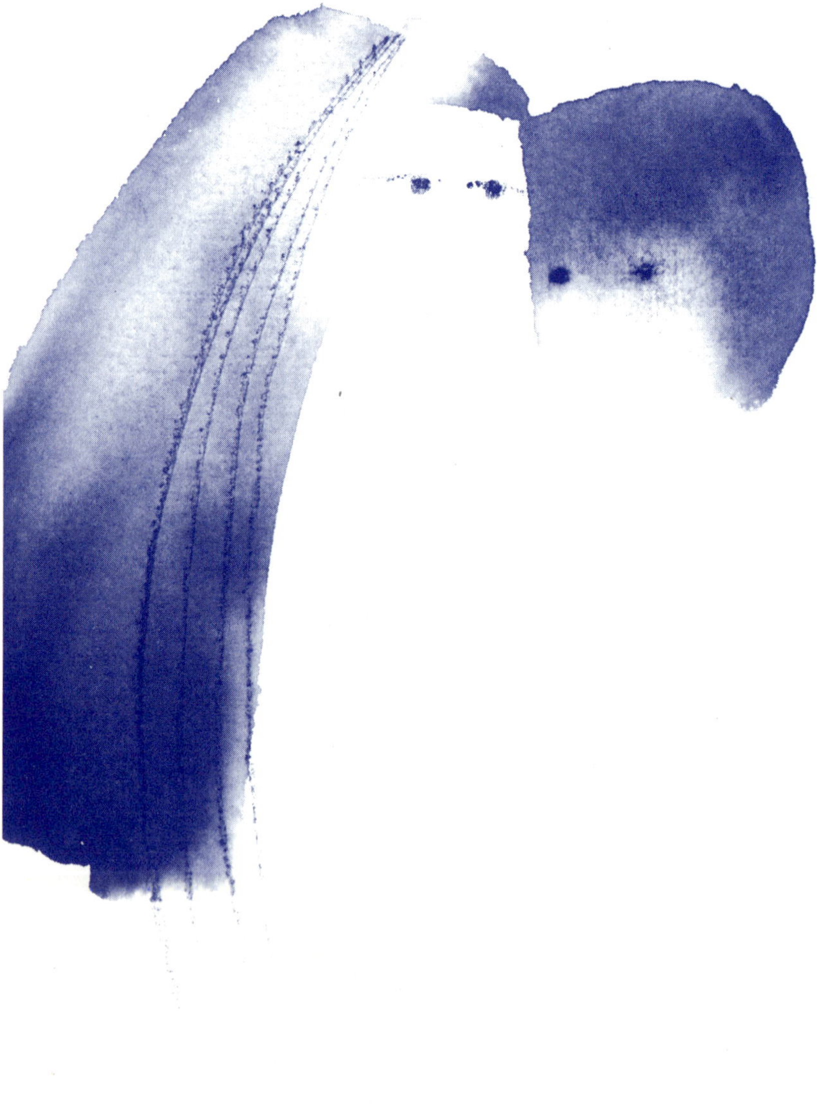

Just You and Me

People often talk about parenthood. But they do not talk much about unfulfilled parenthood. Even the fairy tales that tell about a complicated quest for a child end up with some child, so far I have not found any childless ones.

Our own repeated disappointments, and the fact that I can't fulfil the heartfelt wishes of my close relatives. A feeling of impoverishment that the sense of life is unfulfilled. Sorrow that there is no one to whom we could pass down the good in us, as our parents passed it down to us. (f)
Basically I think that childlessness (unaccepted) can kill a person, an accepted childlessness can lift one to unsuspected heights. I'd even want to say that we would be happy childless, but we would have to finally accept it, to discover joy in childlessness, enter in it, and accept it as a gift. (f)
Be grateful for the fact that you have children. I couldn't have any. I lived only for my husband and he for me. But my husband died several weeks ago, and I've been left completely alone. It's horrible. (f)
I fought along with my husband up to the end of the biological possibilities, we tried all the currently available methods of diagnosis and therapy, including the unconventional ones. Adoption wasn't advised for us. I started to devote myself intensely to my two nieces. Since my brother left the family, I've been a surrogate parent for my nieces, today already adults. I've started a foundation. One must find something that will fill one's life, something that will give her or him the feeling that she or he is needed. (f)
I enjoy my work, we have a nice marriage, plenty of friends, and interests. But sometimes I find that I cannot truly enjoy anything, nothing gives me the pleasure that I used to feel, things seem to me to be pointless and useless. (f)
My husband and I have taken up [caring for dogs]. We go to a dogs' shelter, we give it a lot of time and money. I've discovered that many people who spend their time there are also those who couldn't have a child. (f)
One must learn to live with it. One must find another meaning in life. It is hard, it isn't easy, but there is no other way. (f)

> We've bought a dog, my wife looks after him, she goes out for walks with him, and it seems to me that she has come to terms with the fact that we won't have children. (m)
>
> I used to go a lot to visit my nephew and niece, I was happy with them, and they liked me. But my brother got divorced, and his former wife has broken all contacts with him and our family. She has moved far away from us. So I've lost the children. I have no other children in the family, so there isn't anyone to look after. I am sad. (f)
>
> Childlessness has brought perhaps only the fact that we're going to experience no pain of our children now that we don't have them. But we aren't going to feel their joy and happiness either. (f)
>
> My husband sometimes yells at home, who am I building the house for, only dogs will be left after us. (f)
>
> I am eighty-five years old. I am an old woman...You know God didn't give me children, my husband died a long time ago, so my only pleasure is television... So I hope that the live announcers remain...(a letter from the daily press about the intention of the management of the regional television to stop using live announcers) (f)

A child gives human life a direction, a goal, in other words, a meaning. It is somebody to whom one can devote one's love, one's care, one's abilities, one's time. People who had reserved an important place in their lives for a child can miss such a meaning ('A feeling of impoverishment that the sense of life is unfulfilled' 'Things seem to me as pointless and useless' 'There isn't anyone to look after') and so search for another important goal ('One must find something that will fill one's life'). It can be found in improving the relationship with the partner ('I lived only for my husband and he for me'), in contact with children ('I started to devote myself intensely to my two nieces, my brother's daughters' 'I used to go a lot to visit my nephew and niece, I was happy with them'), in work for others ('I've started a foundation'), in one's profession, etc. Many childless people purchase a dog ('We've bought a dog, my wife looks after him' 'We go to a dogs' shelter'). It is difficult to find a new goal ('It is hard, it isn't easy' 'We would have to finally accept it, to discover joy in childlessness'), often the search takes many years and sometimes it is not successful. Moreover, even this new goal can be lost ('I used to go a lot to visit my nephew and niece, I was happy with them, and they liked me. But my brother got divorced...so I've lost the children' 'My husband died several weeks ago, and I've been left completely alone').

A child is not only the target of one's efforts, the receiver of one's energy. A child is also a source of energy, a source of happiness, joy, ('We aren't going to feel their joy and happiness'), or the feeling of closeness. It is important to add that, of course, it is also a source of worries, suffering, and despair, which is a topic that I am going to discuss later.

In the chapter about the ways of experiencing the unfulfilled desire for a child, we saw that it is a situation which is so traumatic for many people that they avoid anything that reminds them of their pain: contact with pregnant women, mothers with prams, children, toyshops and shops with children's goods, talking about children. Usually this is not a permanent state; after a while, contact with the traumatic symbols is manageable, many involuntarily childless couples in fact search for contact with children.

Some psychologists say that there are certain basic mental needs that must be satisfied. These needs concern not only our childhood, but they accompany us throughout our entire lives and, under normal circumstances, a substantial part of these needs of our adulthood can be fulfilled and satisfied specifically by living with a child[i]. With the natural change of life's stages, the character of what a child brings into it changes as well. It is understandably not as easy to differentiate these changes as I have tried to do in the following paragraph. I do so only for illustration.

The first stage is the pregnancy and the care for the baby. A soft touch is a feeling that is hard to describe, the experience of bodily proximity is difficult to compare with anything. Then you live with a small child. Childless women often say that they have coped with the situation, that they have reconciled themselves with it, that they have many interests and meaningful work, but they cannot enjoy life as much ('I cannot truly enjoy anything'), which is the worst part. It seems to me to be a characteristic feature. A child is spontaneous and can enjoy ordinary things: when we surprise it with a bark, when it finds an earthworm, when it gets a lollipop. As we grow mature, we see things in a more complicated way; the joy is not so transparent, we see the other side of everything. But we have a chance to re-learn spontaneous joy through young children and, thanks to our maturity, we get the chance not to lose this ability even after the children grow up. For those who have no close contact with young children, it is perhaps more difficult to learn to enjoy little things again.

In the next stage, parents try to pass down to the child, in various forms and with varying success, what they have learned and what they think is important ('Sorry that there is no one to whom we could pass down the good in us, as our parents passed it down to us'), and enjoy the successes of their child in coping with the tasks and tribulations of life. Then they have the opportunity to learn from an older child's original, creative approaches to problems, can admire and get to know a different view of the world than their own—even though the parents of adolescent children may not agree with me in this.

In the next phase, children leave home and start their own families, and their parents enjoy the grandchildren. Here the unsuccessful quest for a child transcends a whole generation ('I can't fulfil the heartfelt wishes of my close relatives'). To one's own suffering from the unfulfilled desire for a child, can be added stress from the pressure of family and friends.

Even the last stages of human life are connected with children. It is a human gift that we can recall and re-present our memories and draw joy and energy from them. For many elderly people, the most precious treasure are the photographs of their children and the opportunity to discuss a distant past. The partner leaves, and children, even if far away, are what prevents loneliness ('But my husband died several weeks ago, and I've been left completely alone' 'God didn't give me children, my husband died a long time ago, so my only pleasure is television'). In one episode of a popular series, an actress plays the role of a childless pensioner who lives in a seniors' home. Speaking to the empty bed of a recently deceased companion (in a loose paraphrase), she says: 'You complained all the time that your children would come only when you had something to give them. I would give gladly, but no one comes…'

For a person on the threshold of death, a child is also the one who holds the hope for the future, the hope that life continues in one's children ('My husband sometimes yells at home, who am I building the house for, only dogs will be left after us')

You may find the preceding paragraphs too detailed. But I believe that it is important to show that a child plays a role throughout human life. Sometimes, I am asked the question of whether it is possible to come to terms with remaining involuntarily childless, and if so, how. As a psychologist, I am expected to provide a positive answer and a few miraculous pieces of advice. But my answer is that it is not possible to reconcile oneself entirely. I do not believe that one can come to terms with a life without a child once and for all if one had really desired a child. There are, of course, periods when one feels all right, does not regret childlessness and does not worry.

> A baby was born to my friend who is 36 years old, it is beautiful, healthy, and I was satisfied to discover that, with a one-month-old baby in my arms, I wasn't devastated, really I am serious in saying that I am fine. The talk about pregnancy and birth bores me, and I am interested in cuddling the baby to

admire it for half an hour, and then I want to go away to live somewhere else. I didn't cry in the little blanket, and the idea that I would walk with the pram for more than an hour a week terrifies me—so I am correcting my ideas that I would walk in a park as if I were a young grandmother that I had in the first wave of enthusiasm over her pregnancy—I'd rather be a middle-aged woman in the pub talking with a friend, or on the balcony planting flowers. Age is a terrific thing: ten years ago, I would have gone insane because the baby was not mine. Well, if my tomcat had kittens, that would bowl me over. (f)

However, as life goes on, the involuntarily childless person keeps finding new ways to fill that unfulfilled desire for a child, new ways of enjoying life.

We tried artificial fertilisation unsuccessfully several times—or, in fact, once we succeeded. When I was thirty-eight years old, I carried the child until the third month, then I miscarried... At that moment, something seemed to break down in me. I ended all attempts, I started seeing a psychiatrist, and my husband and I started talking about adoption. But even that was unsuccessful in the end. My husband and I went over the whole situation, and it was a help that he stood by me. He painted the future in rosy colours, and I must say that his forecast has come true. We have a wonderful life, travel and fully do the work that we enjoy. Only sometimes, when we go for a walk and pass a pram with a child in it, my heart aches. I would like to push a pram, but I know that it will never succeed... (f)

I am 42 years old and my quest for a child has finished in the factual sense of the word, although I think that I will keep travelling toward it for the rest of my life, at least in my dreams. I have arrived at the sentence that you wrote—I have done everything I could—and I am finding myself reconciled and calm as much as it is possible. (f)

It follows from the previous chapters that life without a child and the quest for it bring personal growth, patience, peace, a realisation of life's priorities, and empathy. Childlessness also offers a certain freedom, personal, financial, and, to a certain degree, emotional. Perhaps you will now say that the realisation of life's priorities has lead you to the fact that personal and financial freedom does not mean much to you under these circumstances. But I emphasize the emotional freedom ('We're going to experience none of the pain of our children now that we don't have them'), which we often do not realise. When we love someone, his or her suffering hurts us much more than our own. Moreover, we experience a far stronger feeling of helplessness in the situation. A child is not only a source of energy, happiness, and joy, but also a source of worry, suffering and despair, sometimes a very significant one but we, of course, do not think about this aspect when we dream of parenthood.

A ballet master, answering an interviewer's question about whether he regretted his childlessness when he was so good with children, said that he did not regret it, that everything does not always work out well with children and a big disappointment can arrive in the end, as he has seen amongst his relatives.

Everyone has physiological needs, for instance, hunger and thirst. They must be satisfied and it is clear how this is to be done (food, drink). Psychologists have so far not agreed on the definition and enumeration of spiritual needs (for instance the need for security and safety, love, rewards and acknowledgement, self-fulfilment, the need for knowledge and understanding), but it has been recognised that they might be differently developed in each person and that they might even be missing some. You surely know some people who live a meaningful and happy life without children.

> I didn't feel any need to get married and have children. The unsuccessful marriages of my elder brothers had a negative influence on me. I didn't feel loneliness. Then the years were passing by. I don't regret anything. I am happy without children, I've found a different sense of life. (f)
>
> I was never smitten by children, not at 20 and not at 40. I don't know why. I remember that, when my nephew was little, he used to come with my mother to the house, and she put him on the chamber pot in the kitchen where we all used to eat. Everybody was overcome with excitement, but I didn't find it charming that he was doing a job under my nose when I ate my Sunday dinner. But I looked after him without problems, and I think that he wasn't ever bored with me, but then I returned him with joy. I don't know whether I am an egotist but, to tell the truth, I never bothered about it much. (f)

We all live through longer or shorter periods when a certain spiritual need that is especially important for us remains unfulfilled, and we search for possible ways to fulfil it or to reduce it. Fortunately, unlike physiological needs, there are many ways to satisfy our spiritual needs. It depends, above all, on the individual and on whether he or she looks for these ways and wants to find them. If your desire for a child is significant and unfulfilled, you will probably feel the lack of fulfilment as a major thing all the time. Nevertheless, the desire (need?) to have a child is too vague a concept, and it can be described by a great number of individual spiritual needs. Many of these needs can certainly be fulfilled through a life without a child.

> Our sadness lasted only a while because, in my opinion, one must realistically work with the given situation, and shouldn't suffer through what he or she cannot influence. We talked about it at great length with my husband, and we came to the conclusion that we love each other, and want to stay with each other under any circumstances. We definitely became attached to each other. We refused adoption right away, we didn't have the courage to adopt a strange child. I started studying at a university at the age of 35, and my husband threw himself into entrepreneurial activities. My mom was, of course, sad that, as a single child, I deprived her of the chance to have grandchildren, but she never reproached me for it. Also my husband's parents took everything peacefully. You know, I rarely talk about my private life and I'm immune towards the talk of other people, so I actually have no negative input from my surroundings. Anyway, I am not angry about life. One can find a rich meaning in many other things. (f)

When I was summing up the good things that the quest for a child and a life without a child can bring, I intentionally omitted the deepening of the partners' relationship, because I would like to mention this aspect in more detail. Sometimes, one may hear (but not from the involuntarily childless people) that a marriage without children has no meaning and that, for childless partners, there is nothing else to do but get a divorce. From time to time, a contribution to this topic appears in the media; I recently read that a marriage without children (voluntarily or involuntarily) is fated to perish because the man and the woman do not have a common conversational topic. It is true that, in childless marriages, one does not speak much about children, in the voluntarily childless ones perhaps because it is an unfamiliar and alien topic, in the involuntarily childless ones because it is often a painful topic. I refer to the story from this book's introduction: 'But as they were getting on in years, when all the hopes had disappeared, they stopped talking about it, since they felt guilty before each other, and suffered each on their own.' I am not sure whether talking about children should be the only topic of married partners' dialogues, and hence a guarantee of a good relationship. I claim that it should not. I offer the testimonies of those who have children:

> Partners' relations are a) less intense because there is little energy left, b) they are more problematic because we don't agree on the methods of raising children. (f)

> Our relationship developed along with the growth of the child. There were periods when we couldn't agree on the method of the raising of the child, the arguments were sometimes even stormy; [that is how our] relationship developed. (f)
> Sometimes our life together suffers from the arrival of another child. (f)
> With the arrival of each child, I noted first the joy of both of us, then came a more difficult period of the looking after and rushing around the baby, even some alienation appeared in our relations, less time for the solving of problems. I think that my husband suffered more, and felt neglected. (f)
> The arrival of an unwanted child definitely had a deadening influence on the partner's relations. (f)
> Troubles with children have a big influence on the partner's relations, especially tired parents are often very close to a disagreement. One is tired from the children, while the other is tired from work. (m)

Therefore, a marriage with children has a ready conversational topic, but often it is a singular and rather explosive one. An explosion may follow any slightly careless handling of the topic. It is interesting to look at the statistics on how many people are divorced in countries where divorce is permitted. If it is stated, notice how many couples with one, two or more children are divorced. A child is not a guarantee of a fulfilled relationship. Only the wife and the husband can determine whether their marriage is meaningful. Similarly, a child is not a guarantee that one will perceive one's life as meaningful. Believe me that the following testimony is common.

> When I was in college, I looked forward to finding a fine boyfriend, getting married, and having children. Now I have them, not even in my dreams did I imagine them any better than they are. But when I was on maternity leave, I was going crazy, and looked forward to work. When I am at work, I look forward to collecting the girls from the kindergarten and the school. When I am with them, I look forward to their falling asleep, and me having a coffee in peace. During the weekdays I look forward to the weekend, and that we're going to be together with the children and my husband. During the weekend, I am so nervous that I look forward to going to work on Monday. I am always waiting for something, but I actually know that there isn't any point in it. My parents are growing old, they're soon going to be unwell, and I'll have to look after them. And then I will be old; I dread it, I'd rather not imagine it at all. My grandfather is 90, he is quite independent, but he lives alone, last week his last acquaintance died, with whom he used to have coffee and talk. He can walk, but he cannot walk down the stairs, so the three steps make it impossible for him to go outside. He looks

> forward to our children terribly much and, in fact, he lives for the next visit. Whenever I realise this, I eat everything that I find at home to overcome the depression. (f)

The meaning of life is not something that comes to a person all by itself, perhaps in the shape of children, and that one can just wait for. Each one of us has to search for it, it is what one settles on as the highest value for oneself. And perhaps we all have periods in life when the meaning of our lives escapes us.

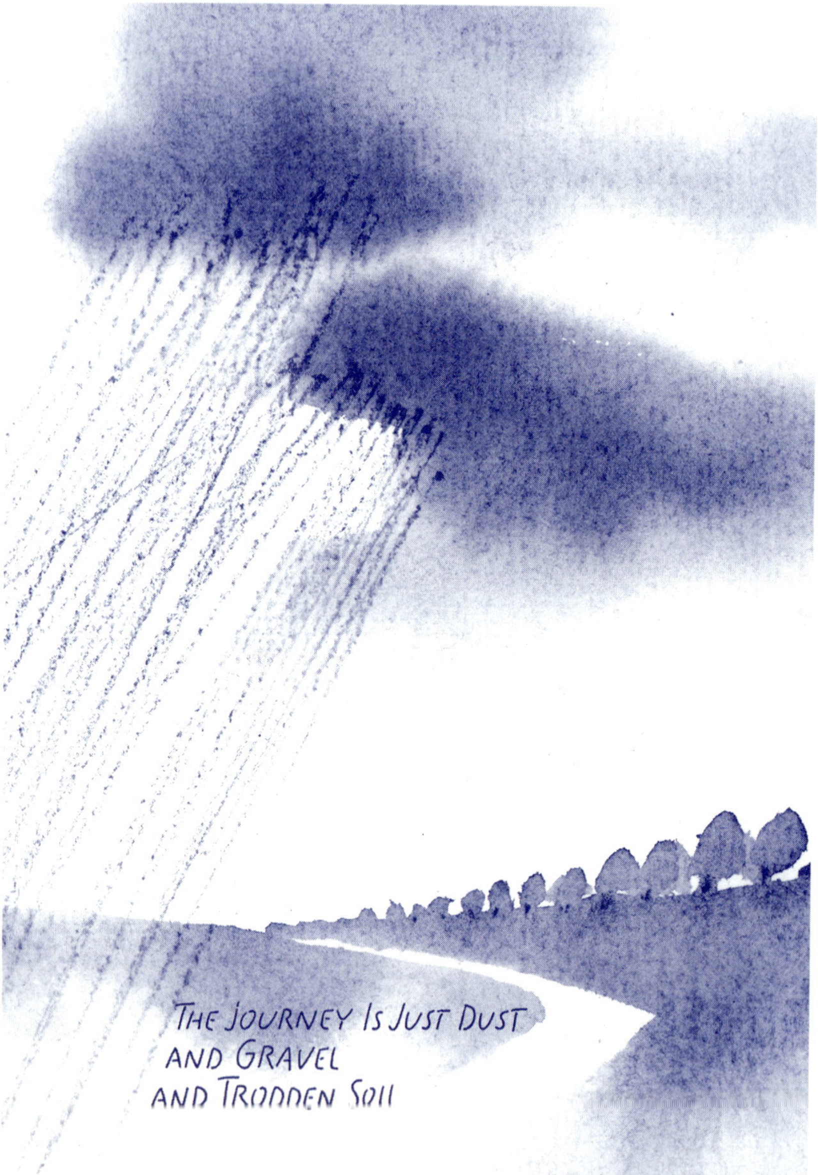
THE JOURNEY IS JUST DUST
AND GRAVEL
AND TRODDEN SOIL

The Journey is Just Dust and Gravel and Trodden Soil

A walk through dust and trodden soil is not a relaxing walk, but it can be coped with even in a mild rain. However, when you imagine meter-high snowdrifts, a windstorm, and freezing temperatures, then the path is virtually impassable. If I keep to the metaphor of a map or plan, the map of the quest for a child was meant to serve as a walking map that shows all the trails and intersections and even the contour lines by which one can assess the terrain. But many other influences affect one's completing the tour. For example, the surface of the trail and climatic conditions. We cannot forget about financial aspects either. The journey will be different for a rich person who will hire a plane, sleep in a hotel, and eat caviar for breakfast, than for someone who will drive an old car, carry a tent along, and eat instant pea soup. The journey will be perceived differently by someone who is athletic and who can elegantly handle the problems on the way, and by someone who loves his or her comfort and is depressed by every blister. Moreover, the journey will be easier with someone who can recognise that you are temporarily at the end of your tether, who can help with the backpack and offer a chocolate, than with a partner who did not want to set out of the walk in the first place, whines all the way and does not want to go any further.

We can, therefore, divide the influences into the outer ones (for example the climatic conditions) and the inner ones (one's personal disposition). The 'map of influences' shows what these can be.

A Map of Influences

Various influences affect different people to different degrees. What is unimportant for one person can have fatal consequences for another.

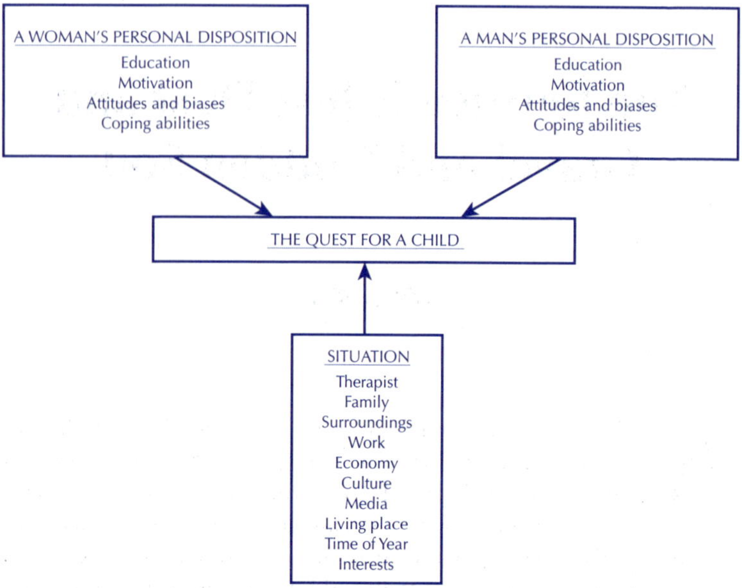

For example, finances do not play any role for a couple who are simply trying to have better nutrition, while a couple who have used up the allotted number of cycles of assisted reproduction covered by health insurance and still need more, or perhaps a donor egg, finances determine the aspect of whether further continuation of the treatment is possible at all. At the same time, for some couples, methods of in vitro fertilisation do not present an obstacle, whereas these methods can be unacceptable for a religious couple. These influences affect the quest for a child, and vice versa. We are going to talk about these various influences in the following part of the book.

My Mama Doesn't Know and She Mustn't Know

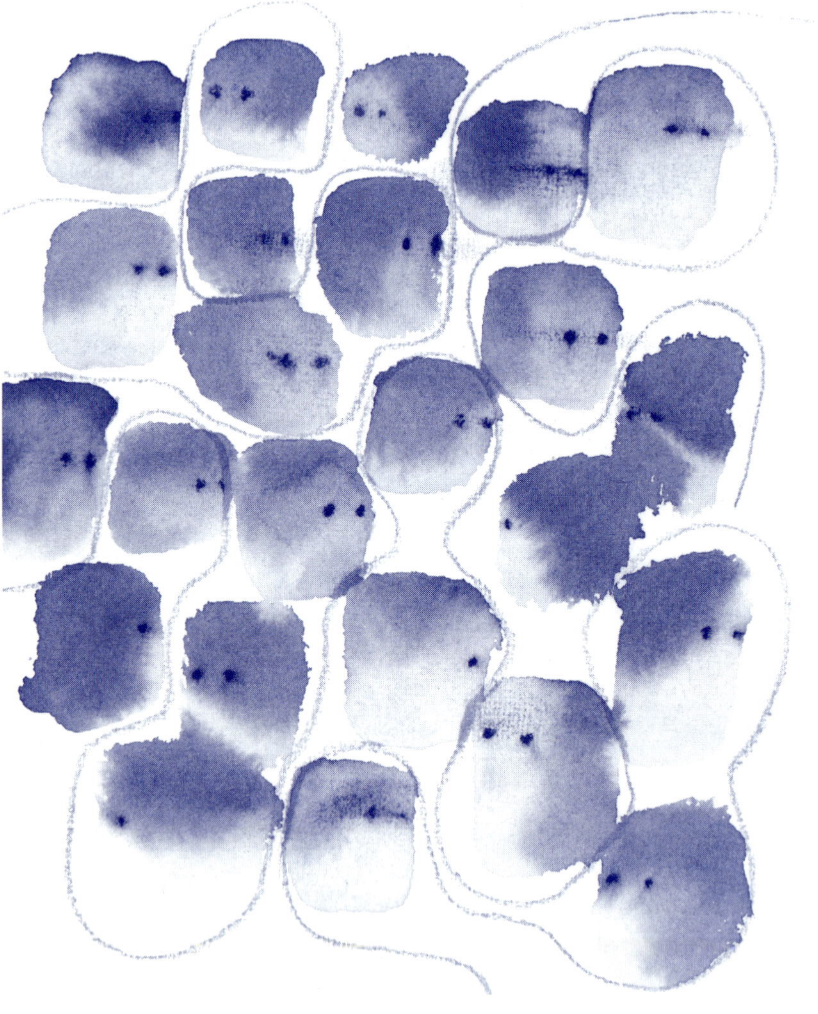

My Mama Doesn't Know and She Mustn't Know

This chapter is concerned in detail with the other influences that affect the quest for a child. First, we will discuss the external influences that appear in the map under situation. The chapter title may give the impression that the situational influences are limited to the influence of one's family, but the content of the chapter is better expressed by the second part of the title, 'doesn't know and mustn't know'. Communication will thus again be at the centre of our attention, this time specifically the communication between the couple and the external influences. The word Mama has its place in the title, too. The most complicated communication usually occurs with one's closest relatives.

Whatever you do, you always influence your surroundings and your surroundings influence you. By surroundings, I do not mean only the people you meet; I also mean the cultural customs of the given region, the legal norms, ethical principles or social behaviour. The influences of the surroundings are then not only of the obvious kind, for example people giving you various kinds of advice. They also include the ethical and financial regulations regarding assisted reproduction or the particular society's view of childlessness. You are influenced by them, and in a certain way, you can influence them.

The Therapists

My physician is a good specialist but he isn't worth much as a human being. (f)

Therapists are in an interesting situation. They are inside, part of the therapeutic process. The success of the therapy essentially depends on their expertise and practical skills. At the same time, therapists influence the situation from the outside, for example through their ability to communicate with their patients. I hear the opening observation often, and a particular therapist's inability to communicate sometimes leads to the patient switching to another therapist.

...and their expertise

Unfortunately, not everyone has the gift of being a good specialist as well as a good communicator and, as you must admit, even physicians are only human beings. You will probably have to settle for a compromise in the performance of the individual roles (specialist or communicator). And unless the therapist's communication skills are unacceptable, you will most likely give preference to expertise and practical skills. But can you recognise a good specialist?

> We went to the second clinic partly through choice (my wife had an exam there and her impression was favourable), partly by accident (it's a short way from home), but also thanks to the list from the medical insurance company. After the first two cycles at the first clinic, I went to the medical insurance company and I wanted to see a list of clinics where they carry out these procedures, what references they have, etc. They gave me a list... Today, if I were in the same situation I was in all those years ago, I still wouldn't know how to decide. Information from this area isn't publicly available, I have a feeling that we were lucky. (m)

Most people choose their therapist or their specialised clinic according to their reputation. Some people follow their intuition. Others, an increasing number of people, compare the information about the diagnosis and therapeutic procedures, which they get from the therapist, with information gained from other sources. For instance, some people go to see several therapists and compare their statements. Others compare the treatment suggested by their therapist with the treatment suggested by the therapist of an acquaintance with the same problem. Still others are influenced by information presented in various magazines, radio, television, etc. Some look up the relevant scientific literature and try to get oriented in it. Many people have recently started using the Internet, where they can access the web pages of various specialised institutions and civic associations, and some people try anonymous online consultation.

...and their communication abilities

'The physician is an important, if not the most important, medical means. Therefore, he should know what effects he has, including the side effects, and should be able to administer the right doses,' says an expert on communication in medicine[13].

Here is an interesting example of the approach of two healers toward couples with fertility problems: We think that it is appropriate to emphasise the important circumstances of our practice. If we want the ill person's cooperation, we must first create an environment in which he or she will feel comfortable. When the patient visits us, we welcome him or her first... We let them tell us what they suffer from. We must be able to listen. We wait until they calm down and start cooperating with us... It is usually women who turn to us about infertility. Nevertheless, the number of cases when both partners in infertile marriages come to us has been increasing. If the woman comes alone, we recommend that her husband come too because, in infertility, we assess and influence the couple as a whole. Married couples usually turn to us only after they have tried everything else. The first thing we have to do is to listen to the couple and calm them down... When we say that, in our treatment, cooperation is necessary, this applies even more to infertile men. In their treatment, it is also necessary to build up their self-confidence. Do you still wonder why people often go to these healers?

> Physicians usually didn't explain the diagnosis to me, and I felt like I was on a conveyor belt: to prescribe drugs and call in another patient. Unfortunately the patients gain more information about treatment in the waiting room than from the physician himself. (f)
>
> Physicians explained to me that, at 27 years of age, I was old, that conception would not occur without problems. (f)
>
> I felt inferior...which physicians reinforced by their statements about my age, statistical probabilities, etc. (f)
>
> I have one child, I cannot become pregnant again. Physicians say they do not know why, but they haven't sent me for any examinations. (f)
>
> We didn't hear any evaluation, any analysis of the failure of IVF. We had an appointment for 1 p.m., but were in the waiting room still around 3 or 4 p.m. [Then for the adoption] my wife went to the appropriate office to collect the forms, and she was told that if we submit them the same week, we have a chance perhaps in the next five years, and if not, then the next chance to submit the application will be in one year and, moreover, the screening criteria will be changed. (m)
>
> In response to my request for more information about the suggested treatment, the physician told me that my partner and I think about it too much and that, if we wanted a child, we must get things going, and do something for it. That she would send us to the centre, they would get us going, and it'd be right away. She refused to invite in my husband, who was waiting in the waiting room, saying that it was useless. (f)

In none of the medical centres that I passed through (mostly the non-state ones) did I have the impression that the highest priority is the effort to help us solve our problem. Never did I meet an effort to analyse the causes of failures, and never did anyone explain to me what the cause of my illness was. It was indicated to me that my questions were inappropriate. (f)

When I asked the doctor in the specialised consultation centre about the undesirable effects of the hormonal stimulation and about how long the whole cycle of treatment can be repeated, he said something in the sense that the undesirable effects would not probably concern me, and that it was obvious that I didn't believe in the success of the treatment. He advised us that we should get ourselves in a positive mood over Christmas and believe in the success of the treatment and, unless we do that, we would not be ready enough to undergo the treatment. (f)

Patients have no patience, they want everything at once. (p)

Doctors won't talk to me, saying that I am old (41), and I have one child. One told me at an examination (I was lying in bed), 'so we have the body here.' I laughed, but only for the sake of form, I didn't find it a good joke. (f)

We have two children, we've been trying to have a third one for nine years. Physicians won't talk to me since we already have two children. (f)

My physician refused to give me a recommendation for the Mojzis method. He said either him or the Mojzis method. (f)

It was also terrible after the miscarriages when I stayed in the same room with women who had had abortions. (f)

Immediately after the most basic examination, the gynaecologist sent us to the assisted reproduction centre. There, they didn't examine us at all and immediately ordered us for IVF with ICSI and PGD. We paid a tremendous amount of money and didn't even know what we were getting into. Then we called that it wasn't successful, but the doctor wasn't at all interested, and only said that we could order it for the next month. (m)

We asked the physician for an analysis of the situation (my wife miscarried four times, she passed through various hormonal treatments). The doctor got offended, we shouted at each other. (m)

The physician told me, after she saw my husband's spermiogram, that she would be surprised if we had a child with such a spermiogram. At the next examination, the spermiogram was normal. Other doctors stated, with certainty, unfavourable diagnoses (myomas, extrauterine pregnancy) that were not confirmed later on. (f)

The doctor was very nice in welcoming me, and even impressed my husband. (f)

Thanks to the approach of the doctor, the nurses, and all the staff, I coped with the failure much better. (f)

It was a new hope for me, after the four failures at IVF, when one doctor said that he would like me to bear with them. (f)

> The physician said to my wife 'you were searching for each other until you found each other.' We both have a reduced fertility. (m)
>
> Nobody talked to me, everything was done in haste. I passed through all the examinations. They didn't find anything. Hours of waiting, then a two-minute-long exam. The doctor said, 'I've wasted enough time with you and your husband.' I've changed my gynaecologist. (f)
>
> The doctors say nothing. I have the worst experience with them. They say nothing, they only shrug their shoulders. (f)
>
> When I came out of the gynaecologist's office after I handed him the result of the spermiogram, the nurse came to me and told me: 'Don't tell your husband anything, cook him fish, encourage him… And get yourself a child elsewhere.' I was in shock! (f)
>
> Physicians don't like sterility cases because they are difficult to treat, it is a long-term and painstaking matter, often without any obvious result. They prefer to treat something that reacts immediately to the treatment. (p)
>
> He told me that they are not miraculous exercises since the patients of Mrs Mojzis were extraordinarily supported by her. He said that the spa had worked only when there had been military barracks there, but otherwise not. (f)

The content and mode of communication varies, depending on the particular medical area. A physician treating a patient after a car accident will not probably carry on an intellectual conversation with him, and not only because the patient is unconscious. In cases of acute medicine, communication between the patient and the doctor does not have such importance. However, the opposite applies to treatment of fertility problems. Minutes or days do not play a role here, and the consequences of unsuccessful treatment are 'only' psychosocial, most of the time (but not always) there is no threat to life as such. The choice of the therapist, the therapy, the schedule, etc. is virtually all in the patient's hands. The doctor's task is to convince the patient about the most effective way of the quest for a child.

What do patients expect from their therapists?

In the first place, people expect human interest and a sensitive, respectful approach. A person seeking medical help is weakened physically and, to a varying degree, also mentally. In the treatment of fertility problems, the mental type of weakening is more important. It is increased by the fact that the patient is in a weaker, inferior, and somewhat helpless position. The patient does not have the therapist's education and so can only trust that the therapist has the expertise as well as the good will necessary to solve the given problem ('In none of the medical centres that I passed through did I get the impression that the highest priority is the effort to help us solve our problem' 'The doctor was very nice in welcoming me, and even impressed my husband'). Sometimes the therapist responds unacceptably ('I've wasted enough time with you and your husband'). A special case is the therapist's attitude toward couples who already have one child ('I have one child...they haven't sent me for any examinations' 'Physicians won't talk to me since we already have two children' 'Doctors won't talk to me, saying that I am old (41), and I have one child'). The therapist can show respect to the patients as an equal, for example by not making them wait hours for an appointment, by giving them enough attention and by showing humane understanding of the psychological context of the problem ('I felt inferior, which the physicians reinforced by their statements about my age, statistical probabilities, etc.' 'It was also terrible when I stayed after the miscarriages in the same room with women who had had abortions' 'And get yourself a child somewhere else' 'Thanks to the approach of the doctor I coped with the failure much better' 'We called that it was unsuccessful, but the doctor was not interested at all').

For the patient, the therapist is the main source of information about diagnostic procedures and results as well as about the suggested treatment and its likelihood of success. Therefore, the therapist should be able to estimate how much information individual patients need and in what form ('The physician told me, on my request for more information about the suggested treatment, that my partner and I think about it too much' 'It was indicated to me that my questions were inappropriate' 'We didn't hear any evaluation, any analysis of the failure of IVF' 'We asked the physician for an analysis of the situation. The doctor got offended, we shouted at each other' 'They say nothing, they only shrug their shoulders' 'Unfortunately, the patients gain more information about treatment in the waiting room than from the physician himself' 'We paid a tremendous amount of money and didn't even know what we were getting into').

The therapist's own conviction about the efficacy of the therapy and his or her belief in it strongly influences how he or she talks with the patient. When the therapist can persuade the patient about the efficacy of the therapy, the patient cooperates better. The therapist should also respect the patient's belief in a given alternative method ('He told me that they are no miraculous exercises since the patients of Mrs Mojzis were extraordinarily supported by her' 'He said that the spa had worked only when there had been military barracks') unless, of course, it is harmful, even though he or she has doubts about its efficacy. Patients often experience feelings of helplessness and any (non-harmful) activity helps them mentally bear the burden of the treatment ('Even when he doesn't believe init himself, he mustn't take my belief away').

A serious communication challenge is often presented when conveying the diagnosis and articulating the prognosis ('They explained to me that, at 27, I was old, that conception would not occur without problems' 'The physician told me, after she saw my husband's spermiogram, that she would be surprised if we had a child with such a spermiogram' 'The physician said to my wife 'you were searching for each other until you found each other.' We both have reduced fertility'). The conclusions are not always communicated orally and in person, it is also possible to send a letter to the address specified by the patient.

> A patient, an ambitious lawyer, asked us to send the documents from our consulting centre for infertility to the work address, without the rubber stamp of the medical centre. I complied with her request, bought a stamp, and sent the letter through a letterbox outside the hospital. (p)
> I consider the conveying of the diagnosis by letter as entirely unacceptable! It was so in my case. In my house there is a person with the same name, so it often happens that the mail is exchanged, sometimes we unwittingly open letters by mistake. (At least such news should come by registered mail!) The second thing is that you are alone for the reading of the diagnosis, without an immediate explanation or support (not that we would get it from the physicians later on). (f)

Many therapists consider it unacceptable to convey a patient's diagnosis by phone.

> A woman phoned me, and asked for information about the results of her husband's examination. I refused to tell her over the phone, and I didn't yield to her strong pressure and insistence. By coincidence, the man was diagnosed with azoospermia. Later on, it turned out that his wife hadn't called, but her mother-in-law. (p)

The forms and circumstances of conveying a diagnosis have been changing. In the context of the treatment of fertility problems, I would like to mention that the conveying of a diagnosis was an interesting legal problem in the past. Infertility is considered an illness of a couple, but in the past it seemed problematic to convey the unfavourable diagnosis of one partner to the other. The author[14] of a book from 1947 emphasises the necessity to think about the legal consequences of the information that could bring about a divorce due to infertility. According to him, there is a contradiction between the duty to convey the findings of the examination and the duty to maintain medical secrecy before the other partner. Nowadays, doctors sometimes legally draw on the marriage formula that usually mentions knowledge of each other's state of health and they convey the diagnosis to the other partner.

> An elderly man asked me not to convey his diagnosis, in case his spermiogram was bad, to his wife. I promised to comply with his wish. Fortunately, it wasn't necessary, since the man's fertility was fine. (p)

What do therapists expect from their patients?

Therapists expect acceptance of their suggestions ('If we want a child, we must get things going,' 'It was indicated to me that my questions were inappropriate'), belief or trust ('To believe in the success of the treatment' 'He said either him or the Mojzis method') them, and patience ('Patients have no patience, they want everything at once' 'He would like me to bear with them').

Therapists are sometimes not accustomed to patients coming up with questions and information from other sources. They often respond with irritation; they feel suspected of lack of knowledge, and are offended by the patients' mistrust. But the relationship between therapists and patients is becoming equal, and patients are being encouraged to bear more and more responsibility for their health. For example, more frequently, the informed consent of the patient is required to perform a diagnostic or therapeutic procedure. The therapist more frequently offers the patient several therapeutic procedures with various advantages and risks and lets the patient make the choice. The patients, even those who were quite happy with the former situation that placed them in a state of passivity and transferred the responsibility for their lives onto others, now have no other choice than to collect their mental strength and search for available information. Many therapists are already aware of this change and they themselves recommend other sources of information to patients, for example: consultation with a colleague, scientific publications, charities concerned with their problems, the address of a web site, etc.

My goal here is not to criticise the therapists—I am one of them—but to map out what you can come across in your dealings with them. I would like to emphasise that it is usually the people who are not happy with the situation who speak about it. We usually take good experiences for granted and, unfortunately, we keep silent about them. So now you should be prepared for the worst, but you can be surprised, and it is likely you will be, when the worst never comes. If you still encounter difficult situations, keep in mind that the therapist is also just a human being, gifted with certain skills and, similarly to the patient, is influenced by his or her state of health, family situation, and by a medical system that does not pay much attention to the psychological side of therapy.

They're Our Family Now, We have to Live with Them

There is probably nothing more difficult than family relations. Every change, every illness, including fertility problems, is projected into the life of the extended family, especially the partners' parents. Not even the parents can avoid the pressure of their friends and acquaintances, who expect their fulfilment of the grandparents' role. Moreover, the parents of a childless couple can feel an even greater helplessness than the couple, since there is no direct way for them to influence the situation.

> My mother's comments that she would like a grandchild are unpleasant (and she already has six). (m)
> My parents take everything easy. We don't talk about it; they are convinced that things need time. Others in the family behave in a normal way, that is they wish us a child on a birthday. (f)
> They wouldn't show anything. (f)
> Everyone wishes that we had a child. They suffer because we don't have any. They don't interfere in our problems. (f)
> Everybody wishes that we had a child, but mostly they don't understand what we are going through, especially my husband's family. When we submitted the application for adoption, the worst opinion was my mother's, who was completely against it. (f)
> My mother-in-law has the opinion that she wouldn't invest any money into IVF. (f)
> They still hope. (f)
> We don't talk with my family about our problems with conception. I don't like saying things to my parents that would worry them. Mother knows about the problem, she recommended a good gynaecologist that has helped one infertile couple. My husbands' parents know nothing. (f)
> My parents have come to terms with the situation, and don't remind me of it in any way. My mother-in-law finds it harder to cope with my childless marriage and from time to time starts a discussion about it. (f)
> My partner's parents didn't know much about the problem, nor did they desire a grandchild. My mother and father were more sensitive about my problems, since they went through some of my states of sadness and crying. They helped me a lot. (f)

They behaved the same; they were interested about when we would have children. (f)

Mom, of course, saw how the unsuccessful attempts devastated me, and she didn't want me to try for pregnancy any longer in any way. Here I definitely needed more support and encouragement. Everybody among the relatives kept their fingers crossed for me, and wished for a child wholeheartedly. (f)

The families couldn't cope with it, even if it was because of them that I fought so much and so long (until the end of fertility). (f)

They were our fans. (f)

They didn't show anything, but it was hard. (f)

There was a great deal of pressure on the part of my mother-in-law, whenever we were visiting them she asked when we were going to have a child, and whether we were trying. I told my husband that I wouldn't go there if my mother-in-law put me under so much pressure. (f)

I don't talk about my situation with my family. I do not want to listen to their chatter. They wouldn't help me and they would only frustrate me. My mother-in-law puts us under pressure, she keeps asking about things, whether we are doing anything. If she could, she would even tell us when to have intercourse. In one situation, my husband told my mother-in-law that we would have a child, even if not our own. My mother-in-law was devastated and she said that no strange person be allowed into her house. (f)

I felt humiliated by my mother-in-law. (f)

My mother-in-law is a widow, a medical worker. First, she told us to go for the artificial, she was searching for the doctors, contributed to IVF, she keeps saving money for it for us. But now she is saying we should give up on it, that perhaps it will happen by itself. (f)

My husbands' parents were not proponents of the idea that we should have a baby right away, and we had a great deal conflict because of that. They had the opinion that we should enjoy life as long as we were young, that a child would tie us down. (f)

There is a great pressure by the mother-in-law on the daughter. She keeps asking what we're doing, she has searched for doctors. So that she wouldn't differ from other people. (f)

Mommy would probably want it (a child). (m)

They are worried they haven't got a grandchild. (f)

The pressure isn't anything special. (f)

The pressure by the extended family; I don't even want to go to visit my grandmother and aunts. (f)

At first, my mother-in-law pressured me so that I would get treatment, she didn't doubt that I was infertile. When they found out that it was my husband, it was a shock for them. They pressure my husband a lot, they keep asking him, they want us to go for artificial fertilisation. They keep giving articles to

> my husband about the latest methods. He is stressed by it. I already told my mother-in-law that she should stop it. (f)
>
> I had a phone call from a woman. She has a daughter, 23-years-old, who got married 9 months ago and hasn't become pregnant yet. The mother is very nervous about it, she asked about what to do. From her talk it followed that her daughter isn't worried about the problem. (p)
>
> A colleague at work couldn't become pregnant, but she coped with it well, she has her interests. But her mother-in-law was beside herself. The husband was from a village, the oldest son, a farm, they waited for an heir. The colleague told her husband to go there alone, that she had no strength to keep answering her mother-in-law's questions about when she had her last menstruation. (f)

Parents experience the failures of their children in the quest for a child in different ways. It depends on how much they long for grandchildren ('Nor did they desire a grandchild' 'Mommy would probably want it (a child)' 'They are worried they haven't got a grandchild' 'They suffer because we haven't got any' 'The families couldn't cope with it' 'They don't mind it'), on how they are able to handle the pressure of their surroundings ('So that she wouldn't differ from other people' 'My mother-in-law copes with my childless marriage worse'), and also on what kind of relationship they have to their adult children ('They wouldn't show anything' 'My parents have come to terms with the situation, and don't remind me of it in any way'). If parents know about their children's fertility problems, they become affected by the situation ('It was a shock for them') and the consequences of treatment ('My mother and father were more sensitive about my problems, since they went through some of my states of sadness and crying'). Sometimes parents see a problem even where there is none ('The mother is very nervous about it...from her talk it followed that her daughter isn't worried about the problem').

As long as the relationship between the parents and the children is a relationship between adults, the parents leave the solution of the problem to the children ('Parents take everything easy. We don't talk about it, they are convinced that things need time' 'They don't interfere in our problems'). But unfortunately that is not always the case and parents often interfere in dealing with the problem. The interference is perceived by the couple as pressure ('There was a great pressure from the side of my mother-in-law' 'My mother-in-law pressured me') that has various goals. The goal of the parental pressure may be to influence the couple's activity in solving the situation as well as the mode of resolving the situation.

The pressure on the couple's activity can lead in different directions: the intensification of the couple's efforts ('Mom's comments that she would like a grandchild are unpleasant' 'From time to time she starts a discussion about it' 'They were interested when we would have children' 'She asked when we were going to have a child, and whether we were trying' 'She keeps asking about things, whether we are doing anything' 'They keep asking' 'To answer her mother-in-law's questions about when she had her last menstruation'), or the mitigation of their efforts ('They are convinced that things need time' 'She didn't want me to try for pregnancy any longer in any way' 'Now she says we should give up on it, that it perhaps will happen by itself' 'That we should enjoy life as long as we were young, that a child would tie us down').

The extended family have their own ideas about resolving the situation, and they convey them to the couple in variously appropriate ways ('When we submitted the application for adoption, the worst standpoint was my mother's, who was against it' 'She wouldn't invest any money into IVF' 'She recommended "a good gynaecologist"' 'If she could, she would even tell us when to have intercourse' 'My husband told my mother-in-law in one situation that we would have a child, even if not our own. My mother-in-law was devastated and she said that no strange person will be allowed into her house' 'She told us to go for the artificial, she was searching for the doctors' 'She has searched for the doctors' 'They want us to go for artificial fertilisation. They keep giving articles to my husband about the latest methods').

The mature response of the family is support ('They wish us a child on the occasion of a birthday' 'Everyone wishes that we had a child' 'She contributed to IVF, she keeps saving money for it for us').

The couple can defend themselves against unpleasant or unacceptable pressure of the family by opting for conflict ('We had much conflict because of that' 'I already told my mother-in-law that she should stop it') or by breaking off contact ('I don't even want to go to visit my grandmother and aunts' 'I wouldn't go there' 'She told her husband to go there alone'). Another kind of defence consists in preventing the occasions for pressure ('I don't talk about my situation with my family. I do not want to listen to their chatter. They wouldn't help me and they would only frustrate me' 'We don't talk with my family about our problem with conception. I don't like saying things to my parents that would worry them' 'My husband's parents know nothing').

What can you do to handle communication about fertility problems with the least damage to your mental health and to the emotions of your closest relatives? In the first place, you need to realise that it is a problem of the couple, just the two of you and no one else, even if your relatives may try to convince you to the contrary. The number of children you want, the planned time of their birth, and the solution of your problems with conception is your own matter.

Next, you should try to predict the response of your and your partner's family. If you expect misunderstanding and trouble, then try to prevent the pressure or, in other words, minimise communication. You can try: 'We want children, but we have not been successful. We are on treatment. We do not want to say anything more about it.' And really stop talking about it. If you do not want to admit that you have fertility problems, then you can tell your family: 'We will not have any children. It is our concern why. We do not want to talk about it any more.' And, again, stop talking about it. If your family still puts you under unmanageable pressure, then you might have to make the hard decision to break off contact until the pressure is off.

It is more difficult if you are planning adoption. Then it is in the interest of the coming child that the extended family be prepared and behaves nicely toward him or her. Sometimes, however, try as you may, you will not be successful in persuading your family.

Even if you have mature relationships within your family and you do not expect trouble, I recommend that you first consider together with your partner how much you will tell the family, and in what detail. One reason for considering the amount of shared information is that it is the couple's problem, and intimate at that, and that it is necessary to respect the wishes of the partner as far as the extent of the communicated matters is concerned. The second reason is the protection of your relatives from unnecessary suffering, also because they are helpless to resolve the situation. Understandably, the situation is different again when you are planning adoption. Then it is necessary to explain as much as possible to the family.

She Said...

> *The Virgin Mary, sprung from the royal stock and family of David, was born in the town of Nazareth... Her father was named Joachim, and her mother Anna. For about 20 years they lived in their own house, a chaste married life, without having any children. Nevertheless, they vowed that, should the Lord happen to give them offspring, they would deliver it into the service of the Lord; on which account also they used to visit the temple of the Lord at each of the feasts during the year. And when the high priest saw Joachim with his offering among his other fellow citizens, he despised him, and spurned his gifts, asking*

why he, who had no offspring, presumed to stand among those who had, saying that his gifts could not by any means be acceptable to God, since he had deemed him unworthy of offspring: for the Scripture said, Cursed is every one who has not begot a male in Israel. He said, therefore, that he ought first to be freed from this curse by the begetting of children; and only then that he should come into the presence of the Lord with his offerings…

'The Gospel of the Nativity of Mary', 1–2

All right, how dare you childless people appear together with those who have children? Perhaps you are not worth having them. The Gospel from which I cite is not part of the usual translation of the Bible, according to a consultation with an expert it is apocryphal—a biblical scripture that is not accepted as part of the canon of the Old Testament or the New Testament. It comes from about the 4th century A.D., and belongs among the newest scriptures. But we are not seeking a theological or historical analysis; we are interested in society's view of childlessness. The extract is from a time in the distant past; has anything changed since then?

The queries of the people around me are sometimes unpleasant. (m)
I guess they take it as it is. Everyone has his or her own problems. (f)
People around me don't pay much attention to it. (m)
People around me keep tactfully silent. (f)
I think that our friends with whom we're in touch wish us a child. We speak about it in an entirely normal way. (f)
At first, we didn't talk about it but now we've been talking about it with everybody openly, even though not with everybody but only with true close friends… I don't intentionally seek out conversations about the topic. Mostly, I talk about it with female colleagues at work. (f)
Largely, nobody knows about it. (f)
Everyone was helping me a lot; they were trying to…distract me. The age bracket of my friends is quite low, so not everyone has children, and they have other problems. (f)
They were interested in when we were going to have children. (f)
The neighbours fortunately don't know much. My girlfriends pitied me and encouraged me, they cried with me, we analysed it from all sides, they kept bringing me information about various treatments, methods, exercises, etc. (f)
The closest ones had compassion for me, the others mostly kept a neutral stand, as I wanted them to. (f)
They didn't know about it. (f)
The closest friends responded in a normal way. People who didn't know us told us: lucky you, go ahead and enjoy life. One mother asked me (I'm a teacher) how I could raise other children when I don't have my own. (f)

Once I heard from one person that our infertility is God's punishment for the fact that I hadn't become a nun. (f)

In the believers' environment, where there is a custom (or there has been one until recently) that a year after the wedding there is a baby, the childless couple soon become conspicuous. First, such people are asked when they are going to have a child but, as time passes, there is mostly silence around them. (f)

Apart from the comments concealed behind your back, the other response of the people around you can be well-meant advice: Go far away for a long holiday, you will forget about everything, and perhaps you will come back with a baby, calm down, stop thinking about it all the time, adopt a child, then you are going to become pregnant. You wouldn't be the first one. (f)

Then there is the other thing, people's views of childlessness: 'She probably doesn't want children, she's making a career', or 'She's lazy, not like our Anna, she has a tougher life, looking after two children, she can't go to the cinema like you', and so on. It is really quite unpleasant, and it is quite difficult to tell people, they don't believe it anyway. (f)

I want people to think a while, to try to sympathise with the concerned couple, and truly admit what they would do in the couple's place. (f)

A girlfriend of mine has not been able to become pregnant for five years. Physicians haven't found any cause. I keep telling her that it is mental, that she should stop getting upset, and it would succeed. (f)

My friends have had a child after eight years of treatment. But, in the village, the people say anyway that the child they have is [adopted]. (f)

I am unnerved when others tell me, 'you mustn't think about it,' 'go out and enjoy yourself,' 'eat well,' (f)

At the request of many subscribers of a magazine for infertile patients , the sender's rubber stamp had to be changed, and the phrase 'Association of Involuntarily Childless Couples' erased. (f)

The fertile and the infertile are two worlds that cannot understand each other. (f)

When a conversation turns that way, I say that I have a daughter after IVF treatment. When people then see her, they look at her as though she should somehow not be normal, and they are surprised that she has both arms and legs, and is pretty. (f)

In our village it isn't a problem, there are about seven families with similar problems. There are also several adopted children, and there aren't any problems associated with this. (m)

There is a young team at work and they keep asking me when there'll be a child. (f)

In the parish, there are several couples with whom we used to be in contact a lot, we married almost at the same time. They are having children now, and I have nothing to talk about with them, they have no time to go anywhere. I am losing contact with people. (f)

People around give me good advice, and claim that I have miscarriages out of mental stress. I hate it. (f)

One relative is envious that we don't have children, and that we can do what we want whenever we want. (f)

First our acquaintances kept asking when it was going to happen, and whatever was going on. Now they don't ask anything, they only stare. That is worse, I'd rather answer questions. (f)

We're isolated. When I meet my girlfriends who have children, there is always 'something' between us. (f)

It is difficult in a village. The neighbours keep asking. We have applied for adoption, but we're afraid of what people will say. At the same time, it is unacceptable for the village that we stay childless. (m)

They kept asking me at work, if and when we were planning a child. I gave evasive answers until they got it, and the director sent me to his acquaintance, a healer. (f)

The mockery of the people around me is much worse than useless pity. For example, husband can't go to the pub. When the guys get tipsy, they mock him that he is good for nothing. (f)

A society that considers the inability to have children to be something denigrating brings up individuals who, when they discover that they themselves are impaired in this way, take up the role of an inferior, by which they incite the condemnation of other people. (p)

I am involved in an association of involuntarily childless couples. When I have an appointment with the authorities (on behalf of the association), I take my six-year-old daughter with me, because I have had the experience that the clerks treat me better. When I go alone, everybody treats me like a 'mentally ill sterile person'; they behave towards me as if I were an inferior person. (f)

My wife's fallopian tubes are both defective, so there's no way we could achieve pregnancy in a natural way. But always, when we go on holiday, our acquaintances advice us to forget about everything, and that for sure we're going to bring a baby back. At first, I tried to explain to them that it is impossible for us, but I have resigned myself, they don't believe me. (m)

My parents were involuntarily childless for 8 years, and they waited another 8 years for the next child... When their wish was fulfilled, under the impact of the lived-through horrors, they made many mistakes in the upbringing. (f)

My female colleagues are fine, they are my fans, and they will support me if it isn't successful again. One colleague always goes to pray for me when I have a transfer. (f)

No IVF is comparable to what one must bear from one's own social environment. (f)

Fortunately, things have changed much over the last several hundreds of years, for example, you can now appear in public even if you haven't given birth to a male descendant. But, as the testimonies show, it is still not a walk through a rose garden either. Since most people are involved in seeking reliable protection against undesirable conception, the reverse problem is often entirely incomprehensible to them ('It is impossible for us, but I have resigned myself, they don't believe me' 'It is quite difficult to tell people, they don't believe it anyway' 'The fertile and the infertile are two worlds that can't understand each other' 'No IVF is comparable to what one must bear from one's own social environment'), they suppose that the partners themselves are somehow to blame for their childlessness.

The childless couple under suspicion ('There is a custom that a year after the wedding there is a baby, the childless couple start soon become conspicuous') are suspected of not having good will. Some people in their social environment refer to it directly, in the previous chapter, we called it pressure on the couple's personal activities ('The unpleasant queries of the people around me' 'They were interested in when we would have children' 'First, such people are asked when they are going to have a child' 'Kept asking when it was going to happen, and what was going on' 'The neighbours keep asking' 'If and when we were planning a child').

If people conclude that the couple have good will, then their abilities come into question. Sometimes the couple are given concrete advice about the act itself. But mostly people speak about the couple's inability behind their backs, that is about the fact that the man is not such a 'stud' as he seemed. Directly, people express their views only under special circumstances ('When the guys get tipsy, they mock him that he is good for nothing'). In women, the cause of their inability is sought in the area of the psyche. Everybody knows nowadays that the source of all evil is stress, so everybody can offer well-meant advice ('Go far away for a long holiday, you will come back with a baby' 'Calm down, stop thinking about it all the time' 'Adopt a child, then you are going to become pregnant' 'It is mental in her, that she should stop getting upset, and it would succeed' 'Others tell me 'you mustn't think about it'' 'Go out and enjoy yourself' 'Eat well' 'People around me give me 'good' advice, and claim that I have miscarriages out of mental stress'). Yet, this is the better case. In the worse case, a deeper cause than stress is sought in the area of the psyche. Often it is said that a child is a gift. A gift is given out of love or as a reward for something. Again, the inability of the couple is at the fore, they are unable to do something ('When I go alone, everybody treats me like a "mentally ill sterile person"' 'How I can raise other children when I don't have my own'), therefore they have not done something right or they are not worthy someone's love, they do not deserve it, and hence they are reprehensible ('They are condemned by the mother-in-law or by the husband's whole family' 'Considers the inability to have children as something denigrating' 'They behave toward me as if I were an inferior person' 'The mockery of other people is much worse than useless pity'), they fail to have children as a punishment ('Our infertility is God's punishment for the fact that I hadn't become a nun'). The couple is ashamed of the problem ('The sender's rubber stamp had to be changed, and the phrase 'Association of Involuntarily Childless Couples' erased'), and may experience feelings of inferiority. As you see, what Joachim and his wife Anna lived through is still familiar to us.

Nevertheless, many people have now come to understand that infertility is an illness like any other and that it presents a difficult life situation for the couple ('I guess they take it as it is' 'In our village, it isn't a problem, there are about seven families with similar problems'). Sometimes they keep silent because they do not know how to respond ('The people around me keep tactfully silent' 'As time passes, there is mostly silence around them' 'Now they don't ask anything, they only stare') or because they sense that the couple are not interested in analysing the topic ('People around me don't their pay much attention to it' 'The others mostly kept a neutral stand, as I wanted it'). The couple can perceive the silence of social environment, no matter what the reasons are, as isolation, a loss of common topics ('They are having children now, and I have nothing to talk about with them' 'They only stare. That is worse, I'd rather answer questions' 'We're isolated. When I meet my girlfriends who have children, there is always 'something' between us'). Others do talk about the topic, it depends on the particular situation ('The age bracket of my friends is quite low, so not everyone has children, and they have other problems') and on their relationship with the couple in question ('At first we didn't talk about it, but now we've been talking about it with everybody openly' 'We analysed it from all sides' 'The closest ones had compassion for me'). Understandably, they also try to help the couple, for instance through encouragement ('They were trying to take the problems easily before me, and distract me' 'My girlfriends pitied me and encouraged me, they cried with me' 'They will support me if it isn't successful again. One colleague always goes to pray for me when I have a transfer') and through sharing information about treatment options ('They kept bringing me information about various treatments, methods, exercises, etc.' 'The director sent me to his acquaintance, a healer'). However, one must be careful, so that the sincere wish to help of others does not become extreme:

> My senior doctor once saw me crying and broken down after the miscarriage and when I explained to her what I was experiencing she decided to help

me. She used her contacts, she managed to set up for us many examinations that would have been almost impossible to arrange by ourselves. And she goes everywhere to see the doctors along with us. It is clear that the physicians deal with her, a physician, in a different way than with us, they wouldn't neglect her because she is assertive and wouldn't give up, she asks about everything. But Ronnie is ashamed in front of her, it is not pleasant for him when she holds discussion about his spermiogram. I was trying to indicate this to her, but she didn't understand it at all, she thinks that we wouldn't manage without her. So I don't know what to do. Of course I am grateful, since she has done a lot for us and she wishes us well, but we can't keep solving this thing in a group of three! (f)

...and she even mentioned childlessness

From the psychosocial viewpoint, childlessness is still difficult to accept for society. People generally expect that, after the wedding, there will be a baby. When it does not come, the couple is suspected of inability, as we have already said, or lack of good will ('People's views of childlessness: "She probably doesn't want children, she's making a career" or "She's lazy, not like our Anna, she has a tougher life, looking after two children"'), and condemned for their selfishness. Some people envy the childless couple ('Lucky you, go ahead and enjoy life' 'One relative is envious that we haven't got children, and that we can do whatever we want whenever we want' 'She can't go to the cinema like you'), or give cheap consolation. In a film, a nurse tells a woman, a teacher who is involuntarily childless: 'Be happy you haven't got your own!'

The pressure of the social environment is difficult to bear even for couples who are voluntarily childless and not because of fertility problems. The situation of a couple who wanted to have a child and could not is all the worse. One sociologist[15] reminds us that a childless woman always keeps encountering the often unarticulated, but permanently present question: does she not want to or is she not able to have children?

We have no children, and I hate the compassionate looks that people around me are bombarding me with. I do not know why they look at me as a useless woman. They consider my life to be wasted when I haven't been able to give birth to a child. Why does no one ask me if I, by any chance, did not decide willingly? I have simply planned my life differently than is common in this country, and I continue to bear the consequences. I have even heard that I am a barren and bitter woman. I can't understand why? Where is the basis for the rule that every woman must give birth to at least one child, and live above all for the family? I think that then I would have been even more bitter. (f)

A childless man is usually still (if there are no doubts about his fertility) seen somewhat differently. He is taken for a bachelor who wants to enjoy life and who does not want to take responsibility for others. It is worse when doubts about his fertility appear. Nevertheless, it must be pointed out that the views of the social environment are, above all, a reflection of the childless person's perceptions.

People usually also have their opinions about what childless couples should fill their lives with when they have not decided for adoption. Mostly people think that childless couples would benefit from some form of work with children, for instance helping in children's homes, organising children's hobby groups or spending time with their friends' children. But it is precisely such contact with children that can be traumatising for some involuntarily childless couples.

> I was on a visit and right on my arrival, they put a baby in my arms. I returned it immediately and rushed out to cry. I don't keep our troubles secret anywhere, so everybody knew that we had recently undergone unsuccessful IVF. It was very cruel of them. How could they have done it? (m)

...and she even shared her opinion on parenting

As I was thinking about the topic of parenting after undergoing therapy for fertility problems, I realised one interesting thing. When people speak about the children or the parenting of someone whose quest for a child was not easy, this fact is emphasised. The testimonies sound approximately like this: she has a little daughter now, after six years of treatment; they couldn't have children, they were on treatment, and now they have twins; over there, little Jane, she is a prayed-for child, her parents didn't even hope that they would live to see her. The child is considered mysterious and strange, and the parents' mistakes in raising the child are not excused by their inexperience, as is common with fertile parents, but are explained by the fact that the child did not come easily ('My parents were involuntarily childless for 8 years... When their wish was fulfilled, under the impact of the lived-through horrors, they made many mistakes in the upbringing').

A quite separate and voluminous topic is society's view of adoption and foster care; here, I refer interested readers to the existing publications in that area. In this book, I would only like to add that, thanks to the activity of the media, the image of adoptive parents has improved significantly and their decision to look after an orphaned child is generally appreciated.

...and you replied

How do you respond to the unpleasant pressure of the society around you, a pressure that can have various degrees of intensity? The extreme solution recommended when there are difficulties in communication with one's family, of breaking off contact, is not possible here. When you move away from one difficult neighbour, it is likely that there is going to be another difficult neighbour wherever you move. You cannot get rid of the people around you, and you will have to come to terms with their reactions. You may keep the social pressure down to acceptable limits in a similar way as in communication with your family: through minimising the communication. It is harder in adoption, it is necessary to prepare the child for the fact that some people are ignorant or plain mean.

Your social environment, however, is not made up only of the gossipy people in the neighbourhood. It also includes the nice people, your friends, and couples dealing with a similar problem. These people can help you in coping with the struggles on the quest for a child. Find someone among your friends with whom you can talk openly about the situation, to whom you can express your feelings, with whom you can cry if need be, and whom you trust that he or she will not immediately share your story with somebody else. But do not forget that it is a couple's affair, yours and your partner's, and an intimate one at that. I recommend that you two first agree on what is acceptable for you both to tell your friends and what is not, and that you respect your partner's wishes.

Adoptive children or children in foster care are sometimes encouraged by diligent neighbours or teachers not to be mischievous and to be grateful to their parents that they have saved their lives. You can probably imagine the effect of such enforced gratefulness on the child. If your child is an object of such pressure, do not hesitate and to tell the child that it is he or she who has saved your life in turn. Is it not so?

A person who is suffering is more sensitive to the interest of other people, to their inquisitive looks, remarks, behaviours. Often such a person cannot stand expressions of pity or sympathy, even if they are meant sincerely. It is natural: the foundations of life are weakened for such a person, it often happens that he or she lives in permanent stress, as if always expecting an attack from somewhere. But one should realise that this tension is a consequence of one's increased sensitivity rather than of other people's spitefulness or malice. It is true that some remarks can be articulated crudely and they hurt, but if you try to distance yourselves from them, probably you will find that there was no malicious intention behind them, just lack of knowledge, false beliefs, misinformation, and sometimes even attempts to gain importance or showing off by offering supposedly wise advice.

No Pain, No Gain

Very few of us belong to the Rothschild family where we can live off a trust fund. Most of us have to go to work. For men the topic of children usually never comes up at an interview. But for women, in seemingly innocuous ways references to motherhood are sprinkled into most conversations. From the employer's viewpoint, this is understandable, from the woman's viewpoint, it is offensive, and from a legal standpoint, it is unacceptable.

The situation of a woman, who is not successful in becoming pregnant, whether she discovers it during her employment or whether she knows it before starting a job, is even worse. Besides the fact that repeated questions keep reminding her of her suffering, there is an additional stress from how to answer the questions about motherhood so that it would not threaten her position at work.

> The treatment of infertility is demanding in terms of time, money, and taking time off work. (f)
>
> For two months every day, I went to a town 50 miles away for a check-up, and every day I went to a town to 20 miles away for an injection. I had to hand in my notice at work. (f)
>
> During one IVF cycle, 4–6 visits plus the operations themselves, it was also a time-consuming affair. (m)
>
> The threat of the complete loss of a professional career (during the IVF treatment). Nowadays, only a few employers are willing to employ a woman who is away from work two months out of a half year because of the therapeutic treatment and, in the remaining months, she rushes around doctors or is on sick leave because she is dealing with the consequences of the hormonal treatment. (f)
>
> A friend of mine also cannot conceive. She is a kindergarten teacher. I told her that at least she is among children, but she said that makes it even worse because she realises all the time that she has no children of her own, she cannot avoid these thoughts. (f)

At first, I was helping my husband with his business. Now I've helped him to stand on his feet and become independent, so I can devote myself to the treatment of infertility. (f)

There is a problem with work, I am set up for a child, I cannot get focused on anything, I don't enjoy it. My boss does not give me major tasks because he expects that I will go on maternity leave. (f)

I work in my husband's business, but I don't enjoy it, I'm isolated from people, often I don't leave the house. But I can't change work because I can't leave it all to my husband, and also there is no employment in which I could afford to go for various examinations and treatments all the time. (f)

Fortunately, I have good work where they let me see the doctor. Otherwise, I would have to hand in my notice. (f)

I haven't worked for five years, my husband supports me. I only go for check-ups, treatments, and to healers. (f)

I wanted to run my own business, but I didn't begin because I was expecting to get pregnant. I have been waiting for 10 years. (f)

I don't have any work, and I am not searching for it in any intensive way, even though we're in such a dismal financial situation. I wouldn't have much occasion to go to work anyway, since I am either having a risky pregnancy or am in hospital. (f)

I had a lot of trouble at work; besides the fact that I didn't enjoy it, there were difficulties with taking time off for treatment. All the time, I kept telling myself that maternity leave would be a solution. It was terrible, every day in the morning for a shot, then the check-ups, and then 14 days of sick leave. My boss does not respect any illness, and he yelled at me. Then he suggested I leave by mutual agreement with severance pay. I welcomed it; now I've been at home for the third month, and I am glad. (f)

At work, they were compassionate at first, but then they were angry that I am on sick leave all the time, and when I came to work, they gave me enormous work loads. At the moment, I have handed in notice, but I am not looking for anything, I must put myself to rights mentally. (f)

At work, they asked all the time if and when we were planning a child, so that they could find a substitute in time. (f)

But I think that, with children (I am a teacher), I was too good and lenient. (f)

One mother asked me (I'm a teacher) how I can raise other children when I don't have my own. (f)

When we went to submit the application for adoption, the social worker wondered why we wanted to adopt a child when we have enough of them at work (we're teachers), she tried to talk us out of it. (f)

I've concluded that, if I'm unable to have my own children, it is perhaps so that I could devote myself better to those entrusted to me (I am a teacher). (f)

Since I was young, I've been terribly interested in children. I had only baby dolls, and I used to walk outside with the prams of all our acquaintances.

> I chose working with children as my profession; I am at the premature babies department. But I've been trying to have my own for nine years, and it has not been successful. I've been thinking that I will have to leave, that I could not bear it. Moreover, we have many premature infants from the IVF, which is also my treatment. I've been rather depressed by work. (f)
>
> My husband is a doctor. A superb doctor. But when it comes to his illnesses, he fails, and does not make any effort to solve anything. (f)

The examinations and the treatment of fertility problems are very time-consuming. Only some of the procedures can be done in one's free time, for many it is necessary to take time off work. The treatment can take a number of years and, if it is successful, the employee leaves for maternity leave. So from the viewpoint of the employer, the prospects are grim in any case.

A woman's desire for a child is usually strong ('I am set up for a child'), and this can be reflected in their losing interest in work ('I cannot get focused on anything, I don't enjoy it' 'I didn't enjoy it'). Understandably, both these aspects lower the women's working efficiency, to which the employer responds ('Nowadays only a few employers are willing to employ a woman who' 'My boss does not give me major tasks' 'My boss does not respect any illness, and he yelled at me,' 'Then they were angry that I am on sick leave all the time, and when I came, they gave me enormous work loads' 'So that they could find a substitute in time').

Some women deal with the situation by leaving work to stay at home ('I had to hand in my notice at work' 'I devote myself to the treatment of infertility' 'I haven't worked for five years' 'He suggested I leave by mutual agreement with a severance pay. I welcomed it' 'I had to hand in my notice'). Others stay in an unsatisfactory job ('But I can't change work' 'I wanted to run my own business, but I didn't begin' 'I am not searching for it in any intensive way' 'I have handed in notice, but I am not looking for anything') and do not try for advancement, not only because their employer is lenient with their absences, but also because they hope that their situation will be resolved perhaps as soon as the next month by their departure for maternity leave ('Because I was expecting that I would be pregnant' 'I kept telling myself all the time that maternity leave would be a solution'). Thus, the consequence is a loss of professional prospects for the woman ('The threat of the complete loss of a professional career'), which may have a great impact on the woman's life ('It's been 10 years that I've spent waiting.').

The professional prospects of a woman on the quest for a child are not rosy at all, and there is no miraculous advice. Sometimes there is really no solution other than to leave the job. If it is possible at all, act as though you are not on any quest for a child, seek employment that is more suitable and get involved in activities that are satisfying for you. Everybody can be replaced, and when you become pregnant, your employer will have to do just that.

For your inspiration, I offer you three possible answers to the question about your plans for motherhood. But you will need to choose the version suitable for you according to your particular situation:

1. I am not planning a child and I do not want it. This is a seemingly advantageous approach in terms of your career, but it provides the basis for frequent queries from your fellow workers about the reasons, for concealed and manifest condemnation of you. Moreover, it is difficult to provide reasons for frequent absences for treatment.
2. I want a child and I am planning to have one, but I have been having trouble getting pregnant. This is an unfavourable answer in terms of your work career. The employer knows that infertility treatment is demanding in terms of time as well as physical and mental strength, and that eventual success would take you away on maternity leave. From the viewpoint of work relations, this response is suitable only for some women.
3. I want a child, but I cannot have it because of a severe, incurable problem. The frequent appointments at the doctor's can be explained by the treatment of this illness. This answer is only partially favourable in terms of your career and in terms of the response of your colleagues. People do not usually ask for details about a severe illness, and they express, directly and indirectly, some sympathy with the person. But not every woman is able to bury her hopes, even if just in pretence, and it is not always easy to bear the sympathy and well-meant help from others (for instance, their bringing articles about the latest methods of artificial fertilisation, the use of a surrogate mother, etc.).

In contrast to women, for men work is a help rather than a stress factor in the process of examinations and treatment.

An interesting question is the impact of fertility problems on a certain profession. You will notice in the testimonies that a special place is taken up by teachers. Due to their frequent contact with children, they may be more intensely aware of the problem ('She realises all the time that she has no children of her own, she cannot avoid these thoughts'), they may think more about the problem in connection with their ability to raise children ('But I think that, with children (I am a teacher), I was too good and lenient' 'If I'm unable to have my own children, it is perhaps so that I could devote myself better to those entrusted to me (I am a teacher)') and they encounter less understanding from the people around them ('How can I raise other children when I don't have my own' 'She wondered why we wanted to adopt a child when we have enough of them at work (we're teachers), she tried to talk us out of it'). This, however, does not concern only teachers. The same applies to paediatricians, midwives, children's nurses ('I am at the premature babies department. But I've been trying to have my own for nine years. I've been thinking that I will have to leave, that I cannot bear it'). Medical workers may find it more difficult to be patients ('A superb doctor. But when it comes to his illnesses, he fails') and they are often more strongly aware of the sadder aspects of treatment ('Moreover we have many premature babies from the IVF, which is also my treatment. I've been rather depressed by my work'). With some overstatement, I sometimes say that the best job for the involuntarily childless is to sell tractors. It has nothing even distantly in common with children and there are usually only men around tractors, so children are not such a frequent topic of conversation.

Behind Everything Look for...Money

The correct wording of the proverb is 'Behind everything look for a woman' and it would be more than logical in a book about fulfilling the desire for a child. But even here, finances frequently play a dual role:

1. In the economic strategy of the health policy of the state. This determines which diagnostic and therapeutic interventions are going to be covered and to what extent by medical insurance companies under basic medical insurance and which ones are not going to be covered at all. Even a reasonably long interview with the patient can be considered a therapeutic intervention. The situation varies from one country to the next and the conditions vary as the legislative framework is currently undergoing many changes.

2. In the financial situation of the couple. The contents of your wallet or the riches in your bank account are, at a certain stage, quite an important factor in deciding about further steps. Your financial situation influences the possibility of treatment through the methods that are not covered by medical insurance companies or are covered only to a certain extent. Repeated treatment through assisted reproduction represents amounts that significantly deplete the family budget. In this area, the couple get into a vicious circle because the assisted reproduction treatments may limit the job options of the woman, and therefore the financial situation of the family, which in turn limits the possibilities of treatment.

The question of money in medicine is somewhat strange, and I understand well that nothing is free... If we'd wanted to persevere in the treatment, I suppose I would have had to visit a financial institution with a stocking over my face. (m)
We were successful on the second attempt, so fortunately it cost us only a few thousand extra for the drugs. But people sell cars and houses, just to have enough money for the next IVF. (f)

Culture...

'I am coming to beg for mercy for my subjects,' the Ant Queen said with a trembling voice, 'We are returning your pupae. Here they are. But we cannot pay the fine for stealing.'

'No, no! We cannot accept that. It cannot be done so cheaply!' Trumbel'nek retorted.

'Really we cannot pay the fine of twenty of our pupae, as you require, simply because we do not have them,' the queen continued almost in a whisper, 'There is poverty at our place. I am old, I cannot lay eggs, therefore there are no new ants being born. The anthill is falling down, we need bricklayers. We are hungry, we need hunters. Our hopes lie with the two pupae that we have left. We hope that there will be two new queens born to us,' she said with tenderness, 'Then we will be saved,' added the queen quietly with glowing eyes. 'The new queens will start laying eggs; the anthill will again have little children and pupae, and from those new ants will be born. Do not be angry that we wanted to steal several pupae from you. There was nothing else we could do. We wanted to help our anthill.' She was now bending with weakness, and quickly one of the servants brought a chair for her. The queen sat down with a shy smile.

'About the Queen Who in the End Sat Down on a Chair',
Andrew Sekora, *The Book of Ferda the Ant*

When I was searching through my bookcase looking for stories related to childlessness for my thesis, it did not occur to me to open *The Book of Ferda the Ant*, I did not expect to find anything there. Only by chance, as I was putting the final touches to this book, I was reading *Ferda* to my children, and the story struck me. I do not know how to explain any better than the queen why living beings, ants as well as people, need to have descendants. Childlessness cannot be perceived with favour, because it threatens the existence of a certain group: an anthill, a pack, a clan, an ethnic group, a nation.

Therefore, probably in all cultures[16], childlessness has been and is still considered a misfortune from an economic point of view, as well as for reasons related to the cult of ancestors. The cause of infertility almost always used to be sought by the woman in spells or magic that she hoped could bring a child. She was treated accordingly until she gave birth. The main obligation was to give birth to at least one son.

In the middle ages in Europe, a woman who did not give her husband a descendant was renounced and she was exposed to contempt and mockery. A woman's infertility was a legitimate reason for untying a marriage in the ruling dynasties and in other high spheres of society where marriage was otherwise a sacred and inseparable bond. In the Muslim world, the social status of women, their dignity and their self-esteem are closely related to their procreation potential; childbearing and child rearing are regarded as family commitments and not just biological and social functions and births of sons remain central to women's well-being. Buddhists traditionally considered infertility as a retribution for past immorality of the man, the woman or even their ancestors. In China, there are historical and current records of the practice of female infanticide; sons are more important to families in that over-populated country. Sons are also important for religious reasons and the traditional family genealogy tree records only the names of males. The traditional cultural norm in old China was unilaterally to divorce women who could not bear a son. In India, there is an enormous stigma attached to being infertile, especially for the woman. And having more than one daughter was a curse, whereas any number of sons was welcomed[i].

Thus, the consequences of infertility used to be quite tragic and even today it does not present a cheerful outlook. That is why people have always searched for all kinds of ways to bring a child (in some places especially a son) into the world.

...Expressed in ethical principles

In polytheistic religions, fertility goddesses and gods are very important and in monotheistic religions, dogmas about reproduction as the basis of life are likewise significant. Some believe that these dogmas form the basis for determining correct and incorrect behaviour, in other words, morality.

It is extraordinarily difficult to write about ethics and I hesitated to undertake it at all, since I am not an expert in this area. However, I consider ethics so important that I cannot omit it. A person on the quest for a child usually seeks all the available means to attain this goal and, in the heat of the moment, does not think much about the possible consequences, be they mental, social, or legal. The following paragraphs are not an expert analysis of the ethics of reproduction; I cannot even ensure the credibility of the sources I have drawn on. I have only one aim: to stimulate readers to think about the broader issues of the quest for a child, to attempt to imagine the countryside beyond the hill that they are climbing at the moment.

The oldest ethical question in parenting is probably the common bloodlines (consanguinity) of descendants. According to historical sources, in ancient communal societies, there existed forms of marriage where the man had an unlimited right to sexual intercourse with all the sisters of his wife, and the woman had the right to intercourse with all the brothers of her husband. In the kinship organisation of certain tribes, it used to be common that women gratified the visiting guests. The tribe and clan were holy institutions that were respected above all; the family did not have such sharp contours. Private property did not exist, and hence neither did the need to establish consanguineous inheritance. The family father was considered the father, and he did not have to be a biological father. From an historical viewpoint, the marriage of a couple is a recent phenomenon, and it was only its arrival that brought the gnawing question about the consanguinity of descendants. Research indicates that, nowadays, it is no longer a question of the need to pass down one's private property of material goods, but the need to pass down one's mental goods.

The other ethical question is the acceptability of external intervention in the reproductive process with the goal to terminate pregnancy. The following information comes from the publication 'Abortion Yes—No'[17]. It is said that, in ancient times, there was no ban on artificial termination of pregnancy. The ancient Greeks even recommended abortion to regulate the population and maintain stable social and economic conditions. Plato recommended abortion to women above 40 years of age, particularly if they had a husband older than 50 years of age. Aristotle also recommended abortion to regulate the size of families.

In ancient Rome, there were virtually no bans on abortion during the whole existence of the empire. The dominant view of the law was that the unborn fetus is part of the woman's body and can be removed at her request and with her consent. In England, there was a law from 1307 to 1803 that allowed women to have an abortion if they asked for it. The regulation followed from the common law that stated that a woman can have an abortion before the 'perceptions of the child' start, and these perceptions meant the movements of the fetus.

According to the above-mentioned book, St. Thomas Aquinas (1225–1274) investigated pregnancy and took as his starting point the structure of the spontaneously miscarried fetuses, and he established that the soul enters the male fetus on the 40th day and the female fetus on the 90th day. In northern Ghana, it is common practice to observe an expectation period until the seventh day after the birth, when the child can finally be identified as a human being. Some Native American tribes ascribe the attribute of humanity only to a child with the skill of sucking from the breast, while premature babies who lack the sucking reflex cannot be identified as fully-developed human beings. The native inhabitants of Taiwan did not punish the killing of a child before its official naming, which did not occur until a ritual was held when the child turned two or three years old. The ethics of abortion and termination of life is bound, therefore, by how different cultures establish the beginning of human life.

You may be wondering why I am discussing such shocking behaviours (whose credibility I moreover cannot guarantee) about termination of life to readers who are more interested in how to conceive life. But the advances in modern reproductive medicine have brought the issue of the ethics of intervention into the reproductive process with the goal of terminating pregnancy extraordinarily close to the issue of the ethics of intervention with the goal to stimulate pregnancy and guide it to a successful fruition. In the past, couples who could not have a child and sought help probably did not worry much about ethical questions. These have been raised by the development of new clinical techniques that enable conception outside the body, but also by a number of other, almost unbelievable, possibilities. On the one hand, these possibilities give hope to childless people, but on the other hand, they raise a very urgent question about the ethicality of such interventions. The main ethical and legal questions include the following areas:

- The moral acceptability of external intervention into the reproductive process
- The moral and legal status of the embryo (reduction, cryopreservation, selection, experiments with pre-embryos)

- The involvement of a third party in the reproductive process—through the donation of genetic material or surrogate parenting

Cultural and religious diversity provides a number of answers to these questions. In regards to the moral and legal position of the human embryo, there are two main spheres of opinion: one attributes to the embryo all the rights of a human being from the moment of fertilisation, while the other, termed 'gradualism', admits that these rights can be gradually acquired during development. With help from specialists in the ethics of ART[18], I will now describe the attitudes of the main world religions. In each of these religions, there are many streams of opinion, and it is no longer possible to formulate precise, holistic attitudes about any one of them. The following are just the views of some of these groups.

- ***Judaism***

The Jewish tradition views an illness as an anomaly. Through the effort to look after an ill person, a human being interferes with the Creator's plans. Generally, Judaism is cautious in its relation to scientific and social development, with certain exceptions. In the Jewish understanding of the world, humans are authorised and even bound to influence and develop the world in all directions that lead to the benefit of humanity. Hence, any activity that contributes to progress in the world cannot be considered contradictory to God's commands. The technology of modern reproduction only uses the factors that have arisen in nature as the result of Creation. If we use, for any reasons, the knowledge that we have, it does not start a new act of Creation. These new technologies do not resolve the mystery of life in any way.

At a worldwide level, there are several different trends in Judaism: the orthodox (about 10% of religious Jews), reform (85%) and conservative (5%) groups. For most groups, all efforts should be exerted to help the infertile. However, the control and guidelines of a limiting codex are indispensable, since assisted reproduction can obscure the feeling of blood relation and it creates thousands of embryos, which are not only a moral, but also a legal problem. The embryo should be respected from the moment of conception itself. It is forbidden to destroy it but, as far as the meaning that lies in the embryo is concerned, its life is not as sacred for Judaism as the life of a person that is in danger. Jewish authorities would allow fetal reduction if it is certain that all the fetuses would be lost otherwise and if prevention fails, in cases of high-order multiple pregnancy. According to the Jewish tradition, life begins with the beat of the heart.

Sperm donation is generally prohibited, because of fear of incest, prohibition of masturbation, disturbance of genealogy and possible problems related to inheritance. But some rabbinical authorities (reform and conservative) permit sperm donation when the donor is a non-Jew. The use of semen from the husband is permissible if no other method is possible for the wife to become pregnant. Egg donation is acceptable, as only the offspring of a Jewish mother may be regarded as Jewish. Jewish religion does not forbid the practice of surrogacy, as indeed the practice is described in the Bible in the case of Sarah and Abraham.

- ***Christianity***

For the Roman Catholic Church, the starting document is the Catechism of the Catholic Church and the doctrinal 'Humanae Vitae' of 1968, issued by Pope Paul VI. This document determines the acceptability and non-acceptability of contraceptives: 'But the most remarkable development of all is to be seen in man's stupendous progress in the domination and rational organisation of the forces of nature to the point that he is endeavouring to extend this control over every aspect of his own life—over his body, over his mind and emotions, over his social life, and even over the laws that regulate the transmission of life.'

A statement of the Pontifical Academy of Life, a consulting body of the Pope states: 'The living human embryo is—from the moment of the union of the gametes—a *human subject* with a well-defined identity from that point begins its own coordinated, continuous and gradual development, such that at no later stage can it be considered as a simple mass of cells.' The church has always had this opinion and has taught that the result of human conception must be guaranteed respect from the very first moment of its existence, since this is a moral duty in relation to the whole totality and the unity of the soul and the body of the human being. It is thus clear that, from the viewpoint of the Roman Catholic Church, the procedure used in assisted reproduction is unacceptable, since the naturalness of conception is interfered with and because of the problem of the superfluous embryos that cannot further develop in a natural way because of the nature of the method.

The specific answers of the Catholic Church are articulated in the Instruction of the Congregation for the Learning of Faith, the 'Donum Vitae':

- Unconditional rejection of all non-therapeutic interventions in the embryo, including freezing (what is therapeutic is precisely spelled out)

- Refusal of heterological (using donor's sperm) in vitro fertilisation (including surrogate motherhood)
- Refusal of homological in vitro fertilisation; even though it is not connected to the elimination of embryos, as in the practice of abortion, or to masturbation. The reason is that it deprives human conception of dignity, which is intrinsic and inborn.

As far as the Protestant and Evangelical churches are concerned, it is almost impossible to describe their position in relation to ART, because there are many different branches. Often they are more lenient in their stance. Fertility problems are considered a serious illness and it is necessary to deal with the difficult situation of involuntarily childless couples. However, the choice of the solution is left to the discretion of the couple who have freedom of conscience and at the same time bear responsibility for their decisions. Some Protestant groups have the theological view that science and technology are, in their essence, a positive force and opportunity for human beings. The development of biotechnologies can then be understood as a gift, a tool that we have received to repair the sins of the fathers (what the previous generations have brought about in nature and in human beings). It is noted that the number of people who cannot have children naturally has been increasing. Interfering with the naturalness of conception is then not a problem for this church. The church considers conception as the start of a human life. In abortion and IVF, which are made possible by modern biology, the church finds itself on the fence between responsible eugenics (selective breeding), euthanasia, and a threat to life. God's gift should be used in harmony with God's will, that is, it should not be misused. Science and technology may be used by humanity for good just as easily as they can for cruelty and self-destruction of humanity. The essential element is that every human being is responsible for his or her own life and for the talents that God has entrusted to him or her. This responsibility cannot be removed by the church. This is, on the other hand, balanced by freedom of conscience. But some other churches are just as authoritative as the Catholic Church.

• *Islam*

According to Islam, incurable diseases do not exist and we must continue to seek treatment. Islam does not know redemption through suffering. One interpretation of the Koran states: 'God's servants, look after yourself. God has not created an illness for which there is no medicine, with one exception—old age.' Scientific work is appreciated by Islam and is seen as an expression of worship. Each individual's responsibility is measured by his or her intentions, which hold more importance than deeds. Public interest stands above any other interests.

Islam encourages marriage, family formation and procreation. Treating infertility, including ART when indicated, is encouraged to preserve humankind within the frame of marriage, in cases of otherwise incurable infertility. The starting premise is respect for life and its sacred character. Only God gives life, and only God can take it away. This corresponds to the generally accepted respect for the individual from the very beginning of life. But there is disagreement as to the beginning of a life: according to some, the soul is breathed into the human being on the 40th day, according to others, life begins with conception. Multiple pregnancy should be prevented if possible. Should multiple pregnancy occur in spite of all preventive measures, then reducing the number of fetuses may be allowed as the choice of lesser harm.

Islam recognises the advantages of assisted reproduction as long as the lineages of the genetic identity of the father and the mother are respected. The basic guidelines for ART in the Muslim world are: if ART is indicated, it is permitted during validity of the marriage contract with no mixing of genes. Recently, the Shi'a guidelines have opened the way to third-party donation, via a Fatwa from Ayatollah Ali Hussein Khomeini in 1999. This Fatwa (or Islamic opinion) allowed third-party participation including egg donation, sperm donation and surrogacy, and is gaining acceptance in parts of the Shi'ite world. All these practices are based on the importance of maintaining the family structure and integrity in the Shi'a family.

In Islam, adoption is not acceptable as a solution to the problem of infertility because of the requirement of purity of lineage and known parenthood of all children; the Koran explicitly prohibits legal adoption but encourages kind upbringing of orphans.

• *Confucianism, Taoism, and Buddhism*

Confucianism is mainly a philosophical and ethical code that teaches humans how to be moral beings. Chinese attitudes to infertility and ART are influenced by three values, in decreasing order of importance: reproduction, preservation of life or promotion of health and pleasure. In general, any intervention in natural reproduction is undesirable because it disturbs the Tao of nature, but it is more acceptable than being childless. Although artificial insemination by a donor is accepted,

Chinese men are reluctant to donate sperm because they think that sperm contains jing or yuan qi, which are indispensable for their health and life.

- ***Hinduism***

ART is perceived as a great scientific achievement among Hindus. There are no laws regarding the use or standards of ART, donor eggs and sperm, or surrogacy in India.

As you can see, it is not at all easy to answer these ethical questions; the topic is a subject of discussion at various conferences.

> *There was a big international conference on the topic of when life begins. The specialists of various professions and religions convened. 'Life begins with the first inhalation of the newborn baby,' said one lecturer. The next maintained, 'Life begins with the merging of the sperm and the egg.' 'Oh no, life begins when the embryo nests in the womb, that is, when a woman becomes pregnant,' explained another. In the end, a very old rabbi stood up and said: 'Friends, life begins when the children get out of the house and the dog dies.'*

...Expressed in acts of law

Law is an expression of cultural customs. Therefore, these ethical debates also instigate arguments in the area of lawmaking. The possible ways of dealing with involuntary childlessness are determined by laws related to adoptive care and by laws regulating to the use of methods of assisted reproduction. The legislative regulation of these aspects is approached differently in various countries. Some have laws that are elaborated very precisely and in detail, others have no such laws at all.

The legal norms often do not resolve problems arising due to continuous advances in medicine. However, informed consent with the diagnostic and therapeutic procedures is required from the people undergoing this therapy.

> People want everything right away, in a hurry, they must have a child now, and they do not read anything about the treatment. Then four embryos get nested, and when they see them at the ultrasound and need to decide on reduction, they break down. (p)

The preceding testimony may sound as if the patients were irresponsible dummies, but finding an answer to these questions is difficult even for specialists who are concerned with the problem professionally. This may also be why it is not easy to work out a legislative framework. I think that it is lucky for many among the medical profession that the ethically problematic interventions are often performed only because the patients take on full responsibility. If you are thinking about a certain therapeutic method, I recommend that you read about it as much as possible, and find your own answers in advance. For instance, the decision about the reduction of embryos can be an insoluble problem for some and may bring you close to a breakdown. You can prevent this situation by being informed about the possibilities and effects and by choosing a specific treatment procedure accordingly; in this case you might allow the implant of only two embryos, not four.

The following international documents can serve as material for thinking about the procedures that would be ethically acceptable for you.

The United Nations Educational, Scientific and Cultural Organization (UNESCO) adopted two declarations related to biomedicine, the Universal Declaration on the Human Genome and Human Rights 1997 (available on the web at http://unesdoc.unesco.org/images/0010/001096/109687eb.pdf) and the International Declaration on Human Genetic Data 2003 (available at http://unesdoc.unesco.org/images/0013/001331/133171e.pdf#page=45)

Another international legal document is the Convention for the Protection of Human Rights and Dignity of the Human Being with regard to the Application of Biology and Medicine: Convention on Human Rights and Biomedicine, negotiated in the European Council in 1997. The complete English version can be found on the web at www.conventions.coe.int/Treaty/EN/Treaties/Html/164.htm. Two other conventions are based on this one. The first is concerned with the cloning of human beings (…168.htm), the second with biomedical research (…195.htm).

In 1985, the International Federation of Gynecology & Obstetrics founded the Committee for Research on Ethical Aspects of Human Procreation. A special international commission was put together to study these issues. The commission consists of obstetricians and gynaecologists, paediatricians, medical workers and lawyers who represent wide geographical, ethnic, cultural, linguistic and religious fields. The newest version of a file of all current recommendations was published in November of 2006 and is available at www.figo.org/docs/Ethics%20 Guidelines.pdf.

The International Federation of Fertility Societies (IFFS) is not a society for individuals like FIGO, but is rather a society for organisations. This organisation also expressed its ideas on ethics. Its last surveillance document was issued in 2007 and is available at the web site: http://eproofing.dartmouthjournals.com/pdfproofing/fns87_4S1_resupply.pdf.

Another important international document is the UN Convention on the Rights of the Child adopted by the UN in 1989. The problem of unfulfilled parenthood is dealt with in the following paragraphs (in full at www.ohchr.org/english/law/crc.htm):

Article 7

1. The child shall be registered immediately after birth and shall have the right from birth to a name, the right to acquire a nationality and, as far as possible, the right to know and be cared for by his or her parents.
2. States Parties shall ensure the implementation of these rights in accordance with their national law and their obligations under the relevant international instruments in this field, in particular where the child would otherwise be stateless.

Another document, this on adoption, is the Convention on Protection of Children and Co-operation in Respect of Intercountry Adoption (www.hcch.net/index_en.php?act=conventions.pdf&cid=69)

Why Don't You Turn the Radio On, Love?

The media (press, radio, television, the Internet) are important sources of information and they create the media image that is the modern view of a given matter, problem, or its solution. I do not study media trends or habits, so my insights here are rather superficial. But I am not attempting a qualified analysis here. The point is to stress that the media influence us and that we should approach their information critically.

I think that the media image of (voluntarily or involuntarily) childless people has improved; there is now more tolerance of a decision to live life without a child. Childless women are no longer depicted as beings with no character, as 'masculine', or as completely powerless things. However, from time to time, there are articles that claim that the fertility problem of one of the partners is the cause of the break up of their marriage or that a childless marriage loses its meaning because the spouses have difficulty in finding a common conversation topic.

The media depict fertility problems as any other illness. There have even been some courageous celebrities who have admitted that they have this problem. You might have read in magazines that difficulties with conceiving a child are not exceptional among members of the emperor's dynasties, either. For example, in Japan they waited for a successor a very long time. The media should be thanked for contributing to a social climate in which fertility problems are not perceived as only women's problems, but also men's problems. As far as information about the causes is concerned, it seems to me that the authors of articles are now more cautious when writing about the mental causes of fertility problems and stress is no longer depicted as the main or only cause of failures in the efforts to become pregnant. I have even seen a magazine headline, 'Through Stress to Pregnancy.'

Thanks to the media, there is an increased general awareness about diagnostic and therapeutic procedures and specialised clinics. Nevertheless, one should be cautious; the data should be compared to other sources. Most of the available information concerns the newest methods of treatment, for example assisted reproduction, which can create the impression that the only successful therapy of fertility problems is this therapy. The consequences of such an impression can be positive (the hope of the couple), but also negative (the lack of appreciation of other therapeutic methods and overestimation of the efficacy of a certain method of assisted reproduction).

There has been a sharp increase in people's awareness about adoptive parenting and foster care, and social attitudes towards this form of parenting and towards adopted children have improved. When I open one of the celebrity magazines, I get the impression that adoption is a common phenomenon: Mia Farrow, Woody Allen, Tom Cruise and Nicole Kidman, Sharon Stone, Madonna, Brad Pitt and Angelia Jolie, all have adopted children.

A Biological Forecast

In the chapter, 'The Journey is Just Dust...' I talked about the influence of climatic conditions, specifically about metre-high snowdrifts, a windstorm, and below freezing temperatures. But climatic changes are not the only factor that influences the quest for a child; each person is influenced by something different, and in a different way.

> Most couples rush to the surgery in spring when mothers with prams teem around. Then we do not know where to start. (p)
> The most sought-for period for IVF is fall, after the holidays. People are relaxed and have the strength to fight. (p)
> I enjoy my work, so I cope with it well mentally. (m)
> The planning of [a trip to] America has helped. (f)
> Perhaps the exercises of Mojzis helped, and also I focused at that time somewhat more on other things than before. (f)
> Before ovulation, I go to aerobics, after ovulation I go swimming so that I do not miscarry because of the jumping in the gym if I were pregnant by any chance. I have also started playing squash, naturally before ovulation. (f)
> During the winter I am calm, I do not rush into pregnancy because I don't want to [be heavily pregnant] in the summer, and give birth in hot weather. (f)
> I was distracted from the suffering about conception by studying. (f)
> I mentally relax by sewing, knitting, and cooking. (f)
> I keep my head above water by music, singing, dancing, and friends. (f)
> We're building a house, and I must look after a German Shepherd, so I'm distracted and have other thoughts. (f)
> I enjoy my work, I find it meaningful. Even if we don't succeed in having children, I won't consider my life useless. (m)
> I enjoy walking in the countryside, I admire its order. There, my worries always start striking me as much smaller than they seem to me in the surgery. (m)
> My wife and I devote ourselves to [the care of dogs], we enjoy being in the countryside. Moreover, I like my work; I stay there until late in the evening. (m)
> I enjoy working in the garden; one can see there that something has grown because of my efforts. (f)
> I have a young nephew who helps me cope with loneliness. (f)
> Walking with my husband helps, as do our dog and reading. (f)
> I vent my stress in sport; I sweat out plenty of sadness. Probably it's true that sport releases certain chemical activators that improve one's mood. (f)
> I travel a lot with my husband and get to know new countries. When one changes one's environment, one has different thoughts. (f)
> When my husband saw how much I suffered that I have no one to look after, he bought a dog. Beautiful. But I am not much into dogs. I am in two minds about it, but, of course, I didn't say anything about it to my husband. I do not want to spoil his joy. (f)

> A colleague at work couldn't become pregnant, but she coped with it well, she has her interests. But her mother-in-law was beside herself. The husband was from a village, the oldest son...they waited for an heir. The colleague told her husband to go there alone, that she had no strength to keep answering her mother-in-law's questions about when she had her last menstruation. (f)

In the area of fertility problems, no influences of the air pressure, the dew point or the ozone layer have been verified, as far as I know, but there certainly is the influence of the season of the year ('Most couples rush to the surgery in spring' 'The most sought-for period for IVF is fall' 'During the winter I am calm, I do not rush into pregnancy'). As you can see, we all perceive the weather differently.

The influence of building a house also varies. It distracts some people from thoughts about the child's non-existence ('We're building a house, so I'm distracted and have other thoughts'), while it reminds others of the absence of children's laughter ('Who am I building the house for, only dogs will be left after us').

The place of residence can be a factor, too. It is obvious that the availability of top-level medical care is worse in smaller places and in places far from a city. The social environment is also different in smaller places where one sees directly into what the other people have on their plates than in anonymous cities ('It is unacceptable for the village that we stay childless' 'It is probably the biggest problem in villages and small towns, where childless couples aren't protected by anonymity' 'The husband was from a village, the oldest son, the farm, they waited for an heir')

Interests help the partners cope with the mental load related to dealing with the situation ('I enjoy working in the garden, one can see there that something has grown because of my efforts' 'I enjoy walking in the countryside, I admire its order. There, my worries always start striking me as much smaller' 'I was distracted from the suffering about conception by studying' 'I have a young nephew who helps me cope with loneliness' 'Sport releases certain chemical activators that improve one's mood'). I have mentioned elsewhere that many childless people have a dog ('I must look after a German Shepherd, so I'm distracted and have other thoughts' 'My wife and I devote ourselves to the care of dogs'). But this may not be a suitable interest for everybody ('But I am not much into dogs'). The interests are in turn influenced by the people's consciousness of being on the quest for a child ('Before ovulation I go to aerobics, after ovulation I go swimming so that I do not miscarry because of the jumping in the gym if I were pregnant by any chance. I have also started playing squash, naturally before ovulation').

For men who are undergoing diagnosis and treatment of fertility problems, employment is a help rather than a stress factor ('I enjoy my work, so I cope with it well mentally' 'I enjoy my work, I find it meaningful' 'I like my work').

JUST AFTER I WAS BORN,
I STEPPED INTO A HOLE,
I NEVER WENT TO SCHOOL,
AND STILL I BECAME A MAN

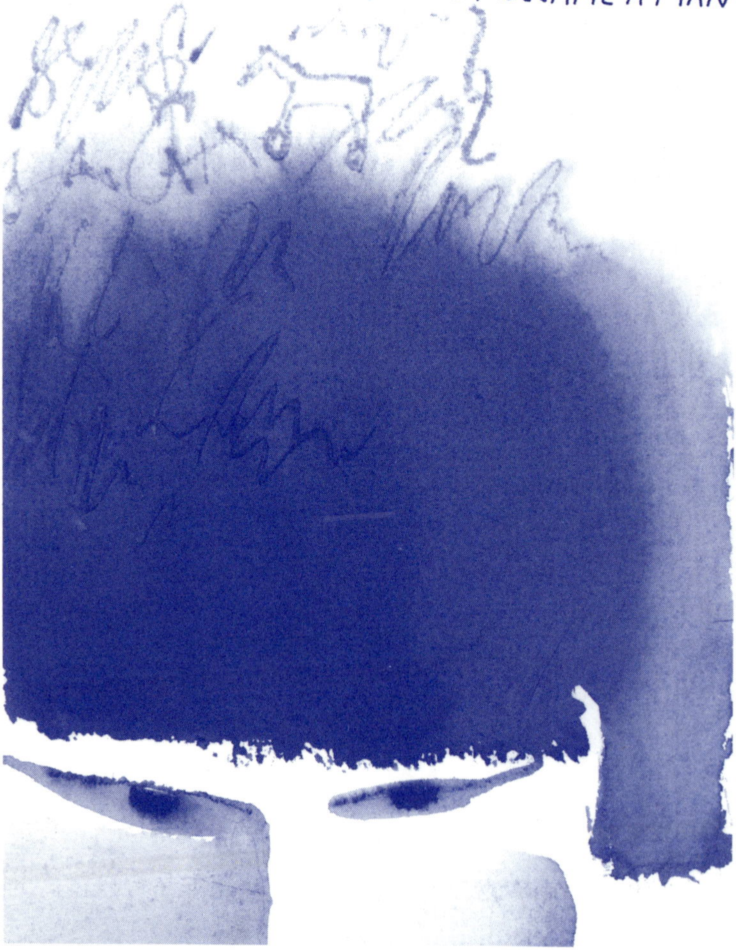

Just After I was Born, I Stepped Into a Hole, I Never Went to School, and Still I Became a Man...

The refrain of the song introducing this chapter is, 'Mom kept me at home and Dad worked hard for me, I could have studied, if only I had wanted to...' We each have a role model who influenced our life. For instance, the hero of the song was affected by his not wanting to study, even though, as he himself admits, he could have easily done so.

That a human being is born with nothing can be said only in reference to material goods. As for bodily goods, if I may call them that, for instance the colour of eyes or the tendency toward certain illnesses, we bring these to the world with us at birth. And the same holds for our mental goods, our personality. There are disputes about how much of these we are born with and how much we acquire through the influence of our social environment (the nature vs. nurture debate), but there is no doubt that both components, the inborn and the acquired, have their say in a person's personality. Nature is considered to influence intelligence or temperament, while it is less involved in the ability to cope with mental stress. Nature most likely has the least influence in motivations, attitudes, and biases. These are gained from models, through one's upbringing by parents, through the influence of the close, as well as wider, social circles, and through the culture into which one is born. The following pages deal with the role of the personality, or character, in the quest for a child.

...with Some Desire for a Child

> *One farmer did not have children. Many times he said to his wife, 'If only God gave us one single child so that I would have someone to love and someone to pass down some tools to. I don't even know for whom I work.'*
>
> 'About Nesyta', B. Nemcova, *Fairy Tales*

People set out on the quest for a child because they want to have one. But why do they want to have one? Are there motives other than those of the farmer?

> I have come to the stage when I wish for children a lot. I like children, and I would like to have my own children with my husband. I understand it as a consummation of, or a logical next step within, a love relationship. (f)
>
> Having a child means to be needed, not to feel loneliness. To make our parents happy—the joy of grandchildren. (f)
>
> I always wanted to have children. It is entirely natural and important. (f)
>
> Perhaps it is natural; I want to pass down something to someone (even if there is the question of whether I have that something). There is simply a desire in me to be a parent and, even long before the wedding; I imagined what it would be like to raise my own children. (m)
>
> I desire to live through pregnancy and motherhood, to see my child that is of my blood, the continuation of kin, to pass down one's love, to create a family community, to give a son to my husband. (f)
>
> I want to fulfil the heartfelt wishes of my close relatives. (m)
>
> To pass down the good in us, in the same way as our parents passed it down to us. (m)
>
> To fulfil the meaning of life. (f)
>
> I believe: without a child there is no complete family, and how can I raise other children as a teacher when I have none of my own. (f)
>
> What remains hard for me is the non-vanishing desire for my own child in the sense of 'bone of my bone'. A wish to live through pregnancy, birth, to experience the continuation of my own blood. Today I think that this desire is something that I will carry in me for a number of years (if not my whole life). (f)
>
> I have a much younger husband who wants to have his own child. (f)
>
> My marriage is about to break down. My husband has a child from his first marriage, and he devotes himself to him a lot. When we have our own child, perhaps it will draw him back. (f)
>
> Sometimes the man wants a child so that his wife has an interest and he can devote himself to his hobbies. (p)
>
> So that we're not alone, so that we have someone to look after. A life with a child is more cheerful. (f)

I frankly don't know. (f)
It's clear. (f)
I can't imagine a life without a child; I need to look after someone, to live for someone. (f)
In my opinion, it is the fulfilment of life. (f)
I miss it. (f)
To have someone to whom we can pass down experience, whom we can look after, and help him or her in life. (m)
We like children; we don't want to live without them. (f)
Because I like children, and I see in them the meaning of my life. (f)
Because it seems to me that the relationship of a married couple is unfulfilled if they stay just two, alone. (f)

Some people do not know why they want a child ('I frankly don't know'), and these are testimonies of people whose quest for a child has not been easy! It may be that they are just unable to express it ('It's clear').

A child is the purpose of our actions, our efforts, and our life on the personal level ('I see in them the meaning of my life' 'I can't imagine a life without a child' 'To fulfil the meaning of life' 'In my opinion, it is the fulfilment of life' 'To have someone to whom we can pass down experience') on the level of the partners' relationship ('Because it seems to me that the relationship of a married couple is unfulfilled if they stay just two, alone' 'I understand it as a consummation of, or a logical next step within, a love relationship' 'I have a much younger husband who wants to have his own child' 'Without a child there is no complete family'), as well as on the social level ('To make our parents happy' 'To fulfil the heartfelt wishes of my close relatives'). At the same time, a child can be a medium for the achievement of another goal ('When we have our own child, perhaps it will draw him back' 'So that his wife has an interest and he can devote himself to his hobbies').

A child is a source of joy and stimulus for personal growth ('A life with a child is more cheerful' 'Joy of grandchildren' 'Not to feel loneliness' 'How can I raise other children when I have none of my own'), but a child is also a recipient, someone to whom we can give our joy, energy, and love ('I like children,' 'So that we have someone to look after' 'To be needed,' 'To have someone...whom we can look after, help him or her in life').

Each life eventually comes to its end, and most people fear death. A child offers the possibility of the continuation of oneself ('To pass down the good in us, in the same way as our parents passed it down to us' 'I desire to live through pregnancy and motherhood, to see my child which is of my blood, the continuation of kin' 'The non-vanishing desire for my own child in the sense of "bone of my bone" ').

I would also like to cite from the results of an analysis of couples from a statistical survey in 2001:[19]

As the important reasons for the decision to have a child, the respondents most often stated three reasons (they were identified as important by 80% of respondents): 'Having children gives one a special feeling of joy,' 'It is nice to see children mature and develop,' and 'Having children is the meaning of life.' As the least important, from the seven stated reasons for the decision to have a child was: 'When I have children, it is less probable that I will feel lonely in old age.'

In the decision to start a family, the desire to secure for oneself care in old age or to ensure the continuation of the clan does not play the main role. Children represent a different value for some parents: above all, they expect the child to provide an enrichment of one's life and pleasure from the child's development, and, especially for women, the possibility to give birth and raise a child is often the main purpose of life.

In their decision to become a father, men emphasise the practical, and perhaps even egotistical, reasons: according to them, a child does not only bring joy, it can also strengthen the couple's relationship; personify the need for the maintenance and continuation of the clan as a way of passing on of one's existence; a child can also stimulate and speed up the parents' personality development.

In their considerations of becoming a mother, women do not think as practically: they expect that a child will be a source of great joy and pleasure, that it will become the purpose of their lives. Women do not think so much about the securities and advantages that children might provide when they return the care and concern they have received.

It is important to understand the broader context, the other side of the issue: the testimonies of those who do not want to have children. American research[20] from 1987 showed the following motives led voluntarily childless couples to not have children (in descending importance): 1) freedom from the responsibility related to the raising of a child, which makes possible greater opportunities of self-fulfilment and spontaneous mobility, 2) happier relations in marriage, 3) regards for the woman's professional career, 4) financial advantages, 5) worries about population growth, 6) general dislike of children, 7) negative experience from one's own childhood that have led to doubts about one's skill at being a good parent, 8) concern about the physical demands of giving birth and physical recovery, 9) fear of bringing children into the kind of world in which we find ourselves today.

The literature[21] mentions the following reasons why a person wants to have a baby:

- Biological motivation—parental instinct and psychological and social motivation. However, there are strong doubts about the existence of parental instinct. If we looked for a special instinct of procreation of children, we would not find it because it does not in itself exist; we do not find it in the animal kingdom either. 'Animals are equipped with a strong instinct of sexual activity which, together with the innate system which commands them to protect and not to eat their own offspring; that is enough procreation to occur naturally. In man, knowledge of the fact that conception does not always have to follow sex has created conditions for the possibility to exclude children fully from the individual's life cycle,' says a sociologist[22] who continues: 'It is true that childlessness is not a massive phenomenon even in modern hedonistic society, which indicates that the existence of children must contain something that fascinates us and leads us to procreate them.' And a paediatrician[23] states: 'The ability to live in a partnership is ideally followed by the ability to assume such an important role in life as parenthood. But this gradual process is not simple and straightforward. It was assumed that it is governed by instinct, that the tendency to genus conservation plays a role here, that the almost omnipresent mother instinct exists, forcing women to feel an irresistible wish to fulfil her life by giving birth to a child. But this simple concept applies less and less in the developed countries and it seems to be more and more masked by powerful cultural and generally social factors. A French sociologist[24] deals with the relationship to a child as an instinct. Based on her extensive analysis of historical materials recording primarily the behaviour of mothers towards children, she concludes that 'Mother instinct is a myth. We have not met any universal and inevitable maternal behaviour...mother love is only an emotion, accidental in its substance as such... It all depends on the mother, on her private history and on history as such... Mother love does not arrive of its own accord. It is extra. Even the...scientific study of the biological basis of...social behaviour in all species...says that man differs among the animals by being governed by culture, i.e. by learned and transmitted impulses.'

> Drives? They are present in animals. I was influenced when my friends started to have children. Then I told myself: the time has come. (f)
> No parental instinct exists. Not in me. I wanted a baby because I was curious to see what it is like to have one's own child. (f)

It is probably not possible to rely on maternal (and what about paternal?) instinct; it does not release the person from the responsibility for the decision of whether to become or not to become a parent. Nothing remains but to think about one's psychological needs and then decide. The decision whether to be or not to be a parent, why, when or how many times, is a free process. That is why it is so difficult. The complexity of this decision is increased by the fact that it is usually a decision of two people.

Psychologists[25] call attention to the fact that some needs are fulfilled by the birth of the child, but other needs are limited at the same time, see table:

When you think about the table, you will find that it is not so that some needs are satisfied and others are limited by a child, but that the same needs are satisfied and limited at the same time. It seems illogical, but it is true. The evaluation of 'satisfaction' or 'limits' depends on a lot of circumstances: on the personality disposition of the evaluator, on his or her life situation, on his or her momentary mood and, last but not least, on the child to which the evaluation is related and to his or her age. Everybody likes a different period in a child's life: one remembers infancy with horror the ever-increasing crying as the answer to questions about the cause of the crying, and is happy with an adolescent who is able to express his opinion; others could not tear themselves away from the helpless baby, but seek therapy because of the adolescent's all-knowing opinions.

But parental experience is not transferable. Therefore, a human being can evaluate the satisfaction or limits of his or her needs only when he or she is a parent; before that, it is only more or less a qualified guess. Therefore, human beings make decisions with a considerable level of uncertainty and, with a high level of risk of making the wrong decision. However, the impact is not fatal in most cases: you can forget an unpleasant holiday, you can leave a wrongly chosen school, sell a bad house and divorce an unpleasant partner. It is true that it is possible to give up a child, but this variant is usually chosen by people whose parenthood did not result from their own decision. The decision not to have a child is just as irreversible as the decision to have a child.

You may have found the analysis of the desire for a child pointless. A person simply wants or does not want a child, and to dissect the reasons why is not good for anything. But it is not pointless to know why

Table 9.1: Having children/not having children.

HAVING CHILDREN	NOT HAVING CHILDREN
1. Stimulation	
A child is a very mobile element, it brings many stimuli in one's life, there is no need of entertainment and worries or anxieties. Without a child, life would be boring, and also marriage would be boring, empty.	A child prevents stimulation. One is bound to it, cannot fully enjoy life—cannot use up one's leisure. A life with a child is monotonous and because of all the worries one cannot enjoy even one's marriage.
2. Learning, the Exchange of the Sensible Stimuli	
Parents bring up children, but a child influences strongly his or her parents. He or she brings unrepeatable experiences to the parents. They mutually complement each other, they grow inwardly. Only a life with children provides specifically humane experience.	A child prevents one from gaining experience it ties one to the cooker, nappies, school homework. One has nothing out of it.
3. Feelings (life certainty, the feeling of security)	
Children receive love, but they return it as well—there is a relationship here. There is someone who is bound to me through the deepest and purest bond. He or she cannot leave me, I will be taken care of in my old age. For the relationship to other people is the best guarantee of life security.	A child brings about a permanent frustration in terms of security needs. I will always worry that something will happen to him or her, that he or she will be evil, that he or she will go astray. Having children means being vulnerable precisely through them. They can put me under pressure, they will not be accepted to university, they will have no job—I am bound and limited by them.
4. Identity (individual autonomy, social status, individual consciousness)	
Having a child gives worth to a person, it provides a woman and a man with a social status. In the relationship to a child we lose anonymity and we are not threatened by the anonymity of a crowd. The child needs me and I need the child.	Having a child prevents one from the attainment of more important social roles. If I had not had a child, I would have achieved more. I would have been in charge of socially more important things, I would have had a higher social status. "Having a child" places me in the anonymous crowd of ordinary people with ordinary worries.

one wants or does not want something, why one does or does not do certain things. When you know why you want a child—even if this is just a guess—you can think about the question of whether the child is really able to fulfil your expectations, whether your wish that your child provide you with a tennis partner is realistic, whether it is the right thing for the child's and your own happiness. When I consider the farmer from the introductory fairy tale, I do not know whether he would now get much gratefulness from his descendants for the inheritance of a few tools. I doubt it. Fortunately, the farmer also wanted a child so that he could enjoy him. But even here, it depends on where you find joy. Would the child's laughter be enough or would you feel joy only after your child's victory in a major mathematical contest. It is important to try to understand the content of one's desires, even for those who have not succeeded in having a child. If they know what they originally expected from the child, it is easier for them to choose a suitable alternative, to find a new goal in life.

...with Some Ability to Handle Stress

We all face variously important forms of adversity every day, and every day we look for ways to come to terms with them. For instance, say you fall in love with someone who does not want you. Each of us responds in a different way. Some people do not care much; they see plenty of other attractive potential partners. Other people despair, cry all the time, and pour their sadness out to their friends. Still others shut themselves off, tell no one about it, and sometimes may even plan suicide. Or they do not give up and seek to gain the partner by any means. Or they find another partner right away, on purpose. Some may choose revenge and harm the one who refused them. The situation of the person who has fallen in love unhappily could be analysed for hours and hours; a whole scientific field has been devoted to strategies of solutions and coping with mental stress and to choices according to one's nature and one's situation.

It is similar in the stressful situation of the unfulfilled desire for a child. It is, of course, important what the desire is like. If you want a baby only a little bit, then you will not worry about the failure and you will come to terms with it easily. It is harder for a person who wants to have a child a lot. What can you do about it? Most probably, you will seek out a specialist. But can you, yourself, do something, too?

One's own activity

The desire for a child is so strong that I will do anything. (f)

On the whole I live in a healthy way, I don't smoke, don't drink, and exercise. (f)

I am trying to fill my free time so that I do not think about only the one thing. (f)

First I had to put on weight, then keep up a certain weight (mental anorexia). Then I went to Mojzis exercises. (f)

Exercises, the sea, creation of a relaxed atmosphere, the effort not to get upset. (f)

One must try everything. (f)

Some reduction in athletic activities, change in food from vegetarian to a mixed diet, exercises. (f)

Alternative medicine, yoga. (f)

Information, exercises. I welcome every little per cent of hope, I'll do anything. (f)

We're searching for information. (m)

I do the Mojzis exercises all the time, it is good for me. I have changed my gynaecologist three times, I'm searching for information on the Internet. It is important for me that I can do something for myself. (f)

I haven't drunk alcohol for a year, I eat healthy food, I avoid smoky areas, I keep up hygiene, I'm searching for the most suitable position for intercourse so that the sperm gets to where it should be, I'm searching for other ways of influencing the situation. I do not feel like swallowing tablets. (f)

I have even been to a herbalist. He recommended some teas to me, I was for some time conscientious in preparing them and drinking them, but probably they were weak, they didn't help. On the other hand, I had at least the feeling that I was doing something, it was better than sitting and waiting. (f)

I drink teas, I do the Bach [flower remedy] therapy, I go for psychotherapy, I have been to a fortune teller, I underwent the regressive therapy, I had an astrological calculation done, I have been to many healers. I follow the recommendation of the herbalist Zentrich, I have used mud tampons. I'll do anything. (f)

I've changed my life; I've found another partner who indicated to me that together we would be perfectly successful. (f)

I use the massage mat and relaxation music. (f)

I do not influence the situation, I do not much know how to. (f)

Patients consider medicine as a service similar to, for instance, a car mechanic. They give the doctor a fee and expect positive results without accepting one's own share in the treatment. They do not have the basic anatomical information, and mostly they are not much interested in the information provided by the doctor. They do not accept even the smallest share

> of responsibility, they want everything to be decided and done for them by the doctor. They refuse to wait, rather they choose the treatment of the symptoms, which promises pregnancy quickly, rather than the causes, where pregnancy is achieved more slowly but a person becomes healthy. (p)
>
> A beautiful young woman came to the infertility clinic and asked for artificial fertilisation. It followed from the interview that her husband is so busy that he isn't at home much, and if he is, he is so exhausted that he isn't interested in sex. She excluded the possibility that her husband doesn't want a child or that he has a lover. (p)
>
> There are many among managers who have reduced fertility. This is due to the character of their work: frequently driving a car, great workloads and the related stress. These men usually refuse to lower their workload for two months and go on holiday; they'd rather have 'their balls pricked'. (p)
>
> A man with azoospermia, the physicians didn't want to treat him, he said. He couldn't stand being inactive, he visited healers, ate healthy food, played sports. It helped him to come to terms with the diagnosis, so that two years later he was able to accept treatment through the methods of assisted reproduction, which was unacceptable for him earlier. (p)
>
> A man with azoospermia who was, in his words, written off by the doctors. He didn't give up, searched for information about treatment, saved money, regularly was seen by healers. Ten years later they had a healthy child in a natural way. (p)

For many people, it is unimaginable not to try to exert their strength and participate in the solution of the problem ('I'll do anything' 'One must try everything,' 'I'm searching for other ways of influencing the situation' 'He couldn't stand being inactive' 'He didn't give up'). The feeling of helplessness, waiting, the impossibility of doing something for oneself, is unbearable for them ('I had at least the feeling that I was doing something, it was better than sitting and waiting' 'It is important for me that I can do something for it myself'). But not everyone is active in the quest for a child, some because they do not know what they could actually do themselves ('I do not influence the situation, I do not much know how to'), others are happy with their passivity ('They expect a positive result without accepting their own share in the treatment' 'They do not accept even the smallest share of responsibility' 'Her husband is so busy that he isn't at home much, and if he is, he is so exhausted that he isn't interested in sex' 'They refuse to lower their work load for two months and go on holiday' 'They are not much interested in the information provided by the doctor').

If you want to keep the situation in your own hands as much as possible, then you should try to orient yourself in it in the first place, to have as much information as possible about treatment possibilities ('Information,'

'We're searching for information,' 'I'm searching for information on the Internet,' 'He searched for information'). According to the gathered information, you should choose a therapist ('I have changed my gynaecologist three times') and the therapy. You can also try to increase the efficacy of the therapy by other forms of individually prescribed therapy, most often the Mojzis method or unconventional procedures, and by trying to keep yourself in the best possible physical shape ('I don't smoke, don't drink, exercise') as well as mental shape ('To fill in my free time' 'The effort not to get upset').

Can I bear it?

In a sandy land where only a little greenery grows, several miles from the Chinese capital where Prince Vetchvoot resided, in the middle of a clay field, next to his potter's oven, there lived a potter with his wife. They were by themselves, childless and lonely. The land all around was as flat as the surface of a lake, dim and monotonous, no tree or shrub was to be seen anywhere. Every day the good people begged heaven to give them a baby so that they would have something dear, but their wish was not fulfilled. The potter decorated all the pots that he made with beautiful little angels' heads and the potter's wife dreamed all night about green meadows and enchanting shrubs and trees among which children were playing: for what one's heart desires, one's eyes can see all the time.

Once the potter made two beautiful objects for his wife's birthday: a gorgeous cradle made from clear white clay, all decorated with angels' heads and roses, and a big pot made from red clay, painted around with bright butterflies and flowers. The potter's wife prepared the little cradle like a little crib and she filled the pot with the best soil that she brought herself from a great distance in her apron, and she placed both gifts next to her bed in the hope that her wish would come true. And so she prayed one evening from the bottom of her soul: 'On my knees I beg you my Lord, give me a pretty baby, we will bring him up in a godly way.'

So did the good woman pray in tears and then she went to sleep. At night, a big storm came, there was thunder and lightning, and at one moment, an especially clear light flashed through the bedroom. In the morning there was gorgeous weather, through the window there blew a cool wind. The good potter's wife still slept and she dreamt in a beautiful dream that she was sitting with her husband under a myrtle tree. Then the foliage rustled around her, she woke up and lo and behold: next to her on the cushion, there was a fresh myrtle twig and the wind moved and played with the tender leaves next to her cheek. Filled with joy, she woke up her husband and she showed him the twig. On their knees, they both thanked God that he had given them something living after all, something that would become green and blossom before their eyes. They meticulously planted the myrtle twig in the beautiful pot and their most beloved task every day was to water the young trunk, place it in the sun and protect it from the harmful dew and rough winds. In their hands the myrtle twig grew and filled their hearts with peace and joy...from the myrtle tree there grew up a beautiful girl.

'About the Myrtle Girl', H.C. Andersen, *Fairy Tales*

The potters did not give up; they did not lose hope that heaven would fulfil their wish. What about the mental strength of others?

I don't give up, I believe that it will turn out well. (f)
The prognosis is excellent, I definitely believe in success. (f)
I cope with it because I believe that everything will turn out well. Without belief one wouldn't handle anything. (f)
Never did we speak about the possibility that we would not have a child. We believed that Ann or Martin would be born. (f)
But you must believe that it will come off. (f)
Always, with new drugs, I was full of hope, and then disappointment arrived. (f)
I'm slowly losing my belief in the success of treatment. (f)
The couple went for the third IVF only because they had an appointment. They entirely gave up believing that it could come off. The woman became pregnant, she has twins. Throughout her pregnancy, she didn't believe it, she didn't preparing any layette. After the birth, she kept looking at the babies, she couldn't believe that she had them. (p)
When I am put on the IVF schedule with another doctor than X, I change the day, I don't believe in another doctor. (f)
I believe in it very much, so I'm not thinking about this fact (adoption). Simply I believe that we will have our own children. (f)
The words of a doctor in a TV program raised new hope in us. (f)
It doesn't depend so much on one's age, as on one's self-confidence. (f)
I'm still hoping that I'll be lucky and will have a child. (f)
I believe in them (healers) a lot. (f)
It raised our hope that we met a cured woman. (f)
The application for adoption keeps my head above water. (f)
I go to see a gynaecologist who is perhaps good as a physician, but fails as a psychologist. When I started doing the Mojzis exercises, he told me that they are no miraculous exercises since the patients of Mrs. Mojzis were extraordinarily supported by her, so then I did the exercises and didn't believe that there was any sense in it. When I came from the spa, I was hundred per cent sure that it must have helped. I was relaxed, and after the baths and mud tampons I truly believed. After the visit to the doctor—a disaster. He said that the spa had worked only when there had been military troops, but otherwise

> not, that it was only the spa doctors who were convincing me that the spa was good. And I clearly realised all this only when I told it to my friend at work. Since then I haven't been to see the doctor, but I'm determined to tell him about it. Perhaps he doesn't even realise what he's bringing about. Even when he doesn't believe in it himself, he mustn't take my belief away. (f)
> I need advice. Is it better to count on and still have hope, or is it better to take it as another failure in advance? (f)

As the testimonies show, in order to have the strength to cope with something, one needs to have faith. The relatively large number of testimonies about something as intimate as faith in something indicates how important faith is for people ('Even when he doesn't believe in it himself, he mustn't take my belief away' 'Without belief one wouldn't handle anything'). What kind of faith? Firstly, faith in success, in a good ending of a certain process ('I believe that it will end up well' 'I definitely believe in success' 'I believe that everything will end up well' 'We believed that Ann or Martin would get born' 'You must believe that it will come off' 'I'm still hoping that I'll be lucky and will have a child' 'It raised our hope that we met a cured woman'), which can include an alternative solution ('The application for adoption keeps my head above water').

In the chapter Do Anything... I said that the process of solving a certain situation does not include only the procedure (for instance a therapeutic one) as a purely technical matter. Important elements of the therapeutic effect, besides the procedure, are also the therapist and the patient. You have faith in a good ending of a specific process when you believe that you can cope with the process ('On one's self-confidence'), when you believe in the procedure or the method ('Always, with new drugs, I was full of hope' 'After the baths and mud tampons I truly believed'), and when you believe in the therapist ('I change the day, I don't believe another doctor' 'I believe in them (healers) a lot,' 'The words of a doctor in a TV program raised new hope in us'). Some researchers maintain that one's belief in some unsurpassable and unfailing power has the biggest effect.

I would like to remind you that I pointed out the importance of an active attitude to the solution of problems and the role of faith in mentally coping with a difficult situation. In other words, I discussed what a person can do in order to survive in good health and without going insane. I did not talk about the influence of activity and belief on the final result, for instance on getting cured. Sometimes I am asked whether it is better, for instance before IVF, to believe one hundred per cent that it will come off or whether it is better not to have any hope at all. Everybody will tell you something different; some people know couples who did not doubt their eventual success and it arrived ('Never did we speak about the possibility that we would not have a child. We believed that Ann or Martin would get born'), others know couples who had given up and it turned out well in the end ('They entirely gave up believing that it could come off. The woman became pregnant'). If you do not have at least a minimum of faith that something will work out, you will stop fighting. On the other hand, a certain amount of humbleness and awareness that not everything has to come off according to your will is important, so that the potential failure does not break you. Frankly speaking: if I said that it was necessary not to doubt a successful resolution, would you really not doubt? And if I said that it was necessary to give up without struggling, would you be able to do that? Well, probably not. A human being is not a robot that can be programmed.

Try to imagine the following joke as an actor's sketch so that you see the full effect:

> *A gentleman comes to a doctor and complains: 'Doctor, I have aches here and burnings there, I can't get any sleep.'*
> *Doctor: 'Mr. Brown, there's a simple solution. Here, take these pills, you're going to take one in the morning and the problems will disappear. Only you mustn't think about horses when you are swallowing the pill.'*
> *Man: 'About horses?! That's easy, I've never ever thought about that.*
> *Mr. Brown comes home, wakes up in the morning, and wants to take the pill. 'Horses!' He puts down the box, walks around the apartment in his pyjamas, looks out of the window, comes to the box, and 'horses!' He reads the paper, comes to the box, and 'horses!' He sings and, returning to the box again, 'damned horses!' So he gets dressed, goes to the bar, returns home tipsy, reels to the box, and 'horses!'*

Let me remind you of the song from one of the earlier chapters: do anything that is, in your opinion, worth doing. The feeling that you have done everything you could is very important in coping with a difficult situation, not excepting the unfulfilled desire for a child. But sometimes you no longer know what else to do, and perhaps you are at the end of your mental strength. Then it is all right to cry, in certain situations that is the appropriate and valid response. And when you go to have an IVF, think about horses!

...with Some Education

I would not entirely underestimate the role of education, as the hero of the introductory song does, even though it is clear that earning even

50 academic and scientific degrees is no guarantee that a person will be able to cope successfully with various obstacles in life. Some understanding of biology and medicine will enable you to communicate better with your therapist, you will be able to orient yourself more easily in various leaflets and specialised publications, and you will be able to sign various informed consents and applications for operations in a more responsible manner. An educated person is more likely to know how to work with information, how to search for it (in a library, on the Internet) as well as how to use it effectively (for example to evaluate its erudition).

...with Some Opinions, Attitudes, and Prejudices

I didn't want to boast anywhere of the fact that I have no child, it was unpleasant for me to speak about it, especially in meetings with my schoolmates. (f)

I am ashamed to buy the drugs necessary for IVF, a friend buys them for me in the neighbouring town. (f)

My sister cannot conceive, she is getting ready for artificial fertilisation, and is horribly ashamed of it. (f)

I got my husband to go for the examination only a year later, he obstinately refused to go. (f)

He didn't want to go for the spermiogram, it was a problem to make him go. (f)

The stimulation before IVF wasn't successful (I didn't have an egg) because my mother-in-law humiliated me, even though she knew that I was preparing for IVF. (f)

My wife miscarried out of joy, and her high fever was also out of joy. (m)

Because we kept putting it off—we were building up the nest—I've missed everything. Now I've become too fixated on the idea of becoming pregnant. (f)

I can't become pregnant because of a bad mother, the lack of love in childhood. (f)

I would even go for adoption, but my husband resolutely refuses, he is unyielding. His argument is the bad genetics in the children on offer, and the [innate] damage that can't be influenced by upbringing. Who is giving up such children for adoption? (f)

I don't think that IVF is against God. In the method, there is so much chance (so that the egg is maintained, so that an embryo develops, so that it nests) that God must be present. (f)

We refuse artificial fertilisation, we are believers, we [disagree with] the manipulation of embryos. (m)

I am afraid of late motherhood, that I'll be an anxious mother. (f)

You may be asking what the preceding testimonies have in common. They all express a certain opinion or attitude towards fertility problems themselves ('I didn't want to boast anywhere of the fact that I have no child, it was unpleasant for me to speak about it' 'I am ashamed to buy the drugs necessary for IVF' 'My sister cannot conceive, she is getting ready for artificial fertilisation, and is horribly ashamed of it'), towards their causes ('The stimulation before IVF wasn't successful because my mother-in-law humiliated me' 'My wife miscarried out of joy, and her high fever was also out of joy' 'Because we kept putting it off—we were building up the nest—I've missed everything' 'I can't become pregnant because of a bad mother, the lack of love in childhood'), towards diagnostic methods ('I got my husband to go for the examination only a year later, he obstinately refused to go' 'He didn't want to go for the spermiogram, it was a problem to make him go'), towards therapeutic procedures ('I don't think that IVF is against God. In the method, there is so much chance that God must be present' 'We refuse artificial fertilisation, we mind the manipulation of embryos'), towards adoption ('I would even go for adoption, but my husband resolutely refuses, he is unyielding. His argument is the bad genetics in the children on offer, and the prenatal damage that can't be influenced by upbringing') or towards parenting after treatment ('I am afraid of late motherhood, that I'll be an anxious mother').

We acquire our opinions, attitudes, and sometimes also prejudices, that is our views of certain problems and the possibilities of their solution, above all from our parents, from our close as well as wider social environment, and from the culture in which we grow up. One of the contributing forces in shaping our attitudes could be, for instance, ancient stories. I have used parts of some of them in introducing some of the previous chapters. How do ancient stories describe the unfulfilled desire for a child and the quest for a child?

Fairy tales

Fairy tales are the first stories that children come across and fairy tales have been related to children's upbringing from time immemorial. Fairy tales generally describe the foundations of humanity, their heroes are archetypes whose complicated fates reflect the difficulties and dangers that nature burdens us with. I intentionally did not search in a public library but only in the fairy tale books belonging to my extended family. I wanted to get a number of fairy tales that would be close to the number that a child might hear from his or her mother, father, grandmothers, grandfathers, aunts and uncles. Most fairy tales begin with the fact that someone (a king or a poor man) had several children (most often one or three). I was curious to find out how many fairy tales related to involuntary childlessness a child might come across. I was surprised. In our home, I found 41 such fairy tales.

My goal was to find the basic structure of the story, the main characters, their experiences and solutions of the situation. A fairy tale about involuntary childlessness usually has the following structure. A man and a woman, it does not matter whether they are royalty or poor people, do not have children and they suffer because of it. They express their desire to have a child, no matter what it may be like. Some higher power hears them and the child is born or comes to them. Often the child is under a spell. There are difficult trials in store for the child, but most of the time everything turns out well in the end.

I was surprised how kind the fairy tales were to the childless. Most of them describe childlessness as a problem of the couple. If they focus on one partner only, then it is more often on the man. A poor man as well as a rich emperor can be childless in fairy tales. The childless couple experience their situation as a very difficult one. In no fairy tale is there an indication that someone would be to blame. The partners in all such tales love each other. The couple most often try to influence the situation in some way, usually by praying to God. In all the fairy tales, except for one, the other people in the community treated the childless couple well. Among the fairy tales that I have found, there was not a single one in which the couple would not eventually have a child. In fairy tales, adoption is common, including the adoption of a young animal or a puppet. Even when the child does not resemble a human being, the parents are happy and look after it, except for two fairy tales. The child is usually very good, clever and, sometimes only after the spell is broken, extraordinarily beautiful. Both the biological and the adopted children escape from various dangerous traps and lures in their lives. Most of the time, the fairy tales have a happy ending. The most frequent ending is that the longed-for child has been freed from the spell or has overcome all the obstacles, has married into a royal family, and has become a king or a queen.

Myths and legends

For the purposes of analysing myths and legends about the unfulfilled desire for a child, I have again used only the books available in my extended family. According to specialists, myths and legends clearly reflect the national character of the culture where they have arisen and existed. I was not very successful in finding myths and legends related to this problem, I found only six of them. The best-known legend was the one about Oedipus, who is a child of two childless couples (he was born to one and brought up by the other). The legend ends tragically: 'Do not have a pernicious wish, contrary to gods, and do not ask to have a son born to you. If he is born to you, he will later kill you, and will take his own mother as his wife. And the whole kin will wade in blood.' Another legend is about the famous Hajj Nasreddin, who was an adopted child. It is said that Hajj Nasreddin is an historical character who lived about 900 years ago.

In all the myths and legends, the childless couple are treated well by the community in which they live. In all of them, it is also obvious that the couple experienced their situation as a very difficult one, but nowhere is one of the partners labelled as the guilty party. Usually a supernatural force has caused the childlessness of the couples. However, unlike fairy tales, about half of the legends end in tragedy, sometimes for the children, sometimes for the couple.

Childlessness in the Bible

In Europe, generally we are influenced by Christian philosophy and culture, whether we are aware of it or not. Hence, the Bible was one of the subjects of my search for people's opinions about childlessness (and a potential source of their attitudes and prejudices). In addition to the Old and New Testaments, I also used the Gospel of the Nativity of Mary. My goal was again to find the basic structure of the story, the main characters, their experiences, and the resolution of the situation.

With some exaggeration, it can be said that those who mean something in the biblical stories were born to initially childless parents: Isaac (Genesis chapters 16–21), Joseph (Genesis 30: 1–24), Samuel 1 (1: 1–28), Samson (Judges 13: 2–24), the Virgin Mary (Gospel of the Nativity of Mary 1.1–3.11), John the Baptist (Luke 1: 5–58).

Childlessness is not God's punishment; to the contrary, God stands up for the childless, 'They [who do not know God] prey on the barren and childless woman, and to the widow show no kindness' (Job 24: 21). God promises to the childless: 'Sing, O barren woman, you who never bore a child; burst into song, shout for joy, you who were never in labour; because more are the children of the desolate woman than of her who has a husband' (Isaiah, 54: 1).

In contrast to the fairy tales where the bearer of the childlessness is not designated, in the Bible the childless (except for the Gospel of the Birth of the Virgin Mary) is a woman (Sarah, Rachel, Anna, Elizabeth, Hannah). The 'therapy', if I can call it that, is always a prayer. Women often become pregnant in old age (Sarah is said to have become pregnant at 90 years of age) when they are beyond the fertile age ('Sarah had ceased to have her monthly periods'). Biblical women and men cope with their barrenness with much difficulty ('So Hannah rose up after they had eaten in Shiloh, and after they had drunk. Now Eli the priest sat upon a seat by a post of the temple of the Lord. And she was in bitterness of soul and prayed unto the Lord and wept sore', 'When Rachel saw that she was barren she was envious of her sister'). Women perceive their childlessness as a insult (Rachel after the birth: 'God has removed my defamation', Elizabeth in the fifth month: 'This has been wrought by God...so that he removes my defamation among people'). Biblical marriages do not disintegrate because of childlessness, to the contrary, the barren woman is often much loved by her husband and he consoles her ('For he loved Hannah; but the Lord had closed womb'... Elkanah said to her: 'why are you weeping? Why don't you eat? Why are you downhearted? Don't I mean more to you than ten sons?').

In contrast to fairy tales, in the Bible neighbours and family appear cruel and denigrate the behaviour of others ('her rival kept provoking' 'And when the high priest saw Joachim...he despised him, and spurned his gifts, asking why he, who had no offspring, presumed to stand among those who had... Cursed is every one who has not begot a male in Israel').

Folk wisdom

By the term folk wisdom, I mean a description of a particular situation, a description that expresses an experience or an idea of something. For instance, a proverb comments on a certain phenomenon, a myth explains it, and a ritual demonstrates it in practice.

In all cultures, posterity is a question of being or not being. That is why there exist many myths to explain infertility and many rituals to ensure fertility or cure infertility. Some of them are very beautiful.

> When a woman on the Barbarian Islands wants to have a child, she invites a man who is the father of a large family to pray for her to Upuler, the spirit of the sun. From red cotton, a puppet is made, which the woman cradles in her arms as though she wanted to breastfeed it. The father of many children takes

> a chicken, holds it by its legs near the woman's head and says: 'Oh, Upuler, take this chicken from me. Let it fall, let a child descend, I beg you and plead with you that a child falls down and descends into my hands, into my lap.' Then he asks the woman: 'Has the child come?' And she answers: 'Yes, it is sucking.' Then the man holds the chicken on the husband's head, and mumbles a formula. In the end, the bird is killed and laid with some betel at the household's offering place. When the ceremony is finished, the word is spread around the village that the woman has given birth, her friends come and congratulate her. The pretension that a child has been born is a purely magical ceremony by whose imitation it is to be ensured that a child will eventually be born. The participants also try to increase the efficacy of the ritual by prayers and offerings.
>
> — *(Frazer 1994).*

A Buddhist monk venerable Bhikkhu Kusalananda told me how infertility is traditionally treated in Sri Lanka. The treatment is holistic and it encompasses centuries-old methods of various traditional specialists. Each illness is part of a life problem that is first discussed with the village astrologist and ayurvedic doctor who are often the same person. As with other problems, the first step is to modify the diet and administer phytotherapy. Especially in the psychotherapy of functional infertility, the Kahlu-Kumahra-Tovil ritual is also used. The main goal is to help the patient to accept her human predicament and shape her life in accordance with Buddhist ethics. Moreover, there is a ritual for infertility treatment in which temple dancers, invited from a distant village, take an active part. These become possible donors of sperm during the overnight ritual. In this way, the possibility that the cause is in the man is attended to. Complete amnesia of the participants is important (meaning that they do not remember anything), imposed on the whole proceedings of the temple ritual, which excludes the rise of possible ethical or mental difficulties entailed in the treatment procedure. It could be said that this is a practical implementation of the proverb 'what the eyes don't see, the heart does not mind.'

Here are some references to folk wisdom from closer to home, Europe:

> A rice shower that welcomes them at the exit from the church should bring fertility to the new marriage.
>
> Every married woman is obliged to wear a scarf, otherwise she will not be able to carry the baby to full term.
>
> In the last part of the wedding ceremony, when the wreath was removed and replaced by a cap, the bride was hidden by 'koutnice' (a 'koutnice' was a sheet that isolated a woman in labour and later during the puerpera from the other members of the family).

When a child was not coming, treatment rituals were carried out:

> A certain couple in a village was childless for a long time, which made them sad. The woman set out, without saying anything to her husband, for advice to a witch in another village. The witch, after having performed her ritual, told the woman that a certain woman was to blame, her husband's former mistress, who, when they were on their way to the wedding in the church, arranged it that they had bones from the dead in their bed, which were really found there later on. In addition, the witch advised the woman to grate a piece of a stag's horn and a piece of the belt from her husband's trousers, to boil both in hare's milk, and they should take that drug together. They obeyed, and within a year and a day, God blessed them with a baby.
>
> — *(Bartoš 1906).*

Childless couples also have their own patroness, St. Anne. She is the patron saint of pregnant women (and women in labour), she is often prayed to for the health of ill children and in childless marriages for the missing descendant.

Well, many a reader will perhaps say, the author was just trying to add more pages, that is why she is annoying us with wisdom that is over and done with and has nothing to do with life today. But that is a mistake! I will gladly show you that we are still in the same boat as our predecessors many years ago. There is a spa town, in the Czech Republic with a statue of young St. Francis, which has a shining penis that is visible from a large distance. The woman who touches it is said to be ensured of posterity. (I touched it, too, when I was visiting there some years ago. One never knows, right? And, as they say, it's better to be safe than sorry. In fact, I could now claim that I have children precisely thanks to that ritual.)

> I recall that we also made a sacrifice in Tokyo, to a goddess of fertility. We always stopped somewhere when we were travelling. We even bothered the Black Widow of Montserrat, who can be seen for about three seconds. We imagined how all these gods meet once a year at an ecumenical party and decide who is going to take care of what. (f)

At some weddings, people still throw rice over the newly married couple. Until recently, I thought that this ritual was to ensure plenitude inside the wallet, but an ethnologist has explained to me that the plenitude concerns the cradle. I was also searching for proverbs and old sayings that could be related to the quest for a child.

'A marriage without children is like a needle without a thread' is a proverb that will not encourage childless couples. But because you have now read about the influence of the quest for a child on the partners' relationship, I am sure that you will not let yourself feel dejected by it; your marriage can be just as meaningful with or without a child.

When I was a girl, an older girlfriend taught me that men are either studs or asses, and she explained that if I marry a man who is attractive and capable, he will most likely be unfaithful all the time. If I want someone who is loyal and devoted to his family, I will have to be content with someone uninteresting, unattractive, an incapable dummy, simply an ass. My personal experience has not confirmed this theory, but I remembered it at one professional conference where half of the contributions were concerned with research on boar sperm. When I asked why, at a conference on human infertility, people are talking about boar sperm, I learned that they are ideal for research because they are similar to human ones, and a boar has many of them. Now this could be a possible origin of prejudice: we assume that attractive men are fertile, while those who are unattractive are, in our opinion, incapable, impotent, and uninteresting. Sometimes I think to myself, if only there were a famous, successful and attractive man, known for being a man's man who would be capable of admitting, with self-assurance and nonchalance, that he was infertile, he would accomplish the work of hundreds of psychotherapists.

Often it is said that a child is a gift, or God's gift. The saying is probably supposed to indicate that we are not automatically entitled to have children and that we should be very grateful for our parenthood. But some people may believe that a gift is given out of love and so can feel unloved. Others may understand the saying as claiming that if something is a gift, then it must be someone's will to give or not to give this gift. And they may be wondering what guidelines the donor observes: Merits? Moral qualities? Potential ability to raise a child? The balance in one's bank account? The size of one's shoes?

> I don't have a child because I haven't deserved it yet. I must work on myself so that I deserve it. (m)

I also searched for references to the views of older civilisations regarding unfulfilled parenthood in historical demographic texts.[26] I found that, for the civilisations of the Near East, 'the most cruel punishment that could befall a human being was childless'. Childlessness was mentioned even in the military oath of the Middle-Eastern generals: before addressing the troops at the roll-call, the commander would come and take malt in his hands, with the following words, 'as infertile as this malt is, and just as it cannot be used for planting or baking bread, so infertile will be the woman and the cattle of the man who breaks his oath.' In the pre-Columbian era, it is said that childless women were in scorn. Among Jews, dying without children was such a terrible phenomenon that it was listed among God's punishments for committing a sin and the causes of miscarriage were supposed to include not following prescribed sexual hygiene and mental health issues. As Paracelsus in the 16th century says: 'a woman's imagination reflects God's might and her wants will show in her child.' Sources describing the situation in Central Europe in the early modern ages (around 1650) say that only with the first child was the function of a marriage fulfilled and only then did a woman become a full and valuable member of society. Some time ago, I read a statement in the newspapers by an oncologist saying essentially that health was not a reward and illness was not a punishment. A fertility problem is an illness like any other, but it is surely not a punishment.

Nowadays, it seems to be the norm to be in a low mood or depressed. But usually the people who speak about their low mood or depression describe it as a temporary condition and they usually know what has caused it: a certain situation or event. That is to say, they have their low mood or depression more or less under control. They know that they are going to get out of this condition eventually and they have a good idea of how. Simply, when one wants, everything is possible. And it is precisely the impossibility of control, the entire independence of one's will, that differentiates depression from a low mood. What is the connection between fertility problems and a low mood? They are both often understood by the general public as mental illnesses, that the consequences of the illness are 'only' mental, it is only the soul that suffers. Additionally, both are often believed to be rooted in psychological causes: insufficiency, inability, unwillingness. 'We are weak in the body, but strong in the mind,' says a song. It suggests that we, who are weak in the body, are still worthy, not like those weaklings, who are frail in the mind. They do not have good will, they do not want to, that is why they fade away! But good will is insufficient for the removal of the causes of depression as well as of fertility problems.

However, it is not only wisdom that is clearly expressed and conveyed within the framework of various cultures. There are also the opinions and attitudes shared by smaller groups, for example generations, special interest or family groups, and the opinions and attitudes that are personal and that are very often difficult to identify, so that one is not even aware of them.

I did not want to make light of wisdom, whether the kind passed down from generation to generation or the personal kind. It is very important and most often encouraging and helpful. But, in some situations, wisdom can only be quite ordinary and we need to keep a critical distance. We need to ask ourselves whether our opinions and attitudes towards infertility, towards its causes, towards the possibilities of treatment, towards adoption, and towards childlessness are really a reflection of our current life experience and our current knowledge, whether we can stand by them, draw from them.

For a long time, I wasn't able to accept the possibility that the only treatment for me is artificial fertilisation. It seemed to me against nature, I minded it terribly, and I was preparing myself for the possibility that we would remain without a child. But then I had second thoughts. My bad fallopian tubes are also against nature. (f)

We have one child thanks to the methods of assisted reproduction. We want a second one but, in the meantime, we have become believers, and artificial fertilisation is now unacceptable for us due to the manipulation. (f)

First we refused adoption, we were afraid what the child might be like. Then, by chance, we met a family who has an adopted, beautiful, and clever little boy. We stopped being afraid, and submitted an application. (f)

The worst type of social pressure can sometimes be exerted cruelly against ourselves.

A woman contacted me after an invitation to the seminar 'Hormones and Fertility Problems' led by a doctor from the centre of assisted reproduction (the invitation was broadcast on a radio with a Christian theme). She didn't even notice the title of the seminar, she was drawn by the term 'centre of assisted reproduction'. She said that doctors designated IVF as the last chance for her after a long unsuccessful treatment. She perceives IVF as a big hope, and an almost sure success. (But she didn't have any information and only a distorted idea about its efficacy; she was greatly surprised that sometimes the embryos won't nest). In her way to this 'almost sure' success, there stands, for her as a believer, the Pope's prohibition of the utilisation of these methods. From our discussion, it followed that she had, in fact, decided to go for IVF, and she was looking for someone who would

remove the responsibility from her for transgressing the ban. The best would be a doctor who is a believer, performing assisted reproduction. (p)
'They all think that, if I don't want to adopt a child, that I would be a bad mother to my own child, too,' a woman told me. To my question who specifically is saying this and what precisely is being said, she answered: 'Directly no one says anything, but everybody thinks it, because they look that way.' (f)

SOME OF THOSE WHO'VE TASTED THE DISTANCE,
THOSE WHO UNDERSTAND,
LET THEM TELL YOU...

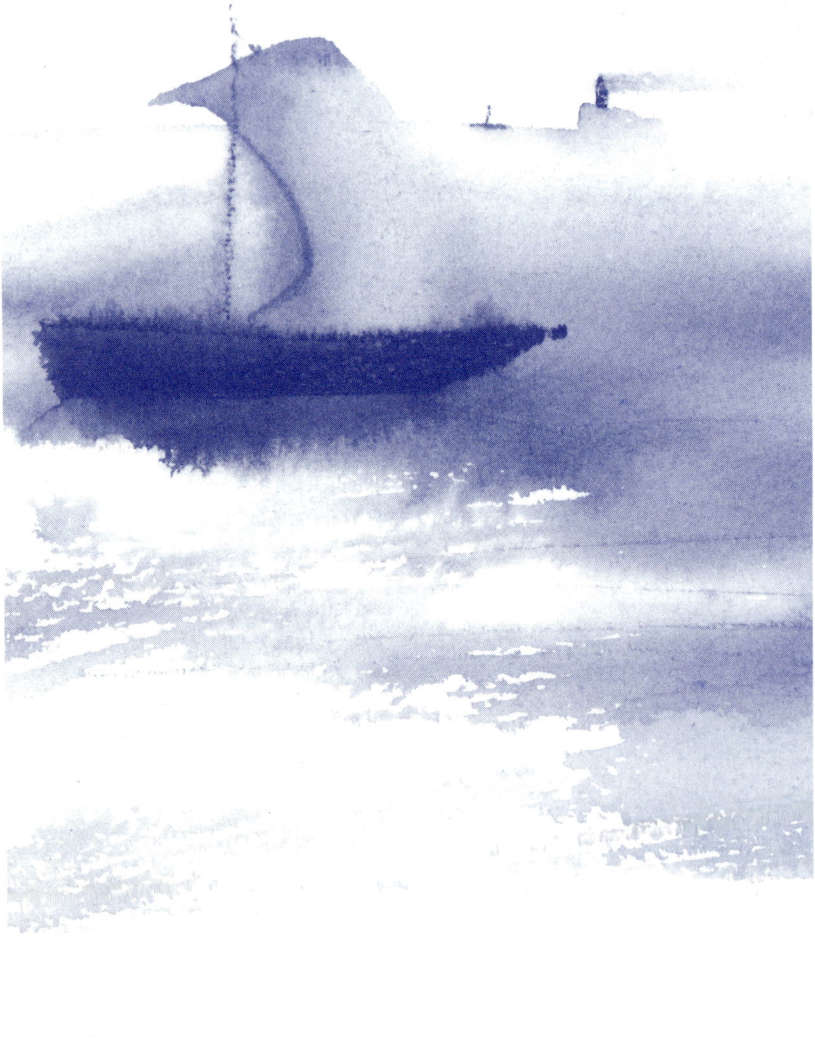

Some of Those Who've Tasted the Distance, Those Who Understand, Let Them Tell You...

This chapter is made up of the stories of people who have 'tasted the distance' of the quest for a child personally and who have left a part of their life in it, sometimes an essential part. They are going to tell their own stories, they are those 'who understand'. Know that it was not easy for them to recall their memories and experiences, often very painful ones, and put them into words.

The stories are anonymous, the names are made up. Some stories are written by both partners, then they are called by similar names, for instance Jane and John.

Other, non-anonymous stories can be found, for example, in the book *I Want to Have a Child, Whatever It Takes!* (in English and Spanish), by the author Carmen Martinez Jover, and in the article entitled Mourning My Miscarriage and book named *Looking for Daisy* by Peggy Orenstein (in English).

Madeleine

My story with a happy ending started at the beginning of the 1990s when I lived for the first time through the endless waiting for a baby. After we learned the diagnosis, which was my husband's infertility, we decided for artificial fertilisation with the utilisation of donor semen.

It took four long years before I was able to conceive, but the pregnancy proceeded without complications and one day I had under the Christmas tree the most precious gift—the girl Madeleine. She grew, becoming prettier and smarter, until she started desiring, according to the pattern of her girlfriends in kindergarten, a sibling. And her parents had already been toying with the idea of having a son as well. The next series of examinations at the fertility clinic started. This time, I became pregnant on the second attempt and lived through nine unproblematic months of happiness. The birth was more difficult, taking 20 hours, and then I heard the longed-for information—it is a boy—and lived through three seconds of euphoria. Then there was a silence without the first expected cry, my thousands of questions, and the evasive answers of the medical staff. Billy came into the world with multiple developmental defects and died in the first minutes after his birth. It was an unusual set of defects that are impossible to discover in the ultrasound and so unique that, even after the autopsy and a thorough genetic analysis, it was not clear whether it was a hereditary disease or an accidental influence of the environment. The probability of my giving birth to another healthy child was set at 50%. Nonetheless, we tried again a year later. I underwent eight unsuccessful inseminations, after which the IVF method was supposed to be used. For some organisational reasons, the ninth insemination was completed and was successful. But the 18 weeks of hope ended unexpectedly. During the amniocentesis examination, the doctors discovered that the fetus had not been living for several weeks. The question of whether the two cases were linked was obvious, but even this time it was not possible to answer it. According to the autopsy report, the baby, a little boy, again had some malformations, but only distantly similar to the first case. Moreover, some doctors thought that they could be caused by the changes in the body after the death of the child.

After the previous sad birth, I nodded my head benevolently in agreement to the nurses' words about another pregnancy and I thought I would never do it again (but the truth is that this resolution lasted only a single day). This time, I decided to struggle on immediately. I got the blessing of the genetic clinic where they said that I could try in vitro fertilisation. I had undergone two unsuccessful attempts when the doctor called me and said that she saw a certain link each time and she recommended I reconsider the situation. She said it carefully and I accepted it calmly.

A few days earlier, during a holiday trip, I hesitated in a bookshop over the purchase of a book that was to change my life. Thanks to it the myth was dismantled that the legal system of my country enables the donation of sperm or eggs but not both at the same time (and possibly the donation of embryos). The doctors at one of the centres of reproductive medicine where I was treated had believed this myth, too. Fortunately, they responded in a very flexible way, and almost instantly they added the transfer of donated embryos to their programme. Technically, it was a matter identical with the second phase of in vitro fertilisation; the new parts were the considerations about the legislative and ethical viewpoints. It was necessary to find suitable donors among couples who did not intend to use all their embryos and to perform genetic tests on these embryos. The first attempt with the implantation of one embryo did not end up well and, maybe for this reason, the doctors decided to implant four embryos as the next step. It was somewhat risky, because I would not have liked to have to think about potential reduction after all the preceding difficulties. But double luck was with me this time. I carried one baby and, for the 10th birthday of my daughter, I gave birth to her beautiful, healthy, and wonderful brother Andrew.

Since it was thanks to my case that a complicated procedure, which changed the policy of the reproductive centre (before me, they had allegedly rejected several parties interested in the same procedure), got under way. I did not have time to deal with possible doubts, but this decision, of course, brings up many questions. I had never thought that I would have a problem with the fact that he is not my biological descendant and, after he was born, I knew that he was mine. In this, men are worse off; the mother has a much better opportunity to live together with the baby during the pregnancy and birth.

The harder part is the thought that one does not know almost anything about one's child, about his or her genes, requirements, predispositions, or inclinations. Even though psychology is not able to determine the precise role of upbringing and of inheritance in the shaping of a human being, it is supposed that genes can play a major role. In this respect, I see room for much improvement in the practice of the donation program in my country. I do not think that the interested parties should be choosing from a database of donors according to photographs and data related to all kinds of things, including religious denomination, as I saw in an American documentary. However, I think that the future parents should learn more about the biological predecessors of their child, more than the colour of the eyes, the height, weight, and the blood group. But I believe that everything is developing and that, even in the area of reproductive medicine, which is still the subject of various taboos, many things will improve in time.

Our longed-for and fought-for beautiful baby is proof enough for me, my daughter, my husband, as well as for our relatives and friends, who discouraged me from having more children right after the first failure, that one should not give up on one's dreams. I thank everyone who has helped me on my quest for a child.

Judith

This serious problem has touched my life, too. I got married very young, but I did not have to. My husband and I loved each other, but we planned to have children later on. However, when my girlfriends had their first children, my desire for a little one started to grow. At that time, we started to work on it. When we had no success (for approximately two years), I went to see my gynaecologist and asked her for an examination. That turned out well. Then it was my husband's turn. They found that he does not produce any sperm. Even today, I still do not like to remember the moment when my husband told me. He was in shock himself. He wanted to solve the situation by getting a divorce. I could not accept his proposal, because we loved each other a lot. I showed the result of his examination to my doctor, who was kind and was trying to help us. (At first, we were thinking about adopting a little infant.) I need to add that this was almost 40 years ago.

The doctor told me about the option of fertilisation by donated sperm. My husband agreed with that, and so we underwent other phases of the examinations in the fertility clinic. My husband was examined again, and the result of 100% infertility was confirmed. For both of us, it was a big mental strain, especially for my husband. He liked children a lot and suffered enormously by the thought that we would have none because of him.

As we kept this fact hidden from our relatives and co-workers, it was quite demanding. I myself had to listen to frequent advice from the members of my family and my friends, cutting remarks from malicious inquisitive women, but also 'offers' from male colleagues at work, even though they did not know the precise cause. This made it even more difficult to explain why I needed time off on certain days. As my boss and other co-workers suspected that I was probably under treatment, they had lots of understanding for me. They accepted the news about my pregnancy with much delight, as if the problem concerned them as well.

Before I became pregnant, I underwent the procedure of insemination by donor's sperm about five times. I measured my temperature, I monitored the most fertile days and, during that time, I had to go to fertility clinic in a city many miles away. Thanks to the airline services, I was sometimes able to make it there and back in one day. It worked out and eight years after the wedding, we had a child. Today we have beautiful grandchildren.

At that time, we already lived in our own family house. The midwife (she was an elderly woman), when she came to give a bath at our place, always said: 'This is as it should be, first the nest, and then the young ones into it.' But if she had known how much effort, disappointment, nerves, crying, and money it cost! My husband and I were willing to sacrifice everything we had for the birth of our child.

As we did not want our child to be an only child, after five years we decided for another attempt. Medicine had made progress by that time, so I did not have to go to as far away, insemination was done in smaller towns as well. I became pregnant right on the first attempt. We were all looking forward to having the baby, especially our first child. When I left for the birth clinic, I had prepared a little bed with everything, a complete layette, and I should not have done that. We were struck by terribly bad luck, the child was born with a severe defect, and died soon.

This was another big blow for my husband and me! I was 32 years old; I was looking forward to staying at home and enjoying just being with the children for a while, and suddenly nothing, nothing... But there was nothing to do but keep my wits about me. Didn't I already have one healthy child at home? I took it hard mentally. Even though I swore after the birth that I was finished with it, after a while the desire for a child came back again. Moreover, our child reproached us all the time that others have siblings and she is still alone.

My decision to undergo another in vitro fertilisation was inspired by a television discussion with a respected geneticist. I wrote to him telling my story, and he recommended an examination and a consultation with a particular expert. He treated me hormonally for seven months, so that he could be sure that the egg would be sufficiently mature. The very first intervention by him was successful. I was 35 years old. During the pregnancy, I was hospitalised twice (because there was a danger of premature birth). In the end, everything turned out well. We had another healthy child.

I recommend to all married couples who are facing the obstacle of childless marriage that, in their decision making about their future life, they shed all their anxieties and prejudices, that they listen to the advice of specialists and use the possibilities that modern medicine provides. Each successful attempt at the birth of a healthy little person is worth it!

I would like to tell such concerned young couples that it depends above all on the two of them, on what kind of strength, courage, and responsibility they can find in dealing with this difficult problem. Mainly, they should not listen to people who are uninformed and are burdened by various prejudices.

Thanks to the understanding of my husband, I could try the new method, even though it was an uncertain purchase. After the second, unsuccessful attempt, the gynaecologist advised me to find someone and try it 'the way things happen in nature'. Not that there would not have been men willing to offer assistance, but I could not do it. Probably my love for my husband won, and also my anxiety that our relationship could suffer.

At that time, there was little knowledge among people about men's infertility, which meant that everything was mostly blamed on the woman. And many of those who were not courageous suffered their whole lives. My husband took a very rational stance toward the problem. He accepted the children as his own, he devoted every free minute to them, and he really loved them. And they clung to him, too, they loved him more than me, because I was stricter. For a short time, he could enjoy our grandchildren, he literally gave himself to them. Unfortunately, I am speaking about my husband in the past tense. He died a few years ago. It still hurts, but even this is something that life brings us… I cannot imagine that I would not have children.

As a conclusion, I would like to cite the proverb: 'It is bad enough with children, and even worse without them.' I tested the proverb during the years before our first child was born.

Eve

I worked as a junior doctor at the children's department of the regional hospital and my husband was studying in a city 95 miles away. I would stay in the department even after my shifts; nothing drew me to my rented room. I read books to the children, or once to a nurse, and I played a puppet theatre for the children. After several months my husband got a job as a company lawyer of the local construction company.

This was incredibly good fortune for us, we were together, both happy with our jobs, and we had been promised an apartment. For the time being we moved to a bigger but, as it turned out, also damper room with a wash basin and a stove. We stopped [using birth control], and we were looking forward to having a child. But pregnancy was not coming. The gynaecological examinations were repeatedly fine and, according to the urologist, nothing should have been preventing my husband from making me pregnant. We became a target for various advice. Our friends advised us not to think about our longing for a child and then pregnancy would come of its own accord, or that we should leave for a pleasant environment and repeatedly make love, or that we should change positions when making love. The advice that, in this way, we could resolve our apartment situation was not left out, either.

At that time I did not feel very well, I suffered from insomnia. The frequent night shifts out in the field, the noise at the kindergarten where we rented our room, from 5 a.m. and long into the night, were all to blame. I was among children all the time, at the hospital, at the clinic, and in the kindergarten. When I heard a crying child from the locker room early in the morning, I would get up, calm the child, and help it to change clothes. I started having problems with my back due to the almost daily trips with the outpatient department at the mountain health centres. When part of my husband's parents' apartment became free after the departure of a tenant, we decided to go back to the city.

In the city I started to work at an infectious disease clinic. I liked the work a lot, but I was exhausted by the night shifts, in six months I lost 16 kilos. I was still trying to become pregnant, I followed any advice; I exercised, I repeatedly went to see the gynaecologist, I drank herbal teas. My husband and I were enrolled in the Astra programme, which calculated the days when I should become pregnant according to the stars, and nothing happened. All the monthly expectations and then disappointments again! My husband did not show the disappointment, only several years later did I learn from him how he suffered. At first he encouraged me, gave me hope. When I worked at the hospital, he wanted me to find a job without night shifts, he forced me to eat so that I would gain back the lost kilos.

All my girlfriends and my husband's friends already had one or more children and we still nothing. How many remarks did we hear from friends when we were leaving for a holiday that we should finally start working on my pregnancy! After three years Astra responded that we were among the 5% of couples with whom their method was not successful.

Then I started to work as a chief paediatrician for infants' and children's homes. When I accepted the job, I did not suspect how much the environment of the institutions would affect me. I saw so many orphaned children and I did not have a single one! I went from room to room, I cradled the children, and cuddled them, I could not leave them. In one children's home, I got to know a two-year-old boy who looked as if he were my husband's spitting image. As soon as I returned from this children's home,

I told my husband about the boy, and we went to visit him the next Saturday. My husband was excited, he arranged everything at the local court where he had an internship during his studies, and he took care of all the paperwork related to the adoption. Before this happened, we had not talked about adoption; I learned about the possibility of adoption only after I started travelling around the children's homes.

We went through all the necessary examinations, the administration of the home was very helpful, the local court also, and it looked as if nothing was in the way of having the boy move in with us. And yet! A social worker called to inform us that she would come to our apartment to check up on the suitable conditions for the child. We waited impatiently, we kept going to listen to the door, but she did not come. Instead of her, a letter came that we were not a suitable couple for the adoption of a child. It was terrible, my husband and I discovered that a decision had been made that we were not a suitable couple for political reasons. A few years later, my husband and I applied for adoption for the second time, this time for a six-year-old child. But before the process started, we withdrew our application because my husband's aunt, who had lived with us for a long time and who had raised my husband when his own mother died in his childhood, asked us to let her live her last days in peace and not to bring a child into the apartment.

When I was 39, my brother's wife gave birth to a daughter and, four years later, to another. These nieces were a big joy for us, at first we spent weekends with them, later also holidays. In 1983 my husband died.

In 1990, my financial conditions improved so much that I got to thinking about starting a foundation. As a paediatrician, I understandably thought about a foundation that would help children. However, I discovered that there were many foundations like that. Since my whole life has been marked by an unfulfilled desire for a child and a struggle for it and, as a doctor as well as a patient, I am very well oriented in this area. So it became clear. I decided to help couples who have problems with fertilisation or who repeatedly miscarry. That was the beginning of the Maternal Hope Foundation. I can sympathise with the situation of couples who are longing in vain for a baby and, thanks to my medical contacts and knowledge of the modern methods of diagnosis and treatment (which were not available in my time), I can offer them hope for the longed-for pregnancy.

My desire for a child was fulfilled when my older niece had a little girl, Lucy. Both of Lucy's grandmothers are young and go to work, so I provide almost all the help with the baby for my niece. Only now have

I experienced what a child's hand around my neck means, her joy over my arrival, children's talk and smiles. And so, in the end, what I had desired all my life has been fulfilled.

Peter

I grew up as the oldest with two younger sisters, the younger was eight years younger than I, so I was accustomed to looking after her and from my childhood it was a matter-of-course for me, as it were, that I would have children one day. After my wedding (I was 24 years old), I automatically expected that children would simply appear: first one, then another... I wanted to have a lot of them. When nothing happened for a year and a half, some examinations started (first my wife, then myself) and it still did not occur to me that we could have a problem, that even I myself could have that problem, and that it could be unsolvable. Approximately after half a year we were told the verdict: you will never have children in a natural way. It was said in a very insensitive way, it was told to us separately even though we both waited in the waiting room, simply as a statement of fact, and in a tone like: it should have been clear to you a long time ago. And if you want to, you can come back for more information about in vitro fertilisation. Good bye, next please.

My parents already had two granddaughters from my sister who got married a year before me, and so they, especially my Dad, impatiently waited for us to give them the good news. When we shared our pain it was a shock for them, too.

At first, our infertility was not a big problem for me, I was only 26 years old and there were so many things to do, we could travel or devote ourselves to church activities. Today I would say, in retrospect, that it was not only this, but also the great sorrow of not being able to have my own children, and so I suppressed the problem and the pain deep into myself. Then for several years seemingly nothing happened, we spent two years outside the country and I did not have much time to think about it. After we returned and started to settle down, we started to get in touch with my and my wife's friends again, who had gotten married and had children in the meantime, and my problem started coming to the surface.

I was beginning to realise better (also thanks to the psychotherapeutic training that I was starting at the time) that I had suppressed the problem. I was living through my pain. Our relationship deepened due to the situation, but it took us (especially me) a long time until we were able to speak to each other about our deep pain.

We also felt our loneliness, the 'unusualness' of our situation, and that the close people around us (married people with children) could not fully understand us. My wife and I started looking for people like us, and we started a friendship with a married couple who were suffering from the same problem that has lasted until today.

At that time I had nephews and nieces, and my need for children was in many respects compensated by the time spent with them, but also with the children of our friends and acquaintances. So I enjoyed going to the places and events where this need could be met, which was a source of tension between me and my wife because for her, children (and mothers speaking hardly about anything else) reminded her of our common pain and made it worse.

After a certain time of living through the pain, I started to realise that we needed to decide what to do next, what we would choose as our life's journey, whether we would adopt a child or stay childless. A little later than my wife, I discovered that I would not be happy only at work. I was taken aback by the fact that I was afraid to make a decision, I would have been very happy if someone had done it for me. I tried to find out by all possible means which of the two options (adoption or a life without children) was better, so that I could decide for the better one. In the end I concluded that both ways were equally good, and that I must decide, take responsibility myself. This process took about a year and, in the end, I came to this conclusion: I want adoption. For Pearl, the decision took somewhat longer, and actually, even after the decision, after we went to the social care office for the paperwork, there was about a half-year period when she was still clarifying her decision for herself. I realised in this situation that I could not press her, that I had to wait and hope that we would come to the same decision. Theoretically, I told myself that, if she decided for a life without children, I was willing to submit to that, that I could not force her into something different, but these ruminations were purely theoretical.

Then there were the clerical matters to go through (and a very unpleasant meeting with a psychologist who was assessing our capabilities to be adoptive parents) and the waiting for the child. This was so short that I was not able to reflect on it in any more detail.

How do I perceive our solution? The infertility deepened our relationship, it helped us to get to know each other better, to resolve various things from our past, to mature more, and perhaps become wiser. I see this as a big plus for both of us and for our children—they have parents who are capable of being more fully parents than they were at the beginning of their marriage. It is difficult for me to differentiate and write about 'myself and us'—I think that the problem really made us closer and more united, and I am unable in retrospect to differentiate the two completely.

There was one more question that we were resolving: artificial fertilisation. I was almost immediately and unequivocally against it, and it was difficult for my wife to accept this fact as given. For me, artificial fertilisation is something unnatural, from the 'created' child becomes something like an object that is supposed to serve the parents and gratify their needs. As I understand it, a child is a gift, not something that we have a right to, and we should not play God in this. I think that another under-researched area is how conception in a test tube influences the child. Today there is a lot known about what all a child perceives during pregnancy, and how the various events in the mother's life influence him or her. And how does it influence his or her basic orientation toward life? I think that it is quite a risky experiment. Moreover, the child is conceived anonymously, he or she doesn't have, doesn't know the father or the mother (the donor of the sperm or the egg). Seemingly, it is similar in adoption, but there the child has a chance, and a big majority of children exploit it, to learn about their biological parents (and meet them).

In the last half a year (almost five years after the adoption of our first daughter), I have been surprised that it is hard for me to see pregnant women, especially my and my wife's contemporaries. As if again the pain that I cannot have my own children resounded in me. Perhaps a time has come to deepen my reconciliation with our infertility. At the same time, I want to stress that I am very happy with both of our little daughters, and I have caught myself many times thinking about them as if they had been with us from the beginning and I keep forgetting that it was not always like this.

Pearl

Our desire was to conceive a child about a year after the wedding: we wished to have some time to get attuned to each other without a child and the period of its expectation. At the same time, we did not exactly try to prevent pregnancy. My husband and I wanted a child because it was a matter-of-course for us that we would become parents, that we would link our lives with a new human being.

So we started quite early, about two years after the wedding, to search for what was wrong. First, I underwent some examinations. I took some hormones for a while, although I do not actually know why—I was not told the reason, and I was nervous about everything at the time, I simply trusted the doctor. When my examinations did not show anything, the doctors turned their attention to my husband. The diagnosis was clear, and the report was clear: there is nothing to resolve, a treatment does not exist. You can undergo in vitro insemination or adopt a child. The whole period of the examinations lasted only about half a year, in fact everything happened very quickly.

The suffering and pain of our situation came much later. We lived very active lives, for a certain time it seemed that nothing was lacking. But gradually, as more and more of our contemporaries had babies, I experienced the pain of emptiness more and more. We were surrounded by an environment of young families. I was repeatedly getting dragged into conversations about children, and I repeatedly realised how devastating these conversations were to me. I felt that I did not belong among those women, in fact I felt much more drawn to the discussions of their husbands, but even the there was no place for me. I felt lonely, uprooted, unable to find a way to talk to anyone. There was no activity that could fill my emptiness.

I was angry with God because I had thought until then that he loved me, and now it seemed to me that it was not so, that he could not care less about me. I was angry with my husband as the 'guilty party'. From time to time, we talked about what to do next but we were not very good at it. I think that we did not have the courage to touch each other's pain. It was probably more and more obvious how I suffered, but my husband did not show anything very much. I was convinced that he felt the pain too, but I did not want to hurt him even more. Actually, I reproached myself for my sometimes highly emotional behaviour.

For a long time I thought that we would stay childless. We were very active, and we realised very clearly that a childless marriage can, in fact, be very fruitful. We longed to serve other people, to give our lives to someone: to a child or to other people. Childlessness offered us an immensely wide space. I realised that I had something like a maternal heart, and it was clear to me that I could offer it not only to my children, but also to other people who needed it. For me, a maternal heart means the ability, the gift of consolation, sympathy, support. And so I offered my heart, it helped people, but all the time I felt that this was not it—that the emptiness remained and that the right path may lead elsewhere.

I did not dare to think aloud about in vitro fertilisation. It was clear to me that, as a Christian, the path did not lead this way for me because my church simply says NO. I knew that my husband thought that way, too, so there was really nothing to think about. Nonetheless, I desired this solution, I wanted to have a child at any cost. It seemed to me that my husband did not want to talk with me about this aspect, that for him it simply was not a matter for discussion. It worried me, and it took me a long time until I accepted his stance. I had the impression that I was not being taken seriously, or that my pain was not accepted. I had to cry not only over the fact that I could not have a child with my husband, I also had to cry over the fact that it was entirely impossible. I rationally accepted my husband's reasons, but my soul cried: 'I want a child! I want it!' In fact, we were able to talk about it only much later.

I concentrated my thoughts in the direction of the only possibility left—adoption. I was afraid of it. Although I was gradually starting to accept that giving my love to a 'strange' child could be a way for me and my life, I was anxious anyway. I was afraid that I would not be able to give enough love to a child that had not grown under my heart and whose past I did not know. I was afraid of the complexity of such a relationship, of all the unknowns that the child would bring with himself or herself, in which I might not be able to orient myself. I was afraid that I would not be able to give up the convenience and the freedom in which my husband and I had lived for years. I asked myself whether I wanted to risk this (and much else) at all.

In the end, we submitted an application for adoption and we were offered a newborn girl very quickly. To my astonishment, essentially from the first moments I felt toward her as if she were mine, I felt that I am a mother, I knew that she was mine, that we belonged to each other—despite the fact that I had not carried her, despite the fact that I did not know her past. This intimacy and firmness of the relationship has lasted, and has even strengthened.

Three years later, based on our next application for adoption, we were offered a young boy. From the first moment we met him, we felt a certain uncertainty about him, and we did not know whether he was the one. There were a number of reasons. We took a week to think about it. During that week, we each thought on our own, and then we talked, and mutually explained our positions...and we decided, each in a different way. My husband did not want him and I did. Quite naturally, I accepted that, in this case, it was necessary to respect the decision of the one who did not want to. Somewhere in my soul, I felt it was a good decision, that in me emotional reasons overpowered the rational ones that were necessary to hear out as well. Nonetheless, it was very difficult. It was difficult to cope with the fact that we had the right to refuse, that we had a duty to listen to ourselves. We could not imagine that we would continue living with the knowledge that we left him in the infants' home. Still we refused him after much struggle.

Less than two months after this event, we were offered a young girl; this time, we knew from the first moment that she was ours. In spite of this, my relationship to her was equivocal from the beginning. The feelings of belonging together and affinity came much later, it took me much longer before she grew on me. But it came. The older daughter is much closer to me in her character, I have the impression that I understand her much more easily than the younger one. As if I did not have to work on that relationship, as if everything came freely of its own accord. Nonetheless, they are both mine, I cannot imagine that a child could be more my own than my girls are. I often keep forgetting that, biologically, they are not my own, I think about them as if they were my blood.

I have been trying to talk with the older one who is five now about the way she came to us. So far, everything is clear-cut and beautiful to her. But I feel a certain anxiety, the pain that at some point she will understand that the fact that we are allowed to love her means that someone else had refused her. Naturally, I feel that way toward both girls. I am trying to get used to the fact that they do not belong to me, that they belong only to themselves. That they are a gift for me that I have for a certain limited time, and I must give them enough space so that they can once go their own way, a way that might not be easy for me to accept. In fact, I think that even biological parenthood should be going in this direction. So perhaps it can be easier for me as for an adoptive mother when that time comes. In any event, I realise that I have slightly more worries, and of a different kind, than biological parents.

Nonetheless, I can say that I am happy with my children. I do not know what it would be like if I had biological children, but I do not think that it could be any more beautiful. It is true that sometimes I feel pain because I will never live through biological motherhood, seeing a pregnant woman or a newborn child in a pram sometimes hurts me. But, thanks to my children, I do not have the need to be much concerned with the pain, I do not need to put as much emphasis on it as before, because I am happy.

Olivia

At first, I did not want to have children. I told myself that, if I did not find a suitable daddy, I would rather be childless. When I was about thirty, I eventually got married and started to desire a child.

I suspected that something was not right with me, but the examination at the gynaecologist showed that I should not be anxious. So I became pregnant for the first time, but I miscarried in the second month. The gynaecologist assured me that it was an accident, and that I should not be afraid. Half a year later, we tried it again and the pregnancy was very complicated—I stayed in the hospital for three months, and the child died after a premature birth. Again, I was told that, basically, it was an accident, and that I was otherwise healthy. I summed it up for myself: that if I did not search and try to find the cause of the miscarriages myself, the doctors would not help me very much. Of course my husband had a spermiogram, but he was healthy. It was quite an effort to get him there.

Through exercises, a healthy diet, herbs, and acupuncture I put myself back in shape. But a third miscarriage came. I found out what examinations I could possibly undergo so that I was sure that there was no hitch anywhere. And in the end, I found the cause of my miscarriages and underwent the necessary treatment. My husband wanted a child a lot, but otherwise he did not help me in any way. I had to arrange everything by myself.

Only the fourth time did it turn out well. The fourth attempt was our last one, my husband did not want to try any further.

Of course it was a hard test.

On the whole I kept miscarrying for five years. For five years, I struggled to have a child, knowing that I was not the youngest candidate. But I knew that some women kept trying even longer, and sometimes with no result, so I was not so badly off. In any event, it leaves a mark on a person; at least it did in my case. It was all the worse for me because I did not have help (any help at all) from my mother. There was indifference and remarks like, 'At your age I was raising two children and you keep complaining about something.' It did not matter that I would have gladly been raising them. Only my mother-in-law and my husband came to see me in the hospital. When my child died, my mother did not even see him, and she told me that I was ungrateful and advised me to see a psychologist.

My husband, in turn, when he saw that things took so much effort, would have reconciled himself to the fact that we would not have a child. But I did not give up. And it is true that the last successful attempt was a miracle even for the physician who treated me. Probably nobody believed in it any more at that point.

If someone thinks that a child will save a marriage, it is only half of the truth. I am happy, I have a baby. But my marriage is ripe for divorce. So many duties with the baby make it impossible to think about leisure or devote myself to my husband as it used to be. Added to this could be potential financial problems, and a catastrophe is about to happen.

Today I see the other side, too. If one has a good job, is healthy, and, maybe, also has a good husband, then it is no tragedy if the couple is unsuccessful in having a child. But one must try all the possible avenues, including healers, and also have a lot of time to do it. So I wish all women a lot of resourcefulness and courage in asking their doctors questions.

Theresa

When my husband and I got married, we were the ideal age for starting a family. Of course, we started longing for a child right after the wedding.

But when the child would not come, I was placed in a consultation group for infertile couples. During the treatment at the consultation, I underwent various examinations of the patent fallopian tubes and a follow-up laparoscopy. From the physiological viewpoint, everything was fine. The doctors did not find any health problem in my husband either. Hence, my husband and I were put into the slot of inexplicable infertility.

The bigger our desire for a child, the bigger the burden for my psyche. I started being sensitive to discussions about children, and I started to feel sad that I could not be a normal mother like my girlfriends and schoolmates.

Since I did not succeed in becoming pregnant in a natural way, I started treatment at a centre of assisted reproduction. Here they put me among the IVF patients. Unfortunately, at that time it was not as easy to undergo IVF as it is today. Doctors did not have such a precise assessment of drug dosages, so I had to undergo hormonal treatment several times before they found the right dose. The treatment was also time-consuming, because I had to commute for the check-ups, blood collections, consultations, and ultrasound. Fortunately, I had tolerant employers who understood my situation and tolerated my absence at work. But it did not add to my peace of mind since I knew that, due to my treatment, my colleagues had to do the work instead of me.

My first attempt at IVF did not work out. I was successful in becoming pregnant only after the transfer of frozen embryos. Unfortunately, our great joy from the pregnancy was short lived. The pregnancy proved to be extrauterine. In the fifth week I had to undergo laparoscopy, during which they took away, along with the pregnancy, the right fallopian tube and the endometriosis that arose during the hormonal treatment. Through this unsuccessful pregnancy, my chance of becoming pregnant was again somewhat reduced.

Apart from the treatment at the doctors' offices, my husband and I also tried treatment offered by healers. The first one prescribed drinking a herbal tea for both of us, which did not help in any way. The second healer healed through his energy; he claimed that I was fine and needed only to recharge my energy. I do not know if it was just my imagination, but when he applied his hand, I felt intensive warmth in my lower tummy. We saw the healer several times, but the visits did not help in any way either. However, when longing for a child, one does not want to omit any possibility that may offer a chance of success.

When my husband and I felt that the treatment of sterility would be a long-distance run, we started to admit also the possibility that we would not have our own child. We did not want to stay alone, so we submitted an application for adoption. We knew that the waiting time for an adoptive child was approximately five years, so we did not waste any time putting in the application. At the same time, I was still being treated as an IVF patient.

At a time when another IVF attempt did not work out, we thought it was a miracle that they called us from the social care office that they had an 18-month-old little girl. Our parenthood happened in a split second. We brought the girl home after a week of preparations. When we saw her at home with us for the first time, we fell in love with her. Mainly when she cuddled up to us in our arms. Even though she saw us for the first time, she was not afraid and did not cry. We still have the little stuffed rabbit that we brought to her and that she clasped in her hands the whole way home. At first our parenthood was really hard work, since the girl, at 18 months of age, only knew one word, 'auntie', and we had to teach her to walk, but we managed to make up for all the delays and, when our daughter started going to the day care at the age of 3 1/2, no one noticed any signs of her earlier condition.

It is true that the entrance of a little being into our family interfered a bit with our previous carefree life. We could not go to the cinema, theatre, or to the gym whenever we wanted. But one cannot have everything. We were happy that we were finally a family, that the little girl was making progress, and that she was helping us forget about the failures of my treatment and helping me to relax mentally.

As our daughter was growing up, a thought started to surface that we might try one more attempt at IVF. So, at the age of 33, I underwent one more attempt at in vitro fertilisation. Unfortunately, it did not turn out well, but thanks to our daughter, we did not take the IVF failure tragically at all. Finally, I became reconciled to the fact that the desire for our own child would remain unfulfilled for us.

All of a sudden, a miracle happened. A month after the unsuccessful IVF attempt I became pregnant. I learned about the pregnancy in the sixth week when I went to see the doctor, thinking that I had a cyst. Probably the previous hormonal treatment and the fact that I was mentally relaxed helped. It is true that during the full period of my pregnancy I was more careful and easy on myself than is usual in normal pregnancies. I gave up sports and horse riding immediately. I was afraid I might lose the baby. I was glad for each day when the pregnancy went normally and that brought us closer to the birth of the child. Then, after 11 years, the wonderful day came when we finally held our second daughter in our hands.

And so, after a long time of treatment and mental suffering, we are the happy parents of two little girls who give us much joy.

John

Do not expect any 'story-telling' from me. I do not 'do' stories and parables—not even in communication with my wife. It is difficult for me to recall specific feelings, things that I mind(ed) or that I enjoy(ed), since 'nothing is a problem', right? I live for a goal, for facts, for a system, for order, for the present day. I do not remember what happened, for example, on December 9th, 1998 and how I felt at that time. From my viewpoint, it is not essential! In communication I prefer three minutes on a mobile phone or three sentences by e-mail (facts, procedure, information, performance, target behaviour, system). In the dictionary you will probably find my picture next to the words pragmatism and flexibility. But, fortunately, there are also other words next to it as well.

I will confess to you that, even when writing these lines, I consider the effort to write down this testimony a waste of time—no offence. But I understand that there is a big percentage of people in the population whose personality is completely the opposite of mine and for whom the book with my testimony can be a help in their search for a solution. That is why I continue. Men of similar character—and that is the majority, will probably not read the text. If it is meant for them at all. You can put my name with my address and phone number in the book—I have no problem with that.

I already thought about the fact that I wanted children before the wedding—a natural desire for leaving something to posterity. Gradually, as years have gone by, my opinions shifted, and now they have the character of perceiving the complexity related to raising a child.

When my wife kept miscarrying, I did not take it tragically. I see the problem not as a female one but as a personal or, if you want, an individual one. This is probably caused by the fact that everybody who is concerned with it must cope with it on his or her own. I do not accept problems, life itself is a problem. I place goals before myself, and achieve them. The problems that life brings are not problems in the true sense of the word. They are the conditions of life, of existence, that have been set in advance.

After you have passed through approximately 20 semesters of university statistics in Masters and Doctoral study programs, understood the theory of probability, the theory of games, the theory of catastrophes, the behaviour of biological systems, the theory of stability, the theory of systems, etc., you cannot come to the conclusion that things are not working out or to assess a situation as unsolvable, definite. And not even in situations which 99.9% of the population would assess as definitive. The probability that a specific couple will have a child is different in each couple, and the only question is what options the couple have at their disposal, and, above all—and that is the most important part—what effort they are willing to make to increase this probability.

The fact that there are more and more couples with a reduced probability of giving birth to a child (if we consider the historical data during roughly the last 100 years and compare them with the situation of most couples today) is probably a consequence of the radical transformation of human society and, mainly, of lifestyle over the past 50 years. Personally, then, I do not see the situation as abnormal, but natural. In the next 20 years, we will have to reconcile ourselves to the fact that the effort that couples will have to make to give birth to a child will be very different from what is considered as normal today. (Our poor children!) But it will perhaps still be true in this area that, if you try for something systematically and in a goal-oriented way, when you make a statistically significant number of attempts and try the available and morally acceptable possibilities, you will achieve the goal.

If we take into account all the briefly sketched connections, then you will probably agree with me that the period for which one keeps trying to have a child cannot be temporally limited from above, for instance by the age of the couples. The opinions of the type 'we have tried everything' are erroneous. In the better case they express the attitude of a couple that want to show that the effort that they would have to make would not be adequate for the result. I see going through at least most of today's possibilities as a life-long task (if it is the journey that a childless couple should go through). The fact that nowadays childless couples undergo a certain treatment or therapy and expect to be successful in three months is arrogant in my view.

As can be seen, it is not essential what examinations, where and how many childless couples undergo, but if they succeed in finding the factor (influence) that essentially and significantly influences the conception or the birth of a child, and that is today still just an accident in a significant percentage of the population. The birth of a child is hence a miracle.

I consider myself a stalwart Catholic. I reject in principle the techniques of assisted reproduction, and I believe that I can talk in this respect on behalf on my wife as well, and we have never considered them! My wife and I do not want to recommend them to anyone, and we are, in principle, against them. If some childless couples are convinced that IVF is morally acceptable for them, I am sorry for them! We want children, but not at any cost! The reasons that have led my wife and me to this conviction are very personal, firm, and reasonable.

I have not yet thought about another solution to the situation—adoption. But I have searched out information related to it.

I was not influenced in my experiencing of the situation and the choice of the solution by my surroundings, family, friends, neighbours, or my employer. I am so strong a personality that I influence the surroundings more than the surroundings influence me. But the treatment is greatly dependent on the doctor, that is why we went through several of them until we were satisfied. For me, personally, the decisive element was whether I gained the impression that the doctor's effort to find the causal factor would be adequate to the time spent, the number of attempts undertaken and, above all, the effort we exerted.

Of course, as every situation has its drawbacks and its advantages, there occurred a certain development, a shift, in our relationship, including the sexual aspects. But generally I have a good feeling about it in the spirit of the saying 'what does not kill you will make you stronger'.

My wife's behaviour deserves a 'Cum Laude' diploma. For me it has been a form of compensation for the lack of interest she showed in going to college. During the eight years of our quest, I have left the solution of the situation entirely up to her! Not because it was a female problem, but because finally there was a serious nut to crack for her and it was necessary to make an effort for its solution comparable to the one required for the completion of a college degree. The essential part is not the academic title but whether one has moved forward in terms of personality, knowledge, and intellect. The field is not important. The fact remains that, if I had taken up resolving the situation myself, I would probably not have been more successful; finding the causal factor is still to a large degree accidental. The quicker and the more options you try, the more probable it is that you will succeed. It is the same as with handing in more lottery tickets, with the difference that, on principle, I do not play lotteries because of the low probability of winning. For some childless couples, having their own child is as improbable as the lottery, but the winning is always worth it.

My wife's experience is another thing. Our characters are, to a large degree, opposite. The result of this difference is also a different understanding of experiences by the other. But I am convinced that, over the years, we have been able to overcome this character difference, and to such a degree that we now understand each other in every respect.

How have we resolved the problem? We have a healthy child. I perceive it with a feeling of victory! It means a commitment to the future, responsibility, joy, worry...

Jane

I am going to tell you a story that I have lived through during my eight-year-long marriage.

My boyfriend and I wanted to live together so we got married. I was 20 and my husband was one year older. My husband still had another three years of university studies ahead of him, so we agreed to wait for a while before having children; first for financial reasons, and second so that we could enjoy and raise the children together.

About half a year after the wedding, I became pregnant. My husband and I were surprised but at the same time happy that we would have a baby. The joy did not last long because I miscarried in the 10th week of the pregnancy. It was a serious blow because the pregnancy proceeded without complications and I felt well when pregnant. We had to accept the situation. Even the doctor in the hospital calmed me down, 'one miscarriage, no miscarriage, you are still very young and you can catch up with everything.'

Three years later, I became pregnant again, and I felt some anxiety, what if I miscarried again. In the ninth week, I was told that the fetus corresponded in size to the sixth week, and that the heart was not beating. My gynaecologist recommended hospitalisation and the necessary intervention.

I refused it. I felt fine, and the symptoms of miscarriage did not show. A thought occurred to me, what if they made a mistake and the child was alive. I waited several days. Then problems started and I had to go to the hospital. The ultrasound again confirmed the end of pregnancy. I was very sad about another failure but I was peaceful that they did not take away a living child. I remember that I felt fit soon after the operation. I was kept going by the hope that nothing was finished. Everything would be solved by an examination that would reveal the cause of the miscarriages. And so the phase of searching started. I underwent hysteroscopy (an examination of the womb under complete anaesthesia). Together with my husband, we underwent genetic examinations, but no problem was found. Everything was fine. The strong optimism that I had had until then started to slowly disappear. I found out that it would not be as easy as I had thought. I started to think in a negative way. I began to be afraid of the next pregnancy and worried that we could have a handicapped child.

This period lasted about half a year. It was devastating me, and I suffered until I said, 'Stop, I cannot live in this way, being afraid all the time.' I was trying to erase the word pregnancy and everything that was linked with it from my subconscious. My husband and I agreed that we would wait before trying again. In between, I was pulling together strength for another attempt. The doctor prescribed some hormonal tablets for me so that the next pregnancy would be of quality. I remember that I started doing the Mojzis exercises, we also went to the sea—all of that so that I could carry the child for the full term of pregnancy and give birth to a healthy child.

A third pregnancy followed, again problems and the necessity of hospitalisation. I thought it was the end again. But the ultrasound examination showed that the child was growing and the heart was beating. My husband and I were happy and we had hope. The problem was in the separated placenta. So I stayed in the hospital for a while. The doctors gave me a lot of attention. I had an ultrasound check-up every fourth or fifth day, literally with my nerves in tatters. I expected to hear the painful news that had dug into my heart twice already. Everything was fine, even the placenta. I was happy and I started believing that it would succeed, now for the third time. They let me go home for a weekend. My husband looked after me very well. He cooked, brought me food in bed, he kept asking whether I needed anything, he even carried me in his arms to the toilet. I returned to the hospital and in about two days the ultrasound showed the end of pregnancy. Another painful blow.

I thought I would not be able to cope with it any longer. But, thanks to my closest family, friends, and faith in God, I pulled myself out of it. The feelings in my soul were very, very painful. I often experienced anxiety, sadness, I felt inferior, I was oversensitive, suffered from insomnia, nothing gave me joy, I felt injured, especially when I heard the news that someone close was expecting a baby; I was envious and jealous. I know these are not virtues, but I could not command my heart for a certain period.

There were periods when I minded childlessness horribly. I needed to complain, to pity myself and cry it out. My husband would hug me at that time and he often said 'but you have me' (but it could not be too often, he did not like to see me in tears). I would like to add that he never reproached me that we did not have children. He never blamed me that I was the guilty party.

In half a year, there was another pregnancy and another miscarriage. The doctor did not recommend another pregnancy. He suggested a year-long hormonal treatment and a genetic examination. There was a year-long break and because I could not wait in idleness, I started to look for the cause by myself. My husband left the search up to me (it was sometimes very difficult), but he underwent all the examinations very willingly. I arranged a comprehensive endocrinological examination for both of us, I underwent a month-long treatment in the spa, I asked women who had had similar problems and had children now about their treatment and examinations, I read various articles on the topic of infertility and the tendency to miscarry, we saw a psychologist with whom I needed to discuss my feelings and states. We discovered a contact for the immunobiological laboratory where we both had another comprehensive examination.

In this way it was confirmed that the problem was really in me. Another treatment started. This lasted a year and a half. Sometimes, I felt as if driven by a certain force, that everything was going along easily. The strong will, hope and discovering new possibilities in what we can still try. Sometimes I collapsed in the midst of everything and felt like giving up. Soon after this, I was terrified by the state of doing nothing.

The thought of adoption came to my mind. But we almost did not speak about it at all with my husband. We were not convinced that we truly wanted this option. I did not undergo IVF treatment, my husband and I are not proponents.

How did the winding and steep path of the quest end up? After all the effort we were given the highest reward! The fifth pregnancy led to a successful end in 2001, the birth of our healthy daughter.

I thank all who have helped us to become parents—happy parents!

Margaret

I will try to tell you my story. Some events are painful even years later, that is why I have chosen to tell it in the third person. I need to gain a certain distance and orient myself toward the future, of course a great one…

Margaret was born in the early 1960s. Her parents looked forward to her arrival a lot—they wanted their first child to be a little girl. At the age of eight months, she handled the transfer into the day care centre, and her mother could, though unwillingly, return to work.

Two years passed and another baby announced itself. Margaret was looking forward to it a lot, and she chose a name for it after her first best friend. The girl was born, got the name, but the disappointment: 'so little, I thought that she would play with me!' Margaret was three years old, she grew to love her sister, admired the tender little baby, and later she imagined that this was her baby and she was her Mommy. 'When I grow up, I will also have a baby,' she used to say proudly. She knew she would have to wait a long time, but no one suspected how long and painful the waiting would be.

After the summer holidays of 1971, Margaret's little sister started first grade. With school attendance, a series of illnesses started: pain in the joints, high temperature, high sedimentation levels, loads of drugs. The parents were desperate, the diagnosis uncertain. In the end, her health stabilised and she successfully finished the first year. But the joints stayed swollen, the body weakened. Margaret worried, she helped her sister as much as she could: she carried her bag, they read and counted together. For a year and a half she spent most weekends in hospital hallways, the strict regulations prohibited her visiting the room. At least she sent notes, drew pictures, she even wrote a book. Her mother was successful in arranging an unpaid leave of absence, so she travelled every day across the city to the hospital, and she returned tired in the evening. One day, Margaret returned from school and found out that both her parents were in the hospital with her sister. She stayed with an aunt for the afternoon. Dad and Mom came home by a taxi, in tears and broken—the little sister died. They both held her hand. In two weeks, it was supposed to be her eighth birthday and her mom's 40th birthday… How come? Our little girl…she could not even cry in the first days. Everybody stayed at home and talked quietly about suffering and redemption.

Margaret decided she would give only joy to her parents. She threw herself into studying. In her class, she was considered a swot [studied excessively], she and her schoolmates did not understand each other. She loved playing with small children, she could entertain them and teach them something. She was accepted at a grammar school, and she came out of her reserved attitude and successfully passed the finals. The university entrance exams for were very hard work, she waited for the results for three weeks. She was admitted, her parents cheered. In the study group, there was a good group of friends, they lived through days of intense studying for the exams as well as days full of fun on skiing trips in the mountains, summer courses, and parties...

Among her schoolmates from the elementary school, there were already mothers. From time to time, Margaret would meet them, walk with the pram, and dream about her motherhood. She knitted and sewed baby clothes for her own children.

In the first year, she met a nice man at a college party. The next year, they started seeing each other regularly. She was full of optimism after a long time. She was successful at school, she had a great summer holiday at the Baltic Sea, and in winter she went to the mountains. The first year of working was also devoted to further studies. The goal was the special qualification examination. They were divided by many kilometres, they saw each other irregularly. After four years of partnership, they decided to get married. Margaret got married exactly one month after successfully completing the state exam. She was happy. But the next 10 years resembled a crazy ride on a roller coaster. The chair raced into horrible depths far too often.

For a whole year after the wedding, they did not live together. Margaret stayed in her native city, her husband travelled around the country with a geophysical group. They sometimes met up in the city. Margaret was already 25 years old but, under these conditions, she kept postponing her pregnancy. She decided to leave the city and they started renovating the house where her grandparents used to live. The following year, they started living there together. The work on the house had advanced, she felt more at home there. They planned to start a family, but motherhood was not coming. The candidates for grandmothers and grandfathers became uncertain but they did not interfere in the life of 'the young people'. Two years passed and nothing happened. She told herself it was a question of time and no stress. At a rehabilitation centre, she learned about the Mojzis exercises she practised. Her husband started his own business and invested his first profit into an internship trip. He left for three months to go the

USA. It was 1991 (a nice year for the birth of a first child), and they had lived together for three years. They went on a holiday to the sea to Spain for the first time and planned for the future. But everything turned out differently.

As she was nearing 30, she was struck by the news about her mother's illness. Indigestion, jaundice and it turned out to be pancreatic cancer. The doctor told them that death was only a matter of time. Her mother expressed the fear that she would not live to see her only daughter's children. It was decided: they had to start treatment as soon as possible. Immediately, they made an appointment at the centre for reproduction medicine. After that they spent several hours every month in a crowded waiting room among sad and terrified women. They went through various examinations, but the cause of failure was not found. The doctor was full of wit and optimism, but time was passing by too quickly. Her mother improved after the first surgery, but not for long. At the same time, the reconstruction work in the small house started in full while they were living there: living, business, and reconstruction all at the same time. She found herself between several millstones: the treatment for infertility, her ill mother, her lonely father, her job, problematic construction. She underwent two examinations with hospitalisation: HSG (x-ray of the womb and fallopian tubes) and laparoscopy. Her mother visited her in the hospital and gave her courage. None of the interventions determined the cause of failure. The recommendation was: conservative treatment, idiopathic sterility. And time was passing. She regularly went to the consultation room, always passing the door with the sign 'Obstetrics' and asking the question: When shall I get there? Her mother had another operation ahead of her, the illness was progressing. The second surgery was followed by crises and two hospitalisations. Margaret continued to commute to work (to teach 'strange' children), and she proceeded with the reconstruction of the house. She wanted to manage and achieve more, but how? Why can we not have children, and why is mother being eaten up by a tumour? Soon I will be 31 and I had foolishly planned to have three children before 30.

Then there occurred what she had sensed subconsciously: her husband expressed his fear that she was taking care of her mother too hard, and under those circumstances they could not become parents. Fortunately, he said this only once and for the last time. Later he was very helpful and supportive. The Christmas of 1993 was approaching; her mother was in hospital, her sister-in-law, younger by six years, had a four-month-old son in her arms—the pressure was increasing. There was a breakthrough in the ongoing treatment. Margaret was transferred to the care of the doctors in the IVF team. Finally the ice moved. If only her mother could live to see her pregnancy, but time was short. She longed for children, twins would have been best, and no matter if from a test-tube. Things got going: blood collection and the determination of hormonal levels. The next cycle of hormonal stimulation was followed by insemination. January 1994: a successful stimulation, the results of the ultrasound exam determined 'the day'. The next month the procedure was repeated. Her mother was now in their house, her father was no longer capable of providing care on his own. The worsening of her mother's health made them request hospitalisation...employment, stimulation, commuting to see mother. On February 17th, the insemination was carried out. At the same time, 45 miles away, mother died. But new life did not arise. Not even three months later after the same procedure. They took a break, they went to the sea, she tried mud baths in a spa. Without success, without hope.

Almost three years had passed since her mother's departure. They travelled around the world, especially after Margaret left the sphere of education. A year earlier, she got into the IVF program. The stimulation ended up brilliantly, also the collection of eggs. It must come off this time! It did not! Not even one egg was fertilised. In half a year they got prepared for another IVF cycle. The stimulation worked, the response of the body was appropriate, the collection of oocytes was successful. Two were fertilised, but died. Nature made a mistake: they had three sets of chromosomes instead of two. In the fall of 1996, the third cycle was approaching. Therefore, they postponed an attractive trip to South Africa. The IVF cycle was postponed, it would have interfered with the Christmas holiday. The January cycle was more successful, finally they got to the transfer of embryos. Their expectations were blown apart by the news about her father's illness: a tumour in the pancreas. Again? Unbelievable! Her husband was getting ready for the expedition to South Africa, he was hesitating about leaving. But they agreed that he should take advantage of the opportunity and fly out. Her father was able to cope with the illness for two weeks. Then hospitalisation was necessary. The surgeons refused surgery. Margaret was again drowning in tears and the question: why? In the end, she arranged a place for the father in another hospital where they agreed to do surgery. The operation was successful, but the postoperative care ended too soon. Her husband returned one week earlier from his travels so that he could help her. At the hospital, people did not behave well at all. Her father grew weaker and the doctors had written him off. After talking with her husband, she managed to get the doctors' agreement to take her father home. It was

Easter, Christians were celebrating Christ's resurrection. The miracle was not repeated. She was desperate and did not get enough sleep. Instead of looking after a baby, she was looking after someone else. How can she cradle and bathe this little old man? For the first time she went to buy disposable diapers, but not for her baby. The hopeful Easter recovery was marred by pneumonia. The ninth day of his stay, her Father died at home and surrounded by his loved ones.

After the departure of her sister, mother and father, the pathway into the landscape of her childhood was shut. She found herself in a desert with no relationships: no one in the past generation, emptiness in the present, and the next generation does not yet exist… She ended her sadness by a stay abroad. She and her husband flew to an island in the Mediterranean in the beginning of summer. She sunbathed on the beach, observed the families with children, again she dreamt about her own children and critically assessed the behaviour of actual mothers. She thought that she would be a great mother: smiling, patient, devoted. She was soon to understand that theory and practice were quite different categories.

She started preparing a journal for childless couples, she accepted invitations to the radio and television. During the negotiations, she felt a certain curiosity and embarrassment in her counterparts. As if they were looking for some clearly visible signs of sterility in her, some difference. The fourth attempt at IVF followed, this time it was supposed to proceed according to a more complicated scheme. She went through all the hurdles up to the collection of oocytes. Only six items were capable of fertilisation. The doctors were not very optimistic. In two days, she was told she should come for the transfer. That was an unexpected success! And the shock when they were told that they have five! beautiful healthy embryos. The first week after the transfer, she lay in bed at home and hummed the chant: little babies, I am your mommy. There were still two long weeks that separated her from real success. Even the second week proceeded well, and the summer was so pleasant. They entered into the third week, and tension was growing: will she live to see D day and the pregnancy tests, or will the hope flow away in menstruation blood?. The date of the check-up at the clinic drew near, she examined her body, but she did not find an answer. She could not differentiate the symptoms of a possible pregnancy from the reaction to the hormone injections. At the doctor's, everything happened very quickly. The nurse told her immediately that the test was positive. And so the accidental witnesses knew about her pregnancy sooner than her husband, who was kept out for a while due to a phone call. The doctor congratulated them and prescribed other injections. She had an appointment for ultrasound in another 14 days. The tension remained, she must wait until the time when the screen shows the beating heart, or hearts? The ultrasound exam, where her husband was also present, showed that there were two embryos nested in the womb! A picture to remember, a healthcare recommendation, and off we went home. An unexpected turnabout: four months ago she buried the last member of her family, and now two new members announced themselves! What would her parents say? She kept asking now and many times later. The pregnancy proceeded fine, she underwent various tests and interventions until the hospitalisation before the birth. In the Bastille (this was the nickname that the women gave to the rooms with windows leading toward a wall where it was dark even during the day) she passed the 25 days before the birth of the children. They had known since mid-way in the pregnancy that they would have twins. They arrived two days before the planned date. When she woke up after the drugs wore off, she focused her eyes on the tag by her bed, she could read that the boy measured 49 cm, 47 cm and they were both healthy weights. The nurse brought both babies later. The boy slept, the girl blinked, they did not look alike at all and they looked differently from the way she had imagined. Everything always turns out differently, and will even in the future. On the day of the birth of the twins, it was exactly 11 months after her father's departure. What more can we say?

Soon the twins will be celebrating their fourth birthday. The first two years were not easy at all. The moments of relaxation and happiness were paid for in perspiration. She was mistaken when she had thought that she would manage everything by herself. She had to admit that she was not the perfect mommy she had dreamed about, and the children were not angels either. The arrival of longed-for children is not a panacea for all pains. And now, when we have what we wanted, we like to remember the quiet moments when it was just the two of us. Simply a normal family.

Dominique

My husband and I got married after three years of living together. We had counted on adoption already before the wedding. Not that we would not want to have our own children, but with regards to my basic illness—type 1 diabetes—we decided, I think reasonably, for adoption. Why give birth to a child when there is a good chance that it would not be healthy? I always wanted to have a big family, at least three children. And, with the oncoming years, I feel this even more. Children are a joy, of course also a worry, but mainly it is a natural desire.

Foolishly, we thought that adoption would be a very simple and unequivocal thing. That there are reasons of health that more or less prevent us from conceiving our own child, that we are non-problematic people, that we have a very good relationship. Our extended family is entirely fine, and is acquainted with our situation and our intention to adopt a child. Our parents are healthy people who are looking forward to grandchildren and certainly would be able, when necessary, to help us with the upbringing. Not the least thing is that we are financially quite secure.

After we put together all the necessary documents, a long wait started when you cannot do anything at all. You cannot defend yourself; you can only keep silent and blindly wait. A year and a half later, we received a statement that our application was declined. Paradoxically, for reasons of health—it said that it was probable that, in the future, I would have more health problems and that I already had a disability pension. When people hear that someone is disabled, they usually imagine a person who is not independent, not self-sufficient. That need not be always true. Definitely not in my case. I have no troubles that would prevent me from normal life. When I went on disability, I was significantly worse off. I have had diabetes for 17 years and, after such a long time, even when you follow the doctor's recommendations, complications might start. Then a little increased physical activity is enough, and what would never happen to a healthy person can happen to a diabetic. Both of my retinas became detached, and I was almost blind. But now, after several operations, I can see again. I have stayed on disability because nowadays it is difficult even for a healthy person to find a job and I, despite all of my normality, need certain conditions for my work. I have a secondary school education with specialisation in economics, so I would probably mostly work with a computer. But I must take care of my eyes, and I cannot focus all day on the screen. I work on the PC at home, but only for an hour, at most two hours, then I go and do something in the garden, for instance. I tried to work three years ago, but unfortunately, I had to leave after a month because I could not cope with the exertion. In the evening, my eyes were so tired that they filled with tears and I almost could not see. Unfortunately, the adoption assessment doctor used all this against me in his evaluation of the application for adoption. According to him, since I am unable to work, I am unable to bring up a child. A doctor, who has not seen me at all in my life, just read the brief reports and declined the application wholesale. Even though my optometrist did not have any objection and even though my GP also agreed with the application. Of course, we filed an appeal against the refusal but it did not turn out well for us either.

We submitted another application not quite a year ago. A week ago our second application was declined. We did not have any special requirements for the child, we wanted an older child (pre-school), not an infant because we knew that looking after a baby would be very demanding. We would have even accepted a child with certain health problems and a child of any ethnicity. We wanted to adopt the child or have it in foster care. We stated this in both applications. Now, with the second refusal, we have found out by accident that the possibility of foster care was not taken into account at all. To file an appeal against the refusal is probably our last hope.

My husband and I are taking it very hard. We always wanted to have several children, and now it looks as if we are going to stay alone. I have always said that, if you have a big reason to live (and a child is a big reason), you can achieve incredibly much. I must admit that my state of health is greatly influenced by my psychological wellbeing. The first refusal devastated me, and I could not recover for a whole year. And I think I have still not completely adjusted to it. And now they have declined for the second time. We feel is as a great injustice. Nobody in the world can know what is going to happen to him or her tomorrow, but already a number people 'know' that we are incapable of looking after a child. A worker in the local centre told me 'off the record' that, if we had 10 of our own children and one of us became seriously ill, nobody would hesitate about our ability to bring up the children, but even one adoptive child is a problem. At the beginning, we thought that adoption was not a problem, that it was a sure thing.

Now we are trying, perhaps out of despair, for our own child. We would want it a lot but, at the same time, we are afraid. I have miscarried twice, and that testifies to something. Probably my body does not want it.

We are not giving up so far, but our strength is vanishing. So far the alternative of a life without children is, at least for me, unacceptable.

Dominic

When I met my wife Dominique, I did not think much about the future—not even about starting a family. Our plans did not have a concrete shape, we simply liked being together, and that was enough.

After about two years of seeing each other, I left for a year abroad. Even before my return I started thinking about a common future with Dominique. Yes, at that time marriage and family seemed to me a self-evident continuation of our relationship. A year later we got married.

Of course, I knew about Dominique's health condition and I did not see it as a problem—we had talked about adoption and that was not an obstacle for me. I did not take the first refusal of the application tragically, especially after Dominique and I decided to try to have our own child despite the risks. But when Dominique lost the baby for the first time in the first weeks of pregnancy, I was not so much at peace any longer.

Today, I know that certain things that seemed to me matter-of-fact a few years ago are not so easy. But I think that it is possible to go on living fully. During our quest for a child, we have learned about other possibilities in the care for children than just adoption or foster care. If not even the second application for adoption turns out well, and if we fail to have our own child, we will definitely try other ways of taking care of children, even if short-term ones (for instance to take a child from the children's home for a weekend or for a summer holiday).

Dominique probably feels the impact of all this is a bit more strongly than I do, but that is probably women's fate. But, through our common strength, we will definitely manage to handle all the difficult periods of in our life together.

Marie

I met my husband in 1995, I was 20 and he 25. After four months of dating, we started living together. Of course we thought about a child, but because we lived in our first rented apartment, we did not want to bring a child into uncertain conditions. In the course of time, we moved again and again, until we finally settled down in our little apartment. Then we started furnishing the apartment, we told ourselves repeatedly that the little one must come into a finished place, we wanted comfort and quiet for him or her. When we furnished the apartment and got married three years later, we thought that this was the awaited time to start a family.

My husband comes from a family of four children, I only of two, but we have many nieces and nephews. So we are surrounded by children. It seemed a matter of course to have our own, and we looked forward to it very much. But what a disappointment when I gave up birth control—I had been on it for eight years—and I did not become pregnant. We knew that it could take a few of months so we were patient and kept trying again and again. We got advice from others about how to do it and of course we laughed at this advice but the worm started gnawing, and we felt that something was not right. When I did not become pregnant after half a year, people told me that it was normal after such a long time of taking contraceptives.

But, after a year, it no longer seemed normal to us. We started searching for the cause. First, I had gynaecological examinations, everything came off fine, so they sent us to have a spermiogram. We were told that we should collect a sample early in the morning and bring it to a specialist. It was November, my husband had the flu (no one warned us about that) and we went to the specialist with the sample (it was in my purse, not in my bra, at body temperature, as I learned it should have been later on). The waiting room was shared by several doctors' offices and, when after a long wait, our doctor opened the door, he called across the waiting room, 'Come in, sir! So apparently you are not able to have a family!' At that moment, we were downright ashamed. My husband said later that he would never go there again, only somewhere different. The result was bad. The gynaecologist sent us on to in vitro fertilisation. There, after all the tests, they sent us for a genetic examination because my husband has a congenital eye defect. The elderly doctor was very pleasant and tried to help throughout the visit. But the younger doctor shocked me. After all the tests and genetic examinations I had to come alone (I think I needed my husband there at least psychologically, it is a matter of the whole couple). To my question how the genetic examination turned out, he answered with surprise: 'You want to have a child with your husband?' (It sounded as if he doubted I was normal.) My answer was: 'Of course, and why not?' He shook his head and said that the child could inherit the defect. I need to add that it is possible to treat the defect nowadays—we found this out from a specialist—which I told him. But the conclusion was: they cannot transfer hereditary defects, the risk multiplies. The solution was donation of sperm.

After a discussion with my husband, who, instead of a refusal comforted me that anyway he would be the father because he would raise the child, we agreed with insemination by donor's sperm. I admit I was afraid that he was doing it only so that I would not be unhappy. That probably occurs to every woman. And I was afraid that he could reproach me for that one day. That is why I left the decision up to him. So I went through the hormonal stimulation. On the second attempt I asked, 'Why do I not have eggs in one fallopian tube?' I was told again that first we would try a few attempts and then they would send me to have an examination of the fallopian tubes. That should be done, in my opinion, right during the preliminary examinations. We are not lacking in terms of money, we would give everything for a child, but now I felt like a guinea pig, which I also said to the doctor. Since both attempts came off badly—I started menstruation, vomited, and I got cramps—this was not a good indication, I felt horrible, I went to the gynaecologist again. I asked whether this was normal, and he said yes, that sometimes even hospitalisation was necessary. I thought that I was weak and I could not stand anything, I was psychologically depressed. When I asked my husband what next, he said I must decide myself, that he could not force me into anything.

Making a decision was difficult but in the end it was for the good: to stop in vitro fertilisation, and either adopt, or try for a natural pregnancy. Perhaps it sounded egoistic, sometimes I felt I was a weakling and could not bear anything; that if I wanted a child I had to bear everything. That was also the opinion of other people. But I did not want to place the household on my husband's shoulders and have him take care of me—if I were in hospitals all the time or at home but unable to do anything. He is very good and helps me a lot but I am not probably the kind of girl who would immediately exploit this. My husband fortunately stood by me in my decision, and in the end he told me he was glad—about my ending the IUI—because he did not like to see how it devastated me.

It is interesting but it was he who first came up with the suggestion of adoption. I thought about it in my soul, before the wedding we had even planned to have two of our own children and one adopted, but I did not have the courage to say it out aloud at that moment to force him into adoption. I know from what I hear around me what the opinion of some men is about adoption. And I need to add that we are not believers. We came across this question very often because in our society people are accustomed that only believers adopt children or take them into foster care. My husband encouraged me to go ahead and get the papers at the office. This time we did not say anything to anybody because, with the artificial fertilisation, our problems were becoming almost a public matter, even though we did not share everything at work and at home either. In addition, when someone asked, the answer was, 'We still have time enough and we also want to enjoy life.'

Only our closest friends knew about everything and supported us. When we touched on the topic of adoption at work or at home, we were unpleasantly surprised. We often heard 'Don't even consider it, who knows what genes it would have and what a drug addict's or a whore's child may grow up to be'. We went through hell at that time. When we walked through town during that time, we would always meet, as if on purpose, young children or mothers with prams. At work, colleagues became pregnant, we even went to see them at the birth clinic. (My husband and I work in the same workplace.) In the end I did not even want to go to see the last one. I even took a detour around the square to avoid seeing a young child.

Only the nebulous hope of adoption comforted me. As my husband said: 'One of those little bundles there is waiting for us and needs us.'

At the time when we were arranging the forms for adoption—the state of our health, income, personality, criminal record, the visit of a social worker at our home—my husband took me to his acquaintance, a herbalist. At the time of artificial fertilisation, they treated me also for the growth of the endometrium; she examined me and said that I would become pregnant but it would take time. She gave me herbs for cleansing, advice and, surprise, in one year the endometrium grew so well that my gynaecologist thought I was pregnant. (Of course it made no sense to try to tell the doctor stories about herbs.)

After all the forms, a psychological interview was supposed to follow. We went there with anxieties. But we had a pleasant doctor who discussed with us our opinions, the opinions of our friends and acquaintances, of our family. There were questions that we analysed in detail. For instance, 'Have you reconciled yourselves or accepted the fact that you cannot have a child?' We had to think a lot about that. She explained to us that we should not be ashamed that we would adopt a child, that not every couple is capable of accepting a child as one's own, that an adoptive couple would have a more difficult situation than a normal one. And that even we would eventually get into a situation when we would be proud of adopting and being able to make someone happy, to give love and home to a little bundle. These interviews gave us a lot. It even happened that we started looking forward to these meetings, and we analysed the topics at home as well. As time passed, we got to a stage where we were proud of our choice, and we decided to talk about it at the right time to our family and at work.

My family, especially my mom, has a hard skin, but she has a good core, that is why it takes time until she accepts someone into the family. It took her a long time even with my brother-in-law and my husband. Of course, it was a blow to her. Questions like, 'How come you cannot have a child, everybody among us was healthy, it must be from your father's side,' all came up. I said that I was probably an exception and a black sheep, that we would adopt and stand by it, and if she was ashamed of us or was against it, she could break off contact with us. But I said it was purely our matter and decision, that she would not influence it, that we only came to inform her, so that she would know. Perhaps it sounded and still sounds hard, but I truly think it is the couple's decision. My mother understood our decision and she saw that we stood by the matter. Perhaps it helped us a lot that we lived separately, not with our parents. We told our colleagues at work who were at that time going through difficult personal decisions, so they understood us, in the end we even cried together.

The next phase of the preparation for adoption was group therapy, as we called it. That gave us even more because we met not only couples who had similar problems, but also couples who had adopted or fostered children. We exchanged personal experiences, and we dealt with the questions of when to tell the child about the adoption, what to tell him or her in different phases of development, etc. We realised that it was not easy at all to form an opinion about the biological parents. When a psychologist asked me once what I thought of a mother who would leave a child in front of the institution's door, I came, after all the psycho-tests, to something like this: Probably she liked the child so much that she wanted to ensure it had a much better life than she herself had, and wanted her child to be quickly found. If she had not liked the baby, she could have dropped it into a waste bin. But she probably did not want it grow up in the environment where she herself lived at the moment. What mother would willingly give up her child? And thank God for these women who can make us happy. After these meetings, there followed a preparation workshop for those of us who did not have children. That was in the form of lectures, but again one could learn something new.

Perhaps it (the bureaucracy) can seem long to someone, but the authorities and the psychologists have a lot of responsibility when they give a child to us, we are strangers to them at first. I know what I am talking about. I had a grandmother who was an orphan and because, at the time of World War I, there were none of these authorities, she was moved from one foster family to another. In one, they wanted a small child, in another a boy, in another they needed a maid, in the fourth they did it only for the money and treated her—I would rather not go into describing it. Simply, she lived until her death with the knowledge that she was unwanted and bad because she could not stay put anywhere. Her only joy was later with her own children and grandchildren. My husband and I often remembered her story and it strengthened us in our decision.

The preparation climaxed with us being entered into the register of applicants and a weekend stay in the mountains. We all became very close, and we often call each other and exchange experiences and news. We also went for a visit to the infants' home where each of us had their favourite. Our colleagues from work even sent SMS messages asking whether we were going to bring someone home. They became our fans.

After completing all the tests, my mom asked me whether we were serious about it, she said: 'You know Rosie said—she works in a special education school—that the children from children's homes are a horror.' I explained to her that we would have a young child, from the infants' home. But she said: 'You know, Rosie said that the children from the infants' home go into the children's home.' Again I explained to her that if we adopt a child from the infants' home, thereby the child would not have gone through the children's home. But she retorted again: 'You know, Rosie said you should not get into that, that there are the genes.' I could not control myself, and I told her that I was sorry for her if she did not have her own opinion and only listened to what some Rosie said, that I myself was not interested in some Rosie's opinions. She had not experienced what we had gone through, she had not met such superb people and children. I shocked her a lot, I know, but there was no other way. Simply, most people have not lived through our experiences and pains, so they only live from what someone else said. The other question that she asked me was whether we were going to learn something about the biological parents and whether she would know. My answer was that if we learned something we would not tell her or anyone else because they would form a negative opinion and would not take the child as himself or herself. Mom thought a while, but then she understood what I wanted to tell her. She even told me that I had grown older and wiser after all these pains and experiences and that I was more reasonable than my sister who was five years older. With that she shocked me in turn.

So now we both are looking forward to the little one, and I at least try to help couples who have some chance to have their own child. I have taken a course in the treatment of functional female sterility according to Mojzis, and I experience joy and hope together with my patients. But since I am part of the medical staff, I must say that I am much ashamed of the rude and insensitive behaviour of the doctors toward couples with similar problems. Not that I would wish them the same treatment, but they should at least try to place themselves into the shoes and feelings of these couples and imagine what it is like. Probably they should have stricter psycho-tests at the entrance exams for medical school because the actions and behaviour of the doctor is also part of the treatment.

Marianne

Hello Auntie,

> First I must introduce myself. My name is Marianne, I was born this March and I was in the infants' home right from my birth. I have light brown hair and bluish grey little eyes. Thanks to one kind psychologist,

since Monday I have a new Mommy and Daddy, and a shaggy friend Bobby, who looks after me and licks me like his most precious bone.

My Daddy is just crazy about me; on Wednesday he almost did not leave for work. Every day, after my bath, he rubs my back with ointment and today he even fed me once. He is smitten by me! He said he would get a firearms license for me soon, and that he himself would not be able to make a more beautiful princess.

Mommy takes really good care of me. I have beautiful clothes, super nappies, I love it when she bathes me, and she is going to even arrange swimming lessons in the pool starting in September. Mommy is patient with me, when we do exercises on the balloon or when I did not know what it was like to ride in the pram. Do not wonder, I was lying in bed for four months and I did not know what the sun was. But I have gotten used to it now and we go out twice a day. I have made a lot of progress and I have caught up to 80 per cent. I already weigh 6 kilos.

Everybody says that I take after my Mommy when she was young. Mommy has said I should write you because you are writing a book about adoptions, and Mommy has written our story, so for you to know what changes have happened.

See you,

Marianne.

P. S. Mommy had to write this letter because I am not able to write yet and I had to go to sleep. But I trust her fully.

Mirabelle

I am writing my story with joy, and I hope that it provides hope for couples who are undergoing treatment.

Everything started a short time before the wedding. I was 21 years old, I was getting ready for the big event. I was enthusiastically engaged in the preparations, but shortly before the date of the wedding, my body betrayed me. It looked like a blocked spinal column. As a nurse, I had this problem fairly often, but not so intensely. Instead of the wedding hall, I ended up in the hospital, in a lot of pain, and instead of the vow of marriage, from my doctor came the words that I will never forget: that I have a serious bilateral inflammation of the fallopian tubes, and it might be necessary to remove them. All my plans about the wedding and the future dissolved at that moment.

The antibiotics worked, the puss that was caught up in the abdominal cavity was drained by the doctors, the fallopian tubes were left where they should be, and I was released home after a month of treatment. My partner and I knew what trouble the inflammation could cause. Nonetheless, with the awareness of my potential infertility, he married me two months later.

Right after the wedding, I sought out the doctor who led the regional consultation room for infertility and started treatment. Measuring the basal temperatures, noting down the times of our intercourse in a menstruation calendar, exercises according to Mojzis became my daily duty. Also the dates of various examinations and interventions accumulated. In the end, I underwent surgery of the fallopian tubes, which was supposed to remove obstruction from the fallopian tubes, which had grown together due to the inflammation. It was a demanding operation, followed by spa treatment. Nothing helped. I, of course, tried healers as well. I must admit that some of them established the diagnosis very exactly, but that was all.

I started a new job—by coincidence at a gynaecologist's office. Every day, I met pregnant women. Years were passing by and I, of course, suffered because I kept failing. But women who miscarried repeatedly also came to the office. I saw that that was the real suffering—the hope, several months of uncertainty, and then tragedy! I realised that mine was actually not such a bad case. Thanks to the new job, I had a chance to learn a great deal about infertility and its treatment. I started thinking about in vitro fertilisation and soon I made an appointment in one of the two centres of artificial fertilisation at that time. They set a date for me—in two years! For years I had gynaecological problems—painful intercourse, cysts, inflammations, and mycoses—because of that first inflammation.

My husband and I submitted an application for adoption, we both desired a child, and any way to it seemed good to us. We underwent all the meetings and psychological examinations, sometimes unpleasant and humiliating. Similar to other couples, we were carefully examined, first individually: how we are doing in our marriage, what our relationships in the family and at work are like. Some questions were very intimate. The group meetings that followed were supposed to suggest what problems the applicants can expect to encounter in adoption, and how to solve them. That is certainly useful. When we submitted the application for adoption, we stated that the child (possibly children, siblings) that we were interested in should be as young as possible, white and could have a slight health disability. Of course, a child is not goods, but this had to be stated in the questionnaire. I felt that, during the group meetings, the social workers were trying to work on the applicants so that they could lower their requirements. Otherwise, they would get the impression that the concerned couple were not seriously interested and would not deserve the child. I admit that we did not find the courage to look after [an ethnic] child or a seriously disabled one. I have a great deal of respect for anyone who has that courage. And I wish all the disabled children such parents. Then our employers had to write an assessment. We passed, the last thing was to wait three or more years.

In the meantime, the term for the IVF drew near. I learned that the team that specialised in artificial fertilisation was leaving my hospital. I made an appointment again in the new centre. This time, I did not have to wait so long until they put me in the programme. Stimulations and transfers succeeded, but not the pregnancy. The result of the first attempt was marred by the flu, the second attempt by mental stress. The treatment, commuting, and the frequent absences at work—even though taken from the time of my regular holidays—were too demanding, not only for me, but also for my employer. I had to choose. I gave up my job, which I liked a lot and I became unemployed.

The third attempt was coming up, and I did not want to leave any room for accident. Only now could I handle in peace the demanding commuting to the far-away centre of assisted reproduction. I had the advantage that I could apply the injections myself. At least no one saw my distorted face after the hormone injections (she who has not experienced it will not understand). During stimulation, after the 10th day of the cycle, I had to go 95 miles for the blood collections and to manage this by 8 a.m. We did not have a car at that time, and the connections were complicated. After the blood collection, I had to wait until the afternoon for the results and for the ultrasound. And this several times in a row, until the doctor was satisfied with the number and the size of the eggs. Then their collection followed under short anaesthesia then their fertilisation by my husband's sperm. Then a stay in the city until the second day was prescribed because of possible complications. For several days, we called daily to see whether the embryos were ripe for transfer. It was not until the fourth day that they implanted the embryos in my womb. They gave me further hormonal injections to take home with me and a date when I should come back in case my menstruation did not arrive. I admit that, in the first two attempts, I did not stick it out and did the pregnancy tests myself prematurely; their positive result was influenced by the hormonal drugs. This increased the disappointment when menstruation arrived with several days of delay. I held out in the third attempt.

Eight years of suffering and waiting was nothing in comparison to the endless 10 or 15 minutes spent waiting for the results of the pregnancy test. All the emotions and tears that had accumulated in me during the years came out in full when the nurse told me that the test was positive! But nothing was won yet. The pregnancy was complicated, and also the birth. But eventually we had a baby girl.

In about the sixth month of pregnancy, the social worker called to tell me that they had two siblings for us. I explained to her that the situation had changed, but that our interest in adoption continued even if we had our own child. But that was not possible as there were too many applicants. So we withdrew our application.

I think that my infertility meant an opportunity for me: an opportunity to get to know myself, my husband. It changed our life; we stopped making plans, we became more patient. But it did not change our desire for a child. On the contrary. We tried it once again three years later. There were three frozen embryos left from the first attempt. I underwent the transfer in a state of a complete mental relaxation. Now we have a three-month-old baby boy and a four-year-old daughter. In fact they are twins. Thanks to my infertility I can truly enjoy them.

Martha

That it would be long struggle and last 25 years—one human generation—I could not have suspected. That it would be without result, I fortunately did not know.

I can describe it poetically—it was like other paths—sometimes straight, sometimes taking a turn, sometimes up the hill, sometimes down the hill, sometimes it disappeared, sometimes it appeared again.

I was 23 years old and about to graduate from college and, for the last year and a half, I had been under the care of an allocated school gynaecologist, a rather elderly woman. I had something gynaecologically enigmatic; she tried all possible diagnoses, examinations, drugs, I even underwent a very humiliating examination for gonorrhoea: how ashamed I was that I had to go there, let alone have it! I was young and inexperienced and had no good advice. After two years, I ended up on sick leave, again and again prolonged, which stated that my condition was not improving, is it was getting worse and that I should come back next week. I felt like a squirrel in a cage.

When I return to the reasons why I do not have children, this is where it started. It is not understandable to me that a physician with long working experience could not discover that my problem was endometriosis, and that I did not have much time. Also, my silliness and total trust in the doctor is not comprehensible to me today. I should have known better… but time has run out.

I was saved by the completion of my college degree and my marriage, accompanied by a move to another town—another gynaecologist knew right away and acted accordingly—and one month later the operation was over. It was not successful. Two long years without treatment had done their work. One of my fallopian tubes was removed, the second went through resection. They refused to tell me what my illness meant. When I asked about children, the senior doctor said you are young, you must hope. He did not offer me any treatment. So I decided to hope. I was freshly married and full of optimism.

Slowly I started to look around and to search for information. I worked in the library and, from time to time, there were medical journals and occasionally a description of my diagnosis. I understood. I tried to get drugs imported secretly from abroad, but our financial resources were enough for hardly a quarter of the minimum amount. Thanks to the understanding of a doctor I knew, I got another shipment, now in the required minimum treatment amount. It did not help me to get a child.

I got into a consultation group for childless marriages. I already knew what illness I had, and that my only hope could be assisted reproduction, a child from a test tube. I still think today that the physicians were required to follow an exactly prescribed routine with the patients: x-rays of the womb and the fallopian tubes, cleaning of the tubes, etc. For me it was a waste of time, and pointless suffering, besides the fact that my husband was in military service at that time. I said this in a gentle voice to my doctor, and he responded in an incomprehensible way to me: he yelled at me, threw me out of the surgery and refused to continue to treat me. Later I understood. He wanted to become a senior doctor of gynaecology and my condition and continuing childlessness presented a problem for him.

So I found another gynaecologist (in my life I have gone through the hands of 25 gynaecologists and I hope that the number is not going to increase much more), and he sent me every year to have a laparoscopy for observation to see whether the endometriosis had progressed. It did. I finished with the laparoscopies at the moment when, as I was lying on the operation table during the last one, the doctor asked me right before the anaesthesia: 'and what are we supposed to find in you?' And that was topped off by a senior doctor who refused to let me go home on the third day as in the preceding cases—I understood, he had to improve the socialistic statistics of 'bed patients', but I insisted on my point, I had gone through two laparoscopies before, and I knew I was entirely fine, there were no health reasons for staying in. He got his revenge; he sent me directly to work with the stitches still in. So it was clear that I had to find another way. Through acquaintances, secretly, we found a contact for a doctor in another town who was trying assisted reproduction. They were not very successful. Unfortunately, not even this came off well. Again, I underwent all the examinations, always very painful due to the endometriosis, but the conclusion was again the same: you are young, you have to hope.

And so my husband and I went to apply for adoption to be on the safe side. We were 28 and we began to face attitudes like first an apartment, then a car, and you are too lazy for children, first you want to enjoy, or the alternative—you are lucky, no one jumps on your stomach in the morning—how glad I would have been if someone jumped on me! I was not suffering mentally due to the desire for a child, not at that time, that came later, approximately at the age of 33, but I rationally knew that I wanted a child, that I wished it a lot, that my wish kept growing, and that adoption means five years of waiting if you want a baby. And that was what we wanted. We went through the year-long assessment process from the viewpoint of the appropriate authorities. We were successful, we were found to be suitable future parents. A child was within reach, only some waiting was necessary, perhaps there will be a miracle, everybody said, perhaps you will have your own baby.

It was harder and harder to cope with the questions of our family and friends. I am still proud today that I found the best way (for me) of how to face them. I started saying openly and loudly at the question 'do you have children?' 'No, unfortunately I cannot have children.' And no one went on asking, which was exactly what I needed at that time. I have used it until this day, and I will use it until the end of my life: raised forehead, a look into the eyes, and a smile at the answer. Each time the answer, loudly said, was easier and easier, it rid me of the emotional tension, it made me less vulnerable, until in the end the emotions disappeared completely, and I answered automatically. What a relief.

Years were passing by and then, in one week, my life changed for good. I had thought for six years that I had lived in a very happy marriage, and then my husband stood in the door after a week of an intensive course of English (that was held in another town): 'You know, Martha, I got to know a superb girl and I would like her to go with us on a holiday.' We were divorced in a year, the reason was the childless marriage and my husband did not hesitate to use it.

The paradoxes of fate—the second month after the divorce the social worker called that she had a baby for us, very beautiful, whether we were looking forward to it.

The paradoxes of fate—my husband separated from his love three months after the divorce.

I was 31 years old; I was divorced, childless, and desperate.

Unfortunately not even my parents made it easier for me—they showed me tacitly that, childless and divorced, I was not of full worth to them, and my father wanted to have the family house written over to my sister (also divorced, but she had two children) and to disinherit me.

Of course I was fair game. I became attracted to a married man and I said to myself, out of defiance, why not, I will not love anybody anyway, when my husband could enjoy life, why not me. In three months I found out that I was more in love than ever before in my life. And my boyfriend was in love as never before in his life. After my fresh divorce for the reason of childlessness, I completely refused the idea that he should get divorced because of me and leave his two young children. It looks pointlessly noble, but it was sincere. We were together, with breaks and in secret, for 13 years. We very much wanted to have a child together, and I did not care much about all the morals and ethics. I would have given my life for a child at that time, and it was not just a phrase. My friend found an acquaintance, a doctor who did not want to see the marriage certificate, so we underwent three secret attempts at fertilisation from a test tube. None of them came off. We did not have money for more attempts. I suspect why the artificial fertilisation was not successful: I was worried in my soul by the idea of what I would say when the longed-for child would grow up and start asking where dad was and why he was not with us. I tried hard to suppress it, but I think that the failure was due to my psyche—it did not seem correct to selfishly give birth to a child just because I wanted it and not to have a dad for him or her. My soul struggled with my body and it won. And again the paradoxes of fate—years later my friend told me that if it had happened, he would definitely have wanted to live with us, and he would have. I believe he meant it. His marriage in the end collapsed anyway, regardless of the children.

Today I do not understand how I could bear it, mentally and physically. I was driven by a desire for a child, enormous at that time, I was 38 years old, it was the last chance, I very much wanted a child, more than any other time, and more than anything else. I know that this desire overcomes everything—the morals, truth, lies, shame, anything. To undergo it alone, in secret, without the support of close relatives was often exhausting. My boyfriend and I lived far away from each other, we met for a visit to the doctor midway between our homes, phone calls were not enough for these situations. I could not tell anyone what I was trying to do, why I kept disappearing from work for a couple of weeks, I lied to everyone.

The paradoxes of fate—I remember all the attempts gladly, although that is surprising for anyone whom I tell about it. Everything in the world has its sad and joyful sides. People usually link childlessness and infertility with problems, crying, breakdowns and unhappiness. I was so much in love, I hoped for a child who would have the hands and fingers of my love, or possibly it would be beautiful and superb after him. We were not a husband and wife with a desire cramped and tied up by years of attempts, when the begetting of a child resembles work, deadlines, plans, musts... We very much wanted to get pregnant, it was our reward for the secrets and concealment, it was our unsurpassable motivation. We looked forward to assisted reproduction.

So I underwent everything that was possible to undergo, with all its joys and sadness, the heights of hope and the depths of despair, even the crying and the prams with unknown children in the streets, the avoidance of pregnant friends and those with young children, the imagining in vain what it would be like if a baby grew inside my body, if I was breastfeeding, what it would smell like, whom it would resemble.

I do not wonder at the women who steal a child in the street. I do not know myself how it happened that I did not do it, I think about them with deep understanding and sympathy.

At that time I thought, with each unsuccessful attempt, that life lacked meaning. I felt, and I will always feel, that I am not integral and whole, that I lack one big dimension, a big part of me of which I will never learn what it would be like, one huge experience.

The years have shown me why it was actually good not to have a child. The divorce with the first husband was caused by his denial of homosexuality (he, in fact, never wanted to have children, and I think he would not have been a good father); I separated from my great love, and I cannot imagine how I would live alone with a child and cope alone with his or her upbringing.

I think I underwent everything on my quest for a child, including the acceptance of the two adolescent children of my second husband.

I have taken it as my fate. I say I have done everything that I could. As soon as I was able to formulate it in this way and say it, I felt a big relief.

So everything turned out fine in the end. I am 44 years old, I am reconciled and calm, everything has stopped aching. I have learned so much on my quest for a child which took 25 years! What I take as my biggest victory is that I have learned to love myself and to accept myself as I am. I got to know my worth and strength when I learned to belong gladly to the minority of divorced, childless women. And to belong there and differ is not very easy in my country and perhaps not even elsewhere in the world.

It has been my fate and I am grateful for it; it led me to forgiveness, happiness, relaxation and joy in each new day. I struggled and lost, but I did not run away from the fight and it was a fair defeat. It should have been this way and it is all right—this is my deep conviction.

Caroline

When I was a little girl, I always dreamed that I would have a kind husband and two healthy children. The dream of a happy marriage was enhanced by the divorce of my parents. My husband's parents were also divorced so, before we were married, we often talked about how we valued love, faithfulness, tolerance and mutual understanding between partners.

We were married after we had been going out and living together for not quite two years. Similar to most couples now, we also planned the time when we would truly want children. Our education was completed, we were employed, thus there was no reason why we shouldn't stop taking hormonal contraceptives after the wedding, and we began to 'work' on a baby.

I expected minor difficulties, because my menstrual cycle is irregular so, after three months without hormones, menstruation and or pregnancy, I went to see my gynaecologist. My doctor prescribed some hormones for me that were to adjust my cycle. However, they had little effect and I was soon back at the doctor's. I received new hormones, after which the cycle was regular, but the pregnancy tests were still negative. On the advice of my more experienced women colleagues and mothers, my husband and I tried all kinds of things and studied various kinds of infertility examinations and treatment on the Internet, but there was still no indication that a baby might be in the offing. And so I went back to the health centre again and asked whether they could do an ultrasonic test to see whether I was undergoing ovulation. The doctor performed this test at my request but didn't help me much because she said that she 'couldn't see anything' there. It seemed strange when she collected a fee for this service. Following a conversation in which I told her that I work as a paediatric nurse in a hospital and that I would like to ask an experienced gynaecologist treating infertility, she was happy to give me my medical card stating that, after a year of my failing to conceive a baby, she had no idea what the cause could be.

Therefore, it was that I took my medical card and my expectations and went to the hospital to consult my new doctor, a specialist. I knew from what my colleagues had told me that he had successfully assisted not only in the birth of a number of babies, but also in their conception. The doctor carefully listened to me and examined me. In contrast to my original doctor, he could 'see something' in the ultrasonic image and found that I did not have regular ovulation. He recommended that I have a blood test taken to determine the hormone level; this has to be performed on a certain day in the cycle, which my original doctor probably also did not know. The results of the examination confirmed the irregularity of the cycle. My husband was sent for a spermiogram examination, with which he agreed without problems, but with obvious trepidations. He was told where, when and how he should come in for the examination. My husband's results were all right. Then it was suggested that we could try the method of intrauterine insemination, with which we both agreed. We had to purchase a special catheter, which is available at medical supply centres.

So, equipped with the catheter, instructions, taking vitamin E (for fertility) and my regular hormone treatment and after completion of another vaginal ultrasound, we set out on the day of ovulation for the department where my husband was to provide his sperm. We did not know what to expect, but our ideas of the furnishings of the room for taking the sample probably came out of an American film. After we arrived at the department, we found that, after we rang the bell, everyone knew about us, including the builders who were doing reconstruction work. After brief recording of our history and entering our names, we received a sterile quarter-litre bottle. We were in shock when they closed us in a small toilet, saying that we shouldn't 'let ourselves be disturbed'. After the shock and my husband's question as to whether he had to fill the whole bottle, when we were closed in the toilet, we said they can't mean this seriously and this is the last time we are here. We didn't let ourselves be disturbed, although the banging of a hammer on the wall was neither pleasant nor exciting. However, this was not the end of our tribulations. We were sent to the gynaecological outpatients' department, where we were to arrive in about two hours. We were told that, during that time, the ejaculate would be specially treated and that we should pick it up in the building of the biochemical laboratory.

There everyone knew about us when the nurse shouted out that we were already there. So we set out with a tiny 'bottle of infants' stuck in my brassiere, because it had to be kept warm. The waiting room was completely full, so we waited and waited. I tried to point out to the nurse that I should be admitted preferentially, but was told that the doctor didn't have time because he was performing an operation. So my husband and I gradually ceased believing that this experiment could work. After about an hour and a half, I was admitted. It was probably open doors day at the clinic, because it was certainly not possible to speak of any privacy. However, everything was where it was supposed to be and we could finally go home. Then we could only wait and wait. Subconsciously, we both felt that it would be a miracle after so much psychological strain. And so I cried through my next menstruation.

In the months that followed, I underwent further immunological tests to determine whether I had any antibodies against my husband's sperm. The results were negative. Then I went for a fallopian tube test, which two women colleagues from our department had told me is very painful. I must say that it was certainly unpleasant, but not painful. However, the important thing was that the results were all right—my fallopian tubes are not blocked. So we could keep on trying insemination. When we absolved the process for the third time, there was a change only in that the genetic laboratory had moved, but the sample room was still in the toilet, but in a different building. A completely different doctor arrived for the procedure, accompanied by an experienced doctor, who was to teach him the insemination procedure. Of course, I knew both the doctors from my department, so I was quite embarrassed that the whole gynaecology department would soon know me. My own doctor was sick, which I didn't know, as he had taken an ultrasonic image only two days previously.

Time continued to pass from our efforts and the tests were still negative. At this time, they transferred me to the intensive care department for infants, apparently, so I could conceive even better. However, the opposite results occurred. When I saw all those beautiful healthy babies and pregnant mothers with enormous stomachs, I was not overjoyed. The older nurses told me not to think about it, but that was difficult. Internally, I started to think about adoption, but my husband wouldn't hear of it.

In the framework of thinking of other things, I submitted a university application. I said, if there isn't going to be a baby, then I can at least study; anyway, it was being said that, in the EU, nurses should have a university degree. It was spring and we agreed with my doctor that we would try to introduce children only until the summer. In the autumn, we gradually began to plan artificial fertilization.

We went for the fourth try and, in addition, I was prepared by special hormone treatment, which was to ensure greater success, and was simultaneously warned that several eggs could be released. I was quite worried about this following my experience in the intensive care unit. I had the morning shift that day, which couldn't be changed, because the doctor did the ultrasonic examination the day beforehand and said 'tomorrow is D-day'. My thoughts were somewhat elsewhere, because we had a full department at the maternity clinic. My husband took time off work, which he always received for an absence card with the stamp of the genetic department, so that the gossips at work began to ask if his wife was pregnant and whether they were determining his blood group. A little plan occurred to me that day. I agreed with the laboratory and the doctor that we would leave our bottle there until the doctor had finished operating and would be able to go to the clinic and that they would then call me and I would run down to the department. Our plan worked and I saved two hours waiting and bad nerves at the clinic, which I preferred to spend at work.

We didn't expect any success in my becoming pregnant, mainly because of my work as a paediatric nurse in neonatology. Whenever I looked at the gynaecological histories, I found that few women can become pregnant without problems. I decided that it would be better to concentrate on the university entrance examinations.

Nonetheless, after not quite two years of trying, I finally became pregnant. That might seem like a short time for someone who has not experienced it, but it seemed like eternity to me. We were tremendously happy that we were finally going to have a family. On the recommendation of the doctor, I spent my entire pregnancy on sick leave. Following my experience in intensive care, I was very concerned that the baby be healthy. Nonetheless, after completing the entrance examinations, I entered the university with concerns as to how I would manage it with a baby. However, I received the support of my husband and the future grandmothers, so I said I would try it.

A beautiful, healthy baby boy was born in January 2003 and he is growing rapidly. At the beginning, my father helped enormously by taking leave on the days of my lectures and supported my mother in everything. The only exception was nursing, but I managed even this by excusing myself from lectures. It is increasingly difficult for me to study with our little rascal around, but I know that, if it hadn't been for the school and freeing myself from problems and from thinking only about a baby, he might not even be here. Hopefully we will manage it through to the end. There is only one semester left and then the state final examinations. After I complete school, we would like to have another baby; I only hope I won't have to register for another field of study.

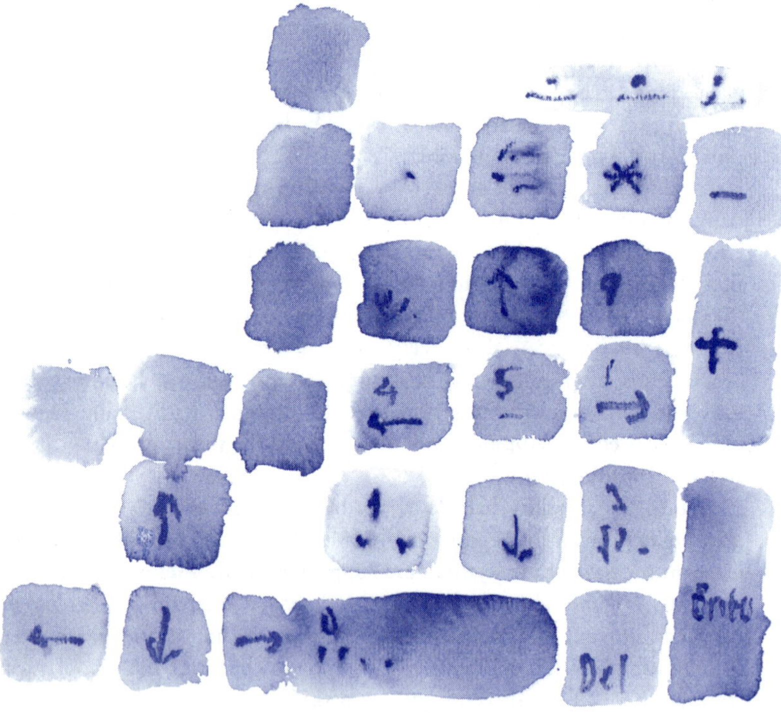

I HAVE COME UP WITH LOTS AND LOTS OF IDEAS

I Have Come Up With Lots and Lots of Ideas

Well, I promised I offer lots of ideas but I am not sure whether I can fulfill my promise. In addition, the song in the title of the chapter continues with 'that make you happy', and this is a very brash promise. But I'll do my best. At the end, such a good idea could consist in a sort of 'minimap' of weapons against what the layman calls stress.

Research work devoted to coping with psychological stress point out that there are two coping resources:

1. Intrapersonal: personality traits, abilities and skills. The ability to deal with unpleasant events consists of several components:

   a) Comprehensibility. The ability to understand the world and one's own position as a comprehensible, recognizable and ordered whole, which functions logically, rationally and with relatively high regularity.
   b) Manageability. The ability to affect, control and manage one's life role and goals in this world.
   c) Meaningfulness. The ability to understand one's life position and activity as worth the attempt to understand and actively manage it.

2. Extrapersonal: financial resources or social support. Social support can be the family, friends, relevant concerned professional and lay organisations, psychologists or a medical team. Social support consists of four components:

   a) Emotional support (provision of important emotions, for example love, faith, empathy)

b) Evaluation support (communication that gives a person self-confidence, self-reliance, a feeling of self-esteem as a human being)
c) Information support (provision of information or advice that assists the person to cope with problems)
d) Instrumental support (practical and substantive material support).

Intrapersonal and extrapersonal resources that assist in coping with psychological stress are not separate, but interconnected: one increasing the other. For example, a human being with certain personality traits and skills more readily seeks social support, and qualified social support substantially affects the use of intrapersonal resources, especially perceiving stress as comprehensible (through information support), manageable (through emotional, information, evaluation and instrumental support) and meaningful (through evaluation and information support).

I hope that, in the previous chapters, I have managed to draw the reader's attention to most intrapersonal and extrapersonal coping resources. However, I have not yet mentioned the following two.

Psychological Help

In many countries, it is still not normal to seek psychological help in coping with one's unfulfilled desire for a child. Could a psychologist help in any way?

> I would not seek out a psychologist. If so, I would like help with the question of how to fill my life in a different way. (m)
>
> No, I talk about it a lot with my husband or with the doctors. I am trying to cope with it myself. (f)
>
> A psychologist could help me if he helped to convince me that it is not a tragedy, and that I have a lot of time ahead of me. (f)
>
> I do not feel so broken down with pain and on the verge of collapse. The psychologist could help me with acceptance of the facts, by advice how to fight the problem, simple venting of emotions, listening. (f)
>
> Calming down, help and advice on how and where to undergo treatment. Learning about the stories of couples who are in the same situation. (f)
>
> From my viewpoint, today I would find it as most reasonable, if he or she convinced me that there are other beautiful things in the world than the hope every month and then absolute despair after the next menstruation. Probably what would help me is what we were unwittingly successful at

planning—another very attractive distant goal and shifting the desire for a child onto a different track. (f)

No, it would not occur to me to seek out a psychologist. (f)

Very often we listen to talks about children and we, too, wish so much to find an 'ear' that would listen to us. (f)

My husband and I know that we must protect ourselves through patience, support each other. (f)

To orient myself in the situation, to plan my strength, and to define the line where we still say 'yes' and where we say 'no longer'. (f)

To boost up my confidence for the negotiations with the doctors, and the assertion of my interests. (f)

I would not seek out a psychologist, it would make me anxious. (f)

The psychologist could give me information in a more understandable form than the doctor could. But he or she would need to have it. (m)

I expect advice on what to do, advice how to convince my husband to listen to me. (f)

My therapist has set a visit at a psychologist as a condition of further continuation of treatment with her. (f)

It is pleasant to talk about the topic with someone. (f)

We are considering turning to a psychologist. (m)

I need to learn how to relax. (f)

We were helped partially by various talks with priests and, especially in me, by participation in psychotherapeutic training. (f)

Many spots in this [thesis] would have helped me some time ago. Mainly the possibility of identification with certain testimonies and a positive and empathetic view, a certain challenge (at least as I understand it) in terms of activity and defiance of certain attitudes or methods of some of the medical staff. (f)

Each thought, each piece of a new information, each personal experience has great value for me, and helps me in my orientation in the very uncertain terrain where I am temporarily finding myself. (f)

A woman told me that she was being treated for infertility. She wanted a contact for the Centre of Adoption and Foster Care. Then she wanted to know what the Maternal Hope foundation does. I told her about the immunobiological examination. She said she underwent one in her own town and asked if the foundation can arrange it. In an hour she called again, and asked what services the immunological institute provides, if they offer some treatment that is unavailable in her town. I answered her, and we talked about the Mojzis method. Then I told her that I am a psychologist, and that I can offer her the possibility to have a quiet talk. She said no, that she is not yet in such a bad state. (p)

During the years that I have been doing the infertility treatment, several of my patients sought out psychological help. Some of them came back terrified,

> that the psychologist told them that they did not have a child because they did not actually want it. (p)
>
> I used to go to a psychiatrist, I was on antidepressants. But I work in medical care, and if someone had found out that I was seeing a psychiatrist, that would have been the end. The psychiatrist was excellent, he understood and did not write it down. The nurse collected the drugs for me in the drugstores outside the district. (f)

Why is it not common to ask for psychological support? ('I would not seek out a psychologist' 'It would not occur to me to seek out a psychologist' 'I am trying to cope with it myself') when, as all the previous chapters have shown, the quest or a child is a very difficult situation? Probably it is due to the fact that psychological help is still considered as an expression of one's inability to cope with one's own problems ('I do not feel so broken down with pain and on the verge of collapse' 'It would make me anxious' 'She is not yet in such a bad state' 'If someone had found out that I was seeing a psychiatrist, that would have been the end'). No one would want to add the feeling of inability to cope with one's own problems to the feeling of inability to beget one's own child.

If it came to psychological help anyway, what should it be focused on? It should be about helping you orient yourself in the problem and the various possibilities of solution ('Help and advice on how and where to undergo treatment' 'To orient myself in the situation, to plan my strength, and to define the borders where we still say "yes" and where we say "no longer"' 'Information in a more understandable form than from the doctor' 'Advice what to do' 'Orientation in a very uncertain terrain,' 'Advice on how to fight the problem' 'To convince me that it is no tragedy, and that I have a lot of time ahead' 'Relaxation') and about helping you find the solutions suitable for you ('How to fill my life in a different way' 'Planning another very attractive distant goal and shifting the desire for a child onto a different track' 'If he convinced me that there are other beautiful things in the world than the hope every month—and then the absolute despair after the next menstruation'). The psychologist can be the person to whom you talk about your troubles ('Simple venting of emotions, listening' 'We too wish so much to find an 'ear' that would listen to us' 'It is pleasant to talk about the topic with someone') and thanks to whose experience your feeling of being isolated and misunderstood can be reduced ('Learning about the stories of couples who are in the same situation' 'Identification with certain testimonies' 'Each personal experience has a big value for me'). The psychologist can advise you about communication principles useful for a balanced contact with the therapist, with the people around you ('To boost up my confidence for the negotiations with the doctors, and the assertion of my interests' 'Defiance of certain attitudes or methods of some of the medical staff'), and with your closest family ('Advice on how to convince my husband to listen to me'). Moreover, the psychologist can teach you techniques for managing stress ('To learn how to relax' 'Relaxation'). Through all of this, the psychologist can encourage you, help you find your lost self-esteem and give strength to continue struggling ('A certain challenge (at least as I understand it) in terms of activity').

It seems that the psychologist's help need not be entirely pointless. However, not to over-praise my profession, I need to add that not every psychologist is familiar with the area of fertility problems and you may not find it easy to talk to some of them. It is necessary for you not to give up and to find the one suitable for you.

Help from Civic Associations and Foundations

In the last few decades, many non-governmental organisations, civic associations and foundations have been established which focus on solving various psychosocial problems, for example alcohol and drug addiction, health disabilities, and the problem of involuntary childlessness. These organisations are usually founded and run by specialists who are professionally involved in the particular area or by people for whom the particular problem was or has been a personal one, and frequently by both.

> The experience of the past years was a strong motivation for me for the utilisation of my strength for those who are currently involved in what I dealt with some time ago. If I can help your foundation in any way, I would gladly do so. (f)
>
> I am also concerned with the topic of childless marriages. If you need any help (in organisation, association, etc.), I offer my whole heart and my hands. Because I know what childless marriage means. (f)
>
> I had worried my whole life that I do not have a child. When the possibility appeared, I started a foundation, so that I could help people with similar suffering. I know what it means. (f)

How can organisations help?

> Perhaps I would benefit from a meeting with similarly handicapped people. On the other hand, I fear that it might be too artificial. (f)

I thank the Internet for information on the topic of infertility; it provided a lot of information that my husband and I needed a lot in the past days. Also, thanks to these articles, we have pulled out of it more quickly. (f)

The appearance of the supplement on the internet was a very good idea. A possibility to gain as much information as possible, and searching for the way towards each other. Luck comes to those who are prepared. We did not know much at the beginning, we were unprepared, and we didn't have luck. I hope that the next generation of infertile couples will be better prepared, and I want to contribute to this. (f)

I am looking for someone who has a positive experience with IVF and wants to share it. (f)

I am very grateful for the appearance of the supplement on the internet that was devoted to infertility. Also thanks to author for his book. (f)

A well-informed couple (or a couple who have had the possibility to talk with other couples who have gone through it) will always be mentally in better shape, they will not have the biases and false expectations. (p)

I was pleased that there is an association that wants to provide information on infertility, its causes, and mainly about the possibilities of treatment. (f)

The information that I have gained, thanks to you, gives me hope that we will not be alone. (f)

It's a pity you are so far away, many times I feel like talking about our problems, and have no one to talk to. (f)

After reading the infertility patient organisation magazine, I got the courage to continue trying our luck. (f)

Thanks to the infertility patient organisation magazine, I read almost all that I needed to know. I did not need to search for various brochures and keep asking the doctors. (f)

The magazine gave me the feeling that I am not alone, and that I have someone to turn to. (f)

I keep telling myself, what would the women 15 or 20 years ago have given for the information in your magazine! (f)

Thanks to the mental support provided by you and your information, I decided to go for IVF. (f)

I was pleased by your magazine and, although I had gone through something, I gained a lot of new information. (f)

After reading the magazine, I'm starting to believe in the efficacy of the treatment. (f)

I am much more balanced and you, as an organisation, have your share in it. You keep my head above water with your letters. (f)

The magazines are superb, and I think they will help other couples to understand their situation. (f)

Organisations are necessary. It would have helped me a lot years ago if I had known that other women on the quest for a child would do anything that would give them a minimal hope. It would have encouraged my realisation that I was not alone, that I was normal. (f)

We have couples in our area who are in the same situation. We meet up with them. At the last treatment, we got to know one couple. We told them what examinations we had passed and these people laughed at what all they had missed. Now we go on holidays together. (m)

I very much appreciate the activity of the foundation. Its representatives communicate with people in a different way from the way we approach people in the surgery. We are simply in a different situation and often we do not have the necessary competence. And the treatment of fertility problems is dependent on communication. (p)

The couple should know about other ways of approaching infertility than treatment. But doctors cannot talk with patients about adoptive care. For one, they do not have the time, and mainly the doctor should be a source of hope in the success of the treatment. By talking about adoption, he or she would not strengthen the belief in the therapy and the motivation in the patient. (p)

We could divide the help of organisations into four areas:

1. Informational help. Organisations can offer comprehensive information about the treatment of a given condition. In the case of involuntarily childless couples, this is information about the causes and the treatment of fertility problems, their financial demands and success rates, about related ethical aspects, about the various clinics providing treatment, about the possibilities of adoptive care and the ways of applying for it, etc. The advantage is that the information can be in various forms (leaflets, magazines, personal letters, references to relevant books, phone contacts), as suits various people. The most effective form of communication is personal contact, which takes place in an informal environment, without the white coats of the doctor's office. The client can, anonymously and without fear, ask the specialist who cooperates with the organisation about things for which there is no time or not enough courage at the doctor's, and in this way the client can gain additional information as well as compare the information from their doctor with information from a second source. This help is needed especially today when the doctor-patient relationship is becoming more equal, patients are often asked for an informed consent with the diagnostic and therapeutic interventions, and sometimes they must even choose among various therapies and drugs. Moreover, organisations

can also provide information that doctors may not offer, not only because doctors may not have enough time but also because doctors are in a different situation.

2. Psychological help. Better information can help people to cope better with a complicated situation. The social support and the feeling of belonging serve to prevent the harmful effects of stress and anger. The opportunity to share one's suffering, to talk to others, is part of psychological hygiene. It is especially effective when it is shared with someone who is or has been in a similar situation. Unfortunately, this form of help is still underestimated, probably for reasons similar to those why people do not to seek out a psychologist.
3. Spreading information about the problem of involuntary childlessness among the general public. Activity in this area vital and various governmental, as well as non-governmental organisations can help by talking to the media and through the publication of information materials. Discussion of a problem can be a particular form of informing the public. An inappropriately chosen form can lead to inflation of the issue and the public perception of the issue can become even worse.
4. Asserting the interests of patients with reduced fertility in medical, scientific, and political spheres, for instance through pressure for changes in acts of law.

Some infertility patient organizations are associated in the International Consumer Support for Infertility iCSi). Its website is: www.icsi.ws, where you can find some interesting information and contacts to individual patient organizations. The iCSi is segmented to four regional alliances: European Infertility Alliance, The Americas Infertility Alliance, Asia Pacific Infertility Alliance and African Infertility Alliance. Another patient project is WorldFAM (www.worldfam.org), a global educational and advocacy community.

Nine Tips for the Quest for a Child

1. The quest for a child is special because both partners must participate. A fertility problem is an illness of the whole couple. Having a child still requires two people. It does not matter whether the cause of the failures is found on the side of the woman or the man, the consequences—involuntary childlessness—affects both. In most

therapeutic interventions, active participation of both partners is necessary, only one solution is being chosen. The presence of both partners should be automatic, at least during the diagnostic and therapeutic consultations and, depending on the situation, also during some of the therapeutic interventions. It will make the couple's communication easier and it can reduce the potential feelings of guilt that may arise in one of the partners.

2. For a couple who have fertility problems, the quest for a child is not a sprint where the whole track is visible and the goal is within reach. It is a demanding long-distance run. It is necessary to accept this fact and to adjust one's pace and output of energy. Those who can achieve this will save themselves mental effort. In other words, it is necessary to set the farthest line for the fulfilment of one's goal (for instance I want a child by 40 years of age at the latest) and work within that timeframe, then the failures and wanderings on the way are not so stressful.
3. Usually people get bogged down in problems because they are unprepared. It is necessary to design one's own map for the quest and know, at least theoretically, where the pathways, roads, hills, dark forests, and steep slopes are, which roads are dead-ends and which are passable. The main source of information is one's doctor, but it is useful to get information from other sources as well. These can be other therapists, organisations dealing with the problem, the Internet, magazines, leaflets, and the experience of current and former patients.
4. Not all roads lead to Rome; not all people will be able to have their own child. It can happen that the hurdles will be so great, and they might not even be known, that it will not be possible to reach the goal. Take time and decide which alternative goal is more acceptable: an adopted child or a life without a child. A blind alley will then not be blind for you, it will have an exit, and the possible failures in the treatment will not be so unexpected and devastating.
5. A fertility problem does not usually have visible symptoms, often it is not perceived as an illness either by the partners concerned or by other people in their community. There is no improvement or withdrawal of the illness, there exists only either/or. The worst part is usually the feeling of helplessness and constant waiting. It is possible to be led on the journey by someone, but it is better to direct one's own steps. There are many options, it is only necessary to realise

what they are: the choice of a particular solution, a particular therapist, a particular method of treatment, of one's attitude toward the therapy, of the strategy of looking for more information, one's orientation in the situation, psychotherapy, healthy lifestyle. It is important that you can say to yourselves, 'we have done all that we could'.

6. The quest for a child is a journey of two people, not any fewer and not any more. The only exception is the case of adoptive care, this journey toward a child can be undertaken by an individual. But it is impossible for more than two people to set out on a quest for a child. It is important to keep this in mind all the time. It depends on the pilgrims, not on anybody else (the doctor, parents, friends, the community) which way they choose to go, what solution they will decide on, and what they will tell others about their quest. It is their quest.
7. The time spent on the journey need not be wasted. It can bring new experiences, better knowledge of one's partner, more intensive experiencing of the relationship, joy from overcoming hurdles together, and discovery of new areas. The examinations and the treatment sometimes considerably limit other activities of the couples, especially of women. On the quest for a child, it is necessary to do everything possible, but not to sacrifice everything. Be interested in other things, too. Biological infertility has nothing to do with infertility in the philosophical sense; it does not mean that your life has no meaning. Life without a biological child can also be rich and fruitful. It is up to you.
8. The quest for a child is sometimes perceived as something inappropriate. We may suppose that when a child does not come of its own accord, we are somehow of lesser value. In families as well as in society, people still sometimes keep this problem secret. The partners are ashamed, they feel isolated, and they lack the opportunity to express their suffering, to share it with someone. Do not remain alone with your suffering, talk about it, express your feelings, doubts, and uncertainties. That is part of psychological hygiene. In addition to your partner, who is the most important one, find someone else in your community who you trust and who can help you bear your pain. A friendship with another couple who are dealing with a problem similar to yours is usually very helpful.

9. Even though the quest for a child is a major life crisis—many pilgrims speak of it that way—only a few of them turn to a psychotherapist. Do not hesitate to seek out a psychologist whom you can trust. The psychologist can help you to orient yourself in the situation, and cope with it in the best possible way. Moreover, the psychologist can be one of the people who will help you keep your head above water during the hardest moments.

NOW WE ASK THE LEARNED ACADEMICS, DOCTORS, AND CLERGY

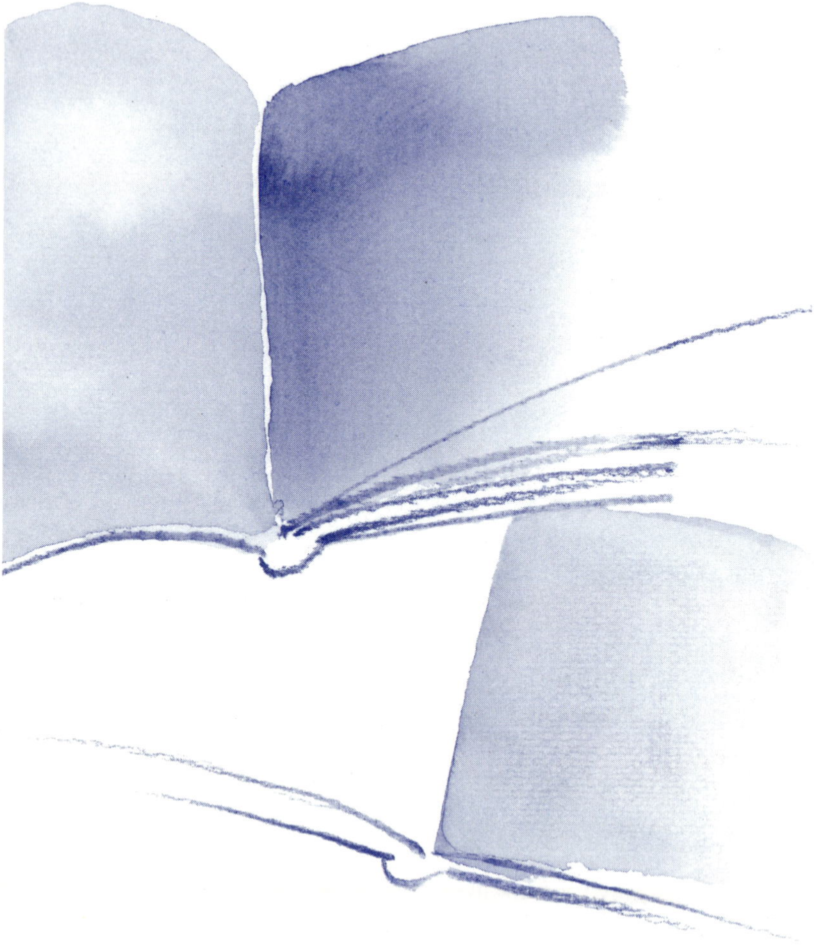

Now We Ask the Learned Academics, Doctors, and Clergy

This book developed from a dissertation in clinical psychology entitled 'Psychological Problems of Infertility' that I defended in 2000. The book has been supplemented by data I have collected since then and by data taken from the ongoing research into the various aspects of parenting (supported by a grant from the Czech Science Foundation No. 406/07/0274). This research has been approached in the same way as the dissertation research.

The dissertation was processed using 'qualitative' methodology. The decision to use processing by qualitative methods was determined by the nature of the researched problem and the nature of the collected data. Therefore, for those who are interested, I would like to outline briefly the manner of processing the data.

Qualitative research has the following characteristics: view from the perspective of the subject, description of the common details of everyday reality, understanding of behaviour and meaning in the social context, emphasis on time and process, preference of open and loosely structured design of the research, and avoidance of conceptions and theories at the beginning of the research. The specific methodology that I have chosen is Grounded Theory.

Data Sources and Collection

In the dissertation, the studied group was a group of people who have or had fertility problems. This was supplemented by the testimonies of therapists of various specialisations and the testimonies of people who are not directly concerned in the problem. It is clear that I could use only data gained from persons who were willing to share their experiences and feelings.

In the course of the research, I found out that I could not do without archetypal stories dealing with infertility, so also I used fairy tales, legends, myths, and biblical stories.

Data gathering methods

To collect the data, I used the following methods: interviews, group discussions, questionnaires, text analysis, and observation.

Types of research used

The types of research used were: analysis of individual case studies, document analysis, behaviour research, and field research.

Materials for the analysis of individual case studies included:

- Narrative interviews with the participants in 'holidays with healers'
- Therapeutic interviews with persons who turned to me with a request for help
- Spontaneous testimonies of people who are resolving or have resolved the given problem and whom I met by accident
- Telephone conversations
- Testimonies from group discussions in seminars for infertile couples about ways of resolving involuntary childlessness
- Testimonies from group discussions (focus groups) in seminars on infertility for mid-level medical staff (nurses and physiotherapists)
- Letters from clients (originals)
- Open-ended questionnaires
- Testimonies of therapists
- My observations
- Testimonies of people who are not directly involved in the problem.

Materials for the document analysis included:

- Letters and stories published in magazines and obtained from therapists
- The study text titled 'When a Child Is Not Coming'

- Stories published in the Internet news, in the documentary 'Micromundus'
- Fairy tales, myths, legends, and biblical stories about infertile couples
- Television series treating the problem of infertility.

Behaviour research

Behaviour research has three goals: to be directly related to specific social problems, to transpose the results into practice during the course of the research, and to maintain equal discourse between the researcher and the researched persons (this means that the researched persons do not feature as experimental persons/objects, but as partners/subjects). For instance, in the course of the research, I organised a series of seminars about the options in the diagnostics and the treatment of fertility problems and about adoptive and foster care. We have also opened a psychological consultation room for the involuntarily childless. In addition, I lectured about the psychological problem related to the unfulfilled desire for a child to physiotherapists and rehabilitation doctors being trained in the Mojzis method.

Field research

Field research means that the subject of the research is examined in as natural a setting as possible, to avoid the distortion that arises from intervention through the research methods and possibly through viewing the subject from an external perspective that is too distant from reality. I collected the data in the natural environment of the participants, that is, in the environment that they chose themselves and where they did not come for research purposes.

I would like to mention the use of written sources. In my work, I used non-expert as well as expert sources. Although, in quantitative research, these materials are not usually used as data sources, in the kinds of research according to the Grounded Theory they play an essential role, complementing the more common interviews and observations.

Data Analysis Methods

In looking for links and meanings in the collected data, I chose the conception of research based on the Grounded Theory. In the Grounded Theory, the analysis consists in three main types of coding: open coding, axial coding, and selective coding. The coding represents operations through which the data are analysed, conceptualised, and again put together in new ways. The analytical methods of the Grounded Theory are designed so that they create a theory rather than simply verify it, they add a critical perspective to the research process, and they help analysts to overcome the prejudices and suppositions that they bring into the research process.

Data Validity Control

In qualitative research, the criteria of the assessment of the results are an immensely important issue from the very beginning. In my research, I used the following techniques of data validity control.

Techniques related to collecting information about the examined phenomenon: triangulation of methods, triangulation of sources, interdisciplinary triangulation, and control of the effect of the researcher. Techniques related to the analysis and interpretation of the collected material: validation by the respondent, feedback provided by non-respondents, presentation of hard data, search for negative cases and discrepancies.

Research Ethics

The goals, tasks, and methods of psychological research must be examined according to ethical criteria to ensure that they serve human ideals, enable implementation of personal values and coping with life, and do not conflict with human rights. Investigating the problem of involuntary childlessness means working with a very intimate topic, and thus it was necessary to consider each step from the viewpoint of ethics.

Only rarely did I ask about topics that the respondents did not bring up themselves, even at the cost of 'poorer' data. The experience of involuntary childlessness is in itself traumatising enough, and so I did not poke into the painful spots. Therefore, a testimony often touched only on a single topic. In the anonymous questionnaires, it was not required that all the questions be answered.

Afterword

The book that you are now holding in your hands gradually took shape over approximately fourteen years; that is how long I investigated, with varying intensity, the terrain of solutions for fertility problems. The changes in intensity were brought about by the four children that I gave birth to during that time. But they also became a big source of energy, the reason why to carry on working. I would like to thank all those who helped me complete this book.

First, I would like to thank my family for the support and for their help with my family responsibilities, especially with taking care of the children.

The main thanks belong to the accidental and more or less anonymous passers-by who are the true authors of the map of the quest for a child. I am only the person who has organised their experiences so that the map would be easy to read and as complete as possible.

Major thanks to the Maternal Hope Foundation based in Prague and to the Brno Centre for Family and Social Care. Without their understanding and their offer of expert as well as organisational support, I would not have been able to devote myself to my work. For personal support, I thank Dr. Eva Domorázková, the chair of the Maternity Hope Foundation, and the director of the Centre for Family and Social Care, Vít Janků.

To orient myself in the problem related to the quest for a child I had to familiarise myself with information from many fields, mainly medicine, psychology, sociology, ethics, law, theology, and ethnography. I thank all of my consultants who are the guarantors of the professional level of this book: the Director of the Centre of Adoption and Foster Care in Prague, the sociologist Dr. Věduna Bubleová, the guarantor of the professional training of the physiotherapists of the Brno Institute for the Advanced Education of Medical Staff, physiotherapist Hana Volejníková, the chair of the Zlín Centre of Reproductive Medicine, the gynaecologist Prof. Ladislav

Pilka, the chair of the Immunobiology Laboratory of the Institute of the Care for the Mother and Child in Prague-Podolí, the reproduction immunologist Dr. Jindřich Madar, and the head of the Centre of Andrological Care in České Budějovice, Dr. Vladimír Kubíček.

In addition, other experts to whom I am grateful for help are the Director of the Psychological Institute of the Academy of Sciences, the psychologist Prof. Ivo Čermák, and the psychologist Dr. Michal Miovský, experts in the methodology of research, the psychologist Dr. Jarmila Koluchová, the psychologist Dr. Maria Poláková, the ethnologist Hana Poláková, the theologian Marie Zelenková, and the lawyer Dr. Ondřej Dostál.

When I was working on the Czech edition of Two Small Wings, I had never written a book before and my long-term maternity leave (at The Maternity Hope Foundation I am just a volunteer) had lowered my professional self-esteem. I waited anxiously for the readers' response. However, my fears soon disappeared as I began receiving wonderful letters that brought me much joy. It was truly gratifying to see that the effort I had invested was not wasted and that the book was doing well.

From reading foreign sources, I have gained the impression that, while the various political, cultural, and economic circumstances do influence the map of the quest for a child, the unfulfilled desire for a child means the same thing everywhere. I got to wondering whether this was really the case, whether my book would speak to readers of other languages, and how such readers—the public as well as the experts—would respond to it. Therefore, I decided to try to find the answers to these questions and publish the book in English. At first, I did not know how difficult it would be to make this plan a reality. Even though I had no idea who might publish the book, I updated the text and had it translated. I would now like to thank those who have supported my project.

The book is based on the testimonies of hundreds of people whose style is varied. Moreover, the theme is interdisciplinary, drawing on terms and concepts from many disciplines. Therefore, the quality of the translation becomes essential. Special thanks go to Jana Poláková, Thomas Pierce, Kateřina Prajznerová, Madaleine Štulíková, Andrew White and Tara Foss who spent many hours with the text. I also thank Dr. Tomáš Mařík for his kind help with the specialized medical vocabulary.

Ms. Karolína Stehlíková with her family, Dr. Eva Domorázková, Prof. Ladislav Pilka, Dr. Tonko Mardešić, Prof. Miloš Velemínský, Ms Renata Brandtnerová, Ms Carmen Martínez Jover and Mr Charles Brady thought that my idea was a bit ridiculous but certainly not foolish.

They not only encouraged me but also helped me look for ways to make it all happen. I am deeply indebted to them, without their support there would be no book. I also thank the Triton publishing house, and for preparing this second, international version, Anshan U.K. for taking the project on.

The book has been sponsored by the ČEZ Foundation Prague and the Maternity Hope Foundation, Prague. I appreciate their support for my work.

I would also like to thank TRIN Třebíč, GMA Stanztechnik Kaplice, NATE Chotěboř, Ludmila Holadová and Ecolab Hygiene. Brno for their support of the Maternity Hope Foundation.

This work has a psychotherapeutic potential whose crucial component is the visual impact of the book. I thank Magdalena Říčná for her kind and clever metaphoric watercolours. I also thank Metoda Brno for the graphic design.

The somewhat ridiculous idea has become a reality. All that is left to do now is to wait to see whether this book will find its readers…

Hana Konečná
October 2007
České Budějovice, Czech Republic
e-mail: materskanadeje@volny.cz

A Glossary of Terms and Abbreviations

On the quest for a child, one comes across many terms that one does not understand. Here is an explanation of the most basic ones. Others can be found in medical or psychological dictionaries.

Adoption – form of adoptive parenting. Couples or individuals accept, as their own, an orphaned or unwanted child and have the same rights and duties toward the child as if they were the child's parents. The relationship between adoptive parents and the child is similar to the relationship between biological parents and their own child. There are two types of adoption, simple and irrevocable.

Androgens – male sex hormones, the most important one is testosterone.

Andrology – field of medicine that deals with the structure, function, and diseases of the male reproductive system.

Anovulation – dysfunction when the ripening and release of an egg in the ovary does not occur.

Assisted reproduction – subfield of medicine that deals with overcoming the obstacles to conception. It enables conception by in-lab modification of the egg, sperm, or embryo. The most common types are IUI and IVF.

Astenospermia – fertility problem in a man. The sperm move too slowly.

Azoospermia – fertility problem in a man. There are no sperm in the ejaculate.

Balneotherapy – various treatment methods used in a spa under the guidance of a doctor, usually during a period of several weeks; usually termed 'going to the spa'.

Basal temperature – temperature of the human body measured after at least six hours of physical calm, usually taken in the morning after waking up.

Biopsy – removal of a sample of an organ or tissue for the purposes of a microscopic (histological) examination.

Children's home – institutional environment for substitute raising of children who cannot be raised in their family for various reasons. Usually from three years of age.

Cryo embryo transfer – transfer of a frozen embryo into the womb.

Cryopreservation – freezing of cells to low temperatures during which all life processes cease. The sperm and embryos can be kept for a very long time, almost without limits.

A deprived child – in children growing up in a collective institution there usually occurs a mental, emotional lack of fulfilment of the need for love and security, possibly also retardation in other areas of development.

A disabled child – child that is physically or mentally disadvantaged in comparison with the child's contemporaries.

Egg (oocyte) – female sex cell.

Ejaculate (the sperm, semen) – liquid flowing from a man's penis during orgasm. It should contain sperm.

Embryo (fetus) – fertilised egg from the moment when it divides into two cells.

Embryo transfer – transfer of the embryo into the vagina.

Endocrine (hormonal) system – system of glands with internal secretion that produce hormones.

Endocrinology – science that deals with the structure and function of the glands with internal secretions, including the examination and treatment of their dysfunctions.

Endometriosis – illness in which the parts of endometrium (the internal mucosa of the womb) are found in other parts of the body, most often in the lesser pelvis.

Endometrium – internal mucosa of the womb.

Extrauterine – outside the womb.

Extrauterine pregnancy – pregnancy that has nested and grows outside the womb, most often in the fallopian tubes.

Fallopian tube – tubular organ connecting the ovary with the womb in which the eggs meet the sperm so that fertilisation is made possible.

Fertility – ability to conceive a descendant.

Fertilisation (conception) – merging of a sperm and an egg.

Follicle – bag in an ovary, filled with liquid. It contains an egg that ripens in it.

Foster care – form of parenting overseen by the state. It ensures sufficient financial security for a child and adequate reward for those who have taken up the care. The foster parent has the right to represent the child and look after its affairs in common matters; for the execution of unusual affairs, the foster parent requests the agreement of the legal representative of the child. Contact between the original parents and the child is not excluded.

FSH – follicle-stimulating hormone. It stimulates the growth of the follicle, in which an egg develops and ripens until ovulation.

Genetics – science of inheritance.

Gestogens – group of female sex hormones (for instance progesterone); they originate in the ovaries and, after conception in the placenta; their function is, amongst other things, the preparation and maintenance of pregnancy.

GnRH – gonadotrophic releasing hormone; it controls the releasing of the FSH and LH hormones.

Gonadotrophines – FSH and LH, the hormones produced through the pituitary gland, they control the activity of the sex glands.

Gravidity – pregnancy.

Gravitest – test to find out (usually from urine) whether a woman is pregnant. It can be normally obtained from pharmacies.

Gynaecology – field of medicine that deals with the structure, function and diseases of the female reproductive system.

hCG (human chorial gonadotrophine) – a hormone produced by the placenta in pregnancy; it stimulates the ovaries to produce the hormones (oestrogen and progesterone) necessary for the maintenance of pregnancy; it is secreted in urine and its increased level in the gravitest is proof of pregnancy.

Hormone – chemical substance; it originates in the endocrine glands and passes to the cells that react to it via blood circulation.

Hormonal therapy – medical therapy by a drug containing a hormone.

Hysterosalpingography – x-ray examination method used for imaging the womb and the fallopian tubes.

Hysteroscopy – examination method enabling direct observation of the uterine cavity, it examines the patency of the genital pathways of a woman and the conditions for the nesting and development of an embryo.

ICSI (Intracytoplasmic Sperm Injection) – the insertion of a sperm into an egg by a needle and a special microscope. The technique is sometimes used in IVF.

Idiopathic – inexplicable.

Implantation – submersion of a fertilised egg in the endometrium.

Impotence – inability to have an erection during sexual excitement.

Immunology – field in medicine that deals with the immune system, its function and diseases.

Indication – reason or set of circumstances that requires a certain therapeutic or diagnostic approach.

Infertility – inability to conceive a child.

Infants' home – institutional environment for substitute upbringing of children who cannot be, for various reasons, raised in a family. Usually until three years of age.

IUI (Intrauterine Insemination) – insertion of the sperm into the womb by a special tool instead of usual sexual intercourse, with the goal of achieving fertilisation and pregnancy.

IVF (In Vitro Fertilisation) – method of assisted reproduction, the in-tube fertilisation, often called by people artificial fertilisation. An egg (eggs) is collected, is cultivated in the lab and fertilised by sperm and, after fertilisation and division, is transferred into the woman's womb.

Laparoscopy – examination of the abdominal cavity via an endoscopic tool (laparoscope).

LH – luteal hormone; it is indispensable for the ripening of an egg and its release.

Masturbation – way for a man to achieve the release of sperm without sexual intercourse.

Menstruation (period; monthly bleeding from the genitals; menstrual cycle) – regular repetitive separation of endometrium accompanied by bleeding, which occurs in non-pregnant women; it is a sign that a woman is in the period of fertility.

MESA – microsurgical collection of sperm from the epididymis with the goal of fertilisation of an egg in a man who has no sperm in the ejaculate.

Micromanipulation – intervention in an egg or embryo (for instance ICSI).

Monitoring of a cycle – hormonal and ultrasonic observation of the follicles in the ovaries.

Myoma – benign tumour in the womb.

Nidation – nesting of an embryo in the endometrium.

Oestrogens – female sex hormones, created mainly in the ovaries. Their level varies in relation to the menstrual cycle.

Oligospermia – fertility problem in a man; not enough sperm.

Oocyte – egg; a female sex cell.

Ovary – oval gland the size of a plum, located on both sides of the womb; it contains a number of follicles where the eggs ripen; it produces the female sex hormones oestrogen and progesterone.

Ovulation – release of a ripe egg from the follicle in the ovary; it is regulated hormonally and occurs approximately in the middle of the menstrual cycle; if ovulation does not occur, pregnancy cannot occur.

Physiotherapy – kind of treatment through physical methods.

Postcoital test – test following sexual intercourse (coitus). Cervical mucus is collected and its permeability for sperm is examined.

Pre-adoptive care – legally established necessary period of three months before the court's decision on adoption, designed for the adaptation of the child and the applicants to the new situation.

Prolonged cultivation – extension of the period of the cultivation of embryos to four or five days through special media, with the goal of distinguishing the good-quality embryos.

Puncture – tapping. For instance, a step in IVF when a ripe follicle is tapped and a ripe egg is aspirated.

Rehabilitation – in a broader sense, the renewal of the independence of a patient, in the narrower sense the renewal of his or her mobility (for instance via physiotherapy).

Reproduction – multiplying.

Social worker – expert in helping people in a life situation when they feel the need of help, or in helping in a life situation when the state requires the social worker's intervention.

Sonography (a procedure better known as an ultrasound) – depiction of the inner organs on the screen via ultrasound.

Sperm – male sex cell.

Spermiogram – analysis of the ejaculate (semen) for examination of all of its components.

Sterility – inability of a couple to achieve pregnancy.

Stimulation – hormonal stimulation of the ovaries with the goal of gaining a larger number of follicles (eggs) before the IVF.

TESE – microsurgical collection of sperm in a man who has no sperm in the ejaculate.

Testicles – part of the male sex organs, they produce sperm and the male sex hormone testosterone.

Testosterone – male sex hormone (androgen). It is created in the testicles and, in a small amount, also in the adrenal glands.

Urology – field in medicine that deals with the structure, function and diseases of the urinary system and male sex organs.

Varicocele – fertility problem in a man. The broadening and lengthening of the venous plexus in the gonaduct; the problem is often innocuous; it can be manifested by pain in the scrotum or by a reduced number of sperm; the treatment is surgical.

List of References

1. Dethlefsen, T. & Dahlke, R. (1995). Nemoc jako cesta [Illness as a Journey]. Praha.
2. Wischmann, T. (2003). Psychogene Fertilitätstörungen. Mythen und Fakten [Psychogenic Fertility Disorders. Myths and Facts]. [Electronic version] Gynäkologische Endokrinologie, 2003 (1), 187–196.
3. Wischmann, T. (2003). Psychogene Fertilitätstörungen. Mythen und Fakten [Psychogenic Fertility Disorders. Myths and Facts]. [Electronic version] Gynäkologische Endokrinologie, 2003 (1), 187–196.
   Klonoff-Cohen, H. (2006). How do psychosocial factors impact IVF/GIFT succes rates? What is new? Where are we going? Course 6. 22nd Meeting of European Society of Human Reproduction and Embryology in Prague.
4. Scholler, J.-E. (1999). Adopcia, vztah založený na slube [The Whole Adoption Book]. Bratislava: Návrat domov.
5. Sobòtka, T. (2004). Postponement of Childbearing and Low Fertility in Europe. Doctoral thesis, University of Groningen. Amsterdam: Dutch University Press; http://dissertations.ub.rug.nl/faculties/rw/2004/t.sobotka/
6. Orenstein, P. (2002). Mourning My Miscarriage. [Electronic version]. www.peggyorenstein.com/articles/2002_mourning_miscarriage.html
7. Barlow, R. & Reilly, P. (2007). Introducing MENSFE.net the Mens Fertility Network. [Poster]. 8th International iCSi Conference: Lyon.
8. Plzák, M. (1986). Gordické uzly rovnoprávného párového dorozumívání [The Gordic Nots of Equal Communication Between Partners]. Praha: Mladá fronta.
9. Schaad, Ch. (1982). Heterologous Insemination and Its Medical and Psychological Indications. In: 6th International Congress of Psychosomatic Obstetrics and Gynecology, Berlin: Springer-Verlag.
10. Matějček, Z. (1984). Rodičovství biologické a psychologické [Biological and Psychological Parenthood]. In: Sborník ze 3. konference o NRP v Olomouci. Praha: MPSV ČSR, Statistické a evidenční vydavatelství tiskopisů.
11. Matějček, Z. & Dytrych, Z. (1999). Nevlastní rodiče a nevlastní děti [Step-Parents and Step-Children]. Praha: Grada.

12. Dunovský, J. et al. (1999). Sociální pediatrie [Social Paediatry]. Praha: Grada.
13. Honzák, R. (1997). Komunikační pasti v medicíně [The Pitfalls of Communication in Medicine]. Praha: Galén.
14. Moudrý, J. (1947). Fertilita a sterilita z hlediska biologických a fysiologických studií [Fertility and Sterility from the Point of View of Biological and Physiological Studies]. Praha: Spolek českých lékařů.
15. Možný, I. (1999). Sociologie rodiny [Sociology of Family]. Praha: Sociologické nakladatelství (SLON).
16. Shenfield, F. & Sureau, C. (eds.) (2006). Contemporary Ethical Dilemmas in Assisted Reproduction. Abingdon, U.K.: Informa Healthcare.
17. Uzel, R., Pekárková, M., Primusová, H., Salajka, M. (2000). Potrat ano–ne [Abortion Yes–No]. Praha: Grada.
18. Shenfield, F. & Sureau, C. (eds.) (2006). Contemporary Ethical Dilemmas in Assisted Reproduction. Abingdon, U.K.: Informa Healthcare.
    Vayena, E., Rowe, P. J., Griffin, P. D. (eds.) (2002). Current Practices and Controversies in Assisted Reproduction. Report of a meeting on "Medical, Ethical and Social Aspects of Assisted Reproduction" held at WHO Headquarters in Geneva, Switzerland 17–21 September 2001. [Electronic version] Geneva: WHO.
    Pilka, L. (undated). Bioetické otázky asistované reprodukce [Bioethical Issues in Assisted Reproduction]. Pracovní text poskytnutý autorem.
    Dostál J. (2007). Ethical and Legal Aspects of Assisted Reproduction. Situation in the Member States that Joined the European Union in 2004. 1st ed., Olomouc: Univerzita Palackého v Olomouci, 143 p. ISBN 978-80-244-1746-2.
19. Czech Statistical Office 2001
20. in: Rabušic, L. (2001). Kde ty všechny děti jsou? Porodnost v sociologické perspektivě [Where Have All the Children Gone: The Birth-Rate from a Sociological Perspective]. Praha: Sociologické nakladatelství.
21. Matějček, Z., Kovařík, J., Bubleová, V., et al. (2002). Osvojení a pěstounská péče [Adoption and Foster Care]. Praha: Portál.
22. Rabušic, L. (2001). Kde ty všechny děti jsou? Porodnost v sociologické perspektivě [Where Have All the Children Gone: The Birth-Rate from a Sociological Perspective]. Praha: Sociologické nakladatelství.
23. Dunovský, J. et al. (1999). Sociální pediatrie [Social Paediatry]. Praha: Grada.
24. Sullerot, E. (1998). Krize rodiny [The Crisis of the Family]. Praha: Karolinum.
25. in.: Dunovský, J. et al. (1999). Sociální pediatrie [Social Paediatry]. Praha: Grada.

26. Horská, P., Kučera, M., Maur, E., Stloukal, M. (1990). Dětství, rodina a stáří v dějinách Evropy [Childhood, Family, and the Old Age in European History]. Praha: Panorama.
Šubrtová, A. (1989). Dějiny populačního myšlení a populačních teorií [A History of Population Thought and Population Theories]. Praha: Ústav československých a světových dějin ČSAV.

Bibliography

Adascalitei, V. (1980). Předu, předu pohádku [Weaving, Weaving Fairy Tales]. Praha: Lidové nakladatelství.

Alexander, F. (1950). Psychosomatic Medicine. London: Norton.

Andersen, H. Ch. (1957). Pohádky [Fairy Tales]. Praha: SNDK.

Assael, M. & Palti, Z. (1974). Post-partum Mental Disturbance Due to Artificial Insemination by Donor. In: The Family, 4th International Congress of Psychosomatic Obstetrics and Gynecology. Tel Aviv.

Badinter, E. (1998). Materská láska od 17. storočia po súčasnosť [Maternal Love from the 17th Century to the Present]. Bratislava: Aspekt.

Badinter, E. (1999). XY. Identita muža [The Identity of a Man]. Bratislava: Aspekt.

Baetens, P., Camus, M., Devroey, P. (2002). Counselling Lesbian Couples: Requests for Donor Insemination on Social Grounds. [Electronic version]. Reproductive BioMedicine Online Vol. 6., No.1. 75–83.

Baetens, P., Ponjaert-Kristoffersen, I., et al. (1995). Ethics and Society: Artificial Insemination by Donor: An Alternative for Single Women. [Abstract] [Electronic version]. Human Reproduction (10), No. 6, 1537–1542.

Baker, R. (1996). Válka spermií [Sperm Wars]. Brno: Jota.

Barlow, R., Reilly, P. (2007). Introducing MENSFE.net the Mens Fertility Network. [Poster]. 8th International iCSi Conference: Lyon.

Bartoš, F. (1906). Deset rozprav lidopisných [Ten Folkloric Essays]. Olomouc.

Baštecký, J., Šavlík, J., Šimek, J. et al. (1993). Psychosomatická medicína. [Psychosomatic Medicine]. Praha: Grada.

Beneš-Třebízský, V. (1941). Pohádky a pověsti [Fairy Tales and Legends]. Třebechovice pod Orebem: Nakladatel A. Dědourek.

Benson, H. & Starková, M. (1997). Moc a biologie víry v uzdravení [Timeless Healing: The Power and Biology of Belief]. Praha: Práh.

Bible. Písmo svaté Starého a Nového zákona. [The Bible]. (1985). Ekumenický překlad. Praha: Česká katolická charita.

Boivin, J., Kentenich, H., Baetens, P., et al. (2002). Guidelines for Counselling in Infertility. [Electronic version]. ESHRE Special Interest Group on Psychology and Counselling in association with Oxford University Press.

Bologne, J.C. (1997). Svatby. Dějiny svatebních obřadů na Západě [Weddings]. Praha.

Bos, G., et al. (1982). The Big Secret: Male Infertility. In: 6th International Congress of Psychosomatic Obstetrics and Gynecology, September 2–6, 1980. [Electronic version]. Berlin: Springer-Verlag.

Brentano, C. (1977). O růžovém keři [About the Rose Bush]. Praha: Vyšehrad.

Brewaeys, A., de Bruyn, J.K., Louwe, L.A., Helmerhorst, F.M. (2005). Anonymous or Identity-registered Sperm Donors? A Study of Dutch Recipients' Choices. [Electronic version]. Human Reproduction, 2005 20. 3, 820–824.

Burcin, B., Ventruba, P., et al. (2004). Demografické souvislosti asistované reprodukce [The Demographic Contexts of Assisted Reproduction], Praktická Gynekologie, 2004 (5), 11–12.

Čapek, J. (1972). Vyprávění o pejskovi a kočičce [Yarns about Doggy and Kitty]. Praha: Albatros.

Carenza, L. & Agostini, R. (1974). Psychosomatic Aspects of Male Sterility. In: The Family, 4th International Congress of Psychosomatic Obstetrics and Gynecology. Tel Aviv.

Čepický, P. (1986). Psychosomatická onemocnění v gynekologii [Psychosomatic Ilnesses in Gynaecology]. Praha: Avicenum.

Čepický, P. (1999). Psychosomatika [Psychosomatics]. Moderní gynekologie a porodnictví, 1999, (8), 3.

Čermák, I. & Štěpaníková, I. (1997). Validita dat v kvalitativním psychologickém výzkumu [Data Validity in Qualitative Psychological Research]. Československá psychologie, 6 (41), 503–512.

Čermák, I. & Štěpaníková, I. (1998). Metody kontroly validity dat v kvalitativním psychologickém výzkumu [Data Validity Control Methods in Qualitative Psychological Research]. Československá psychologie, 1 (42), 50–62.

Chvála, V., Machander, R.A., et al. (1991). Je psychogenní sterilita obranou proti dokončení separace dcery od matky? [Is Psychogenetic Sterility a Defence Against Completing the Mother-Daughter Separation?]. Československá psychologie, 1991 (35), No. 6, 509–511.

Convention for the Protection of Human Rights and Dignity of the Human Being with Regard to the Application of Biology and Medicine: Convention on Human Rights and Biomedicine. [Electronic version] http://conventions.coe.int/treaty/en/treaties/html/164.htm

Coolsaet, B. (2000). Štětec lásky. Život a dílo penisu [The Paintbrush of Love: The Life and Work of the Penis]. Praha: Ikar.

Corbin, J. & Strauss, A. (1990). The Basic Principles of Qualitative Research. London: Thousand Oaks, New Delhi: SAGE Publications.

Daniels, K.R. (2000). A Biopsychosocial Perspective. In: Orgyn, Organon's Magazine on Women and Health, 2000 (3).

Daniels, K.R. & Thorn, P. (2001). Sharing Information with Donor Insemination Offspring. [Abstract]. [Electronic version]. Human Reproduction, 2001 (19), 9, 1792–1796.

Dawkins, R. (2003). Sobecký gen [The Selfish Gene]. Praha: Mladá fronta.

Dethlefsen, T. & Dahlke, R. (1995). Nemoc jako cesta [Illness as a Journey]. Praha.

Domar, A.D., Seibel, M.M., Benson, H. (1990): The Mind/Body Program for Infertility: A New Behavioral Treatment Approach for Women with Infertility. [Electronic version]. Fertility and Sterility, 1990 (53), 246–249.

Domar, A.D., Zuttermeister, P.C., Seibel, M., Benson, H.(1992). Psychological Improvement in Infertile Women After Behavioral Treatment: A Replication. [Electronic version]. Fertility and Sterility, 1992 (58), 144–147.

Dostál, J. (2007). Ethical and Legal Aspects of Assisted Reproduction. Situation in the Member States that Joined the European Union in 2004. 1st ed., Olomouc: Univerzita Palackého v Olomouci. 143 p. ISBN 978-80-244-1746-2.

Dunovský, J. et al. (1999). Sociální pediatrie [Social Paediatry]. Praha: Grada.

Dunson, D.B., Baird, D.D., Colombo, B. (2004). Increased Infertility With Age in Men and Women. [Abstract]. [Electronic version]. Obstetrics and Gynecology, 2004 (103), 51–56.

Dytrych, Z., Matějček, Z., et al. (1987). Mladé rizikové rodiny [Young Families at Risk]. Praha: VÚPs.

Ehmann, R., et al. (1996). Jak je tomu s obrazem člověka v rozporuplné oblasti lidské reprodukce a reprodukční medicíny? In: Medicína dnes a náš obraz člověka [Medicine Today and Our View of the Human Being]. Sborník z 8. Evropský kongres FEAMC (Evropská federace Asociací katolických lékařů) Praha, červen.

Englert, Y. (1994). Artificial Insemination of Single and Lesbian-Mother Women with Donor Semen. [Abstract]. [Electronic version]. Human Reproduction, 1994 (9), 1969–1971.

Eskenazi, B. et al. (2003). The Association of Age and Semen Quality in Healthy Men. [Abstract]. [Electronic version]. Human Reproduction, 2003 (18), No. 2, 447–454.

Evangelium o narození Panny Marie. [The Gospel of the Virgin Mary]. [Electronic version]. www.inext.cz/astrologician/marie.htm

Fenclová, J. (1999). Když dítě nepřichází [When the Awaited Child Is Not Coming]. Studijní texty praxe víry, 1999 (16). Praha: Pastorační středisko při Arcibiskupství pražském.

Ferin, M., Jewelewicz, R., Warren, M. (1997). Menstruační cyklus [The Menstrual Cycle]. Praha, Grada.

Fialová, L., Horská, P., Kučera, M. (1995). Současné a perspektivní proměny rodiny, manželství a rodičovství [Current and Future Transformations of the Family, Marriage, and Parenthood]. Praha: Start.

Foldes, J.J. (1974). Ovulatory Disturbances of Psychosomatic Origin. In: The Family, 4th International Congress of Psychosomatic Obstetrics and Gynecology. Tel Aviv.

Frazer, J.G. (1994). Zlatá ratolest [The Golden Bough]. Praha: Mladá fronta.

Frýba, M. (1995). Psychologie zvládání života [Psychology and Coping with Life]. Brno: Masarykova univerzita.

Gladstar, R. & Jonáš, J. (1995). Přírodní léčba pro ženy. [Natural Therapy for Women]. Praha: TOK ve spolupráci s nakl. Eminent.

Glaser, B. & Strauss, A. (1967). The Discovery of Grounded Theory. Chicago: Aldine.

Golombok, S., Murray, C., et al. (1999). Social versus Biological Parenting: Family Functioning and the Socioemotional Development of Children Conceived by Egg or Sperm Donation. [Abstract]. [Electronic version]. Journal of Child Psychology and Psychiatry, 1999 (40), 519.

Grimmové, J. a W. (1988). Pohádky [The Grimms' Fairy Tales]. Praha: Odeon.

Heřt, J., et al. (1995). Alternativní medicína. [Alternative Medicine]. Praha: Avicenum.

Hewlett, S.A. (2002). Creating a Life. Professional Women and the Quest for Children. New York: Talk Miramax Book.

Honzák, R. (1997). Komunikační pasti v medicíně [The Pitfalls of Communication in Medicine]. Praha: Galén.

Horák, J. (1966). Čarodějná mošna [The Magic Bag]. Praha: SNDK.

Horská, P. (1996). Dějiny obyvatelstva českých zemí [A History of the Citizens of the Czech Lands]. Praha: Mladá fronta.

Horská, P. (2003). Umělé přerušení těhotenství pohledem historické demografie [Abortion from the Point of View of Historical Demography]. Historická demografie, 2003 (27), 225–242. Praha: Sociologický ústav AV.

Horská, P., Kučera, M., Maur, E., Stloukal, M. (1990). Dětství, rodina a stáří v dějinách Evropy [Childhood, Family, and the Old Age in European History]. Praha: Panorama.

Hudec, I. (1994). Báje a mýty starých Slovanů [Old Slavic Myths and Legends]. Ostrava: Vydavatelství Slovart.

Hudeček, P., Ventruba, P., et al. (2004). Terapeutické možnosti asistované reprodukce u perimenopauzálních žen [The Therapeutic Options of Assisted Reproduction for Perimenopauzal Women]. Praktická gynekologie, 2004 (6), 6–9.

Janča, V. (1960). Fysikální terapie a balneologie [Physical Therapy and Balneology]. Praha: SPN.

Jan Pavel II. (1991). Úvahy nad encyklikou „Humanae vitae papeže Pavla VI. [Some Thoughts about John Paul's VI's 'Humanae Vitae']. Olomouc: Cesta.

Jaroš, B. (?). Dítě podle hvězd [A Child According to the Stars]. Časopis Regena, Praha.

Klonoff-Cohen, H. (2006). How do psychosocial factors impact IVF/GIFT succes rates? What is new? Where are we going? Course 6. 22nd Meeting of European Society of Human Reproduction and Embryology in Prague.

Konečná, H. (2006). On the Quest for a Child. Two Small Wings. Praha: Triton.

Konečná, H. (2003). Na cestě za dítětem. Dvě malá křídla [On the Quest for a Child. Two Small Wings]. Praha: Academia.

Konečná, H. & Janků, V. (2002). Rodičovství v 21. stol. [Parenthood in the Twenty-First Century] Unpublished manuscript. Brno: Centrum pro rodinu a sociální péči.

Konečná, H. (2000). Psychologické problémy neplodnosti [The Psychological Problems of Infertility]. Unpublished doctoral dissertation. Palacký University, Olomouc, Czech Republic.

Koryntová, D. (1999). Psychosomatické aspekty sterility [The Psychosomatic Aspects of Sterility]. In Čepický, P. (ed.): Psychosomatické aspekty gynekologie a porodnictví. Sborník prací celostátního kongresu ČGPS ČLS JEP. Praha: Levret.

Kosatík, P. (1999). Devět žen z Hradu [Nine Women from the Castle]. Praha: Mladá fronta.

Kratochvíl, S. (1992). Manželská terapie [Spousal Therapy]. Hradec Králové: Nakladatelství Mach.

Kratochvíl, S. (1991). Sexuální problémy a potíže [Sexual Problems and Disorders]. Praha: Avicenum.

Kubíček, V. (1996). Mužská infertilita a erektilní dysfunkce [Male Infertility and Erectile Dysfunction]. Praha: Galén.

Kubín, J., Š. (1976). Kniha pohádek [A Book of Fairy Tales]. Praha: Albatros.

Kučera, T., Mardešič, T., Žáčková, T. (2005). Úspěšnost mimotělního oplodnění a demografické aspekty neplodnosti v ČR [The Successes of Extrauterine Fertilisation and the Demographic Aspects of Infertility in the Czech Republic]. Sanquis 2005 (39). Praha.

Langmeier, J. & Matějček, Z. (1974). Psychická deprivace v dětství [Psychical Deprivation in Childhood]. Praha: Avicenum.

Leiblum, S.R., Palmer, M.G., Spector, I.P. (1995). Non-traditional Mothers: Single Heterosexual/Lesbian Women and Lesbian Couples Electing Motherhood via Donor Insemination. [Abstract]. [Electronic version]. J. Psychosom. Obstet. Gynaecol. 1995 16 (1), 11–20.

Léon-Dufour, X., et al. (1981). Slovník biblické teologie [Dictionary of Biblical Theology]. Řím: Křesťanská akademie.

Machač, M., Machačová, H., Hoskovec, J. (1985). Emoce a výkonnost [Emotions and Efficiency]. Praha: SPN.

Mardešić, T. (1996). Neplodnost [Infertility]. Praha: Nakladatelství Makropulos.

Matějček, Z. (1984). Rodičovství biologické a psychologické [Biological and Psychological Parenthood]. In: Sborník ze 3. konference o NRP v Olomouci. Praha: MPSV ČSR, Statistické a evidenční vydavatelství tiskopisů.

Matějček, Z. (1994). O rodině vlastní, nevlastní a náhradní [The Biological Family, the Step-Family, and the Foster Family]. Praha: Portál.

Matějček, Z. & Dytrych, Z. (1999). Nevlastní rodiče a nevlastní děti [Step-Parents and Step-Children]. Praha: Grada.

Matějček, Z., Dytrych, Z., Schüller, V., Fischelová, V. (1977). Nechtěné těhotenství a jeho sociálně psychologické důsledky [Unwanted Pregnancy and Its

Socio-Psychological Consequences]. In: Doležal, A., Gutvirth, J. (eds.): Anthropology of Maternity. Praha: Universitas Carolina Pragensis. 321–326.

Matějček, Z., Kovařík, J., Bubleová, V., et al. (2002). Osvojení a pěstounská péče [Adoption and Foster Care]. Praha: Portál.

Mayring, P. (1994). Qualitativ-empirische Forschung in der Psychologie [The Qualitative-Empirical Research in Psychology]. In: Schorr, A. (ed.): Die Psychologie und die Methodenfrage. Studentský překlad pro studenty FFMU, se svolením autora.Göttingen: Hogrefe.

McWhinnie, A. (2001). Gamete Donation and Anonymity. [Abstract]. [Electronic version]. Human Reproduction, 2001 (16), No.5, 807–817.

Mertlík, R. (1968). Starověké báje a pověsti [Ancient Greek Myths and Legends]. Praha: Svoboda.

Michel, G.F., Mooreová, C.L. (1999). Psychobiologie. Biologické základy vývoje chování. [Developmental Psychobiology]. Praha: Portál.

Miltner, V. (1973). Příběhy bájné Indie [Legends of Ancient India]. Praha: Práce.

Ministerstvo práce a sociálních věcí České republiky (2001). Dětská práva a jejich plnění [Children's Rights and Their Enforcement]. [Electronic version]. Zpráva MPSV ČR.

Miovský, M. (2005). Kvalitativní přístup a metody v psychologickém výzkumu. Praha: Grada

Mojžíšová, L., et al. (1990). Children of Your Own: The Mojzis Method. Boulder, Colorado: Richmond Bay Publishers.

Moudrý, J. (1947). Fertilita a sterilita z hlediska biologických a fysiologických studií [Fertility and Sterility from the Point of View of Biological and Physiological Studies]. Praha: Spolek českých lékařů.

Možný, I. (1990). Moderní rodina (mýty a skutečnosti) [The Modern Family: The Myths and the Reality]. Brno: Blok.

Možný, I. (1999). Sociologie rodiny [Sociology of Family]. Praha: Sociologické nakladatelství (SLON).

Mrázek, M. (2003). Umělé oplodnění I. [Artificial Fertilisation I]. Praha: Triton.

Náhradní rodinná péče (1998–2000). [Adoption and Foster Care]. Časopisy z let 1998–2000. Praha: Středisko náhradní rodinné péče.

Niederle, L. (ed.) (1922). Národopis lidu československého I. Moravské Slovensko II [A History of the Czech Slavic People I: Moravian Slovakia]. Praha.

Novotná, M., et al. (1996). Léčebné rehabilitační postupy Ludmily Mojžíšové [The Therapeutic Methods of Ludmila Mojžíšová]. Praha: Grada.

Orenstein, P. (2002). Mourning My Miscarriage. [Electronic version]. www.peggyorenstein.com/articles/2002_mourning_miscarriage.html

Owens, D.J., Edelmann, R.E., Humprey, M.E. (1993). Male Infertility and Donor Insemination: Couples' Decisions, Reactions and Counselling Needs. [Abstract] [Electronic version]. Human Reproduction, 1993 (8), No.6, 880–885.

Pennings, G. (1997). The 'Double Track' Policy for Donor Anonymity. [Abstract]. [Electronic version]. Human Reproduction, 1997 (12), 2839–2844.

Pilka, L. (undated). Bioetické otázky asistované reprodukce [Bioethical Issues in Assisted Reproduction]. Pracovní text poskytnutý autorem.

Plzák, M. & Frýbová, Z. (1981). Do nepohody připraven [Ready for Rainy Weather]. Praha: Naše vojsko.

Plzák, M. (1969). První pomoc při nehodách manželských [First Aid in Marital Accidents]. Praha: Mladá fronta.

Plzák, M. (1986). Gordické uzly rovnoprávného párového dorozumívání [The Gordic Nots of Equal Communication Between Partners]. Praha: Mladá fronta.

Rabušic, L. (2001). Kde ty všechny děti jsou? Porodnost v sociologické perspektivě [Where Have All the Children Gone: The Birth-Rate from a Sociological Perspective]. Praha: Sociologické nakladatelství.

Ratzinger, J. (1987). Donum vitae. Instrukce kongregace pro nauku víry (O respektování rodícího se lidského života a o důstojnosti poznání) [Donum vitae]. Řím: Kongregace pro nauku víry.

Report on Human Artificial Procreation: [Electronic version] www.coe.int/t/e/legal_affairs/legal_co-operation/bioethics.

Řežábek, K. (2004). Léčba neplodnosti. [Infertility Therapy]. Praha: Grada.

Rochebrochard, E., Mcelreavey, K., Thonneau, P. (2003). Paternal Age Over 40 Years: The 'Amber Light' in the Reproductive Life of Men? [Abstract]. [Electronic version]. Journal of Andrology, 2003 (24), No.4.

Roztočil, A., et al. (1998). Vyšetřovací metody v porodnictví a gynekologii [The Examination Methods in Obstetrics and Gynaecology]. Brno: Institut pro další vzdělávání pracovníků ve zdravotnictví.

Říha, B. (1985). Doktor Meluzin [Doctor Meluzin]. Praha: Československý spisovatel.

Sekora, O. (1968). Knížka Ferdy Mravence. [The Book of Ferda the Ant]. Praha: SNDK.

Schaad, Ch. (1982). Heterologous Insemination and Its Medical and Psychological Indications. In: 6th International Congress of Psychosomatic Obstetrics and Gynecology, Berlin: Springer-Verlag.

Scholler, J.-E. (1999). Adopcia, vztah založený na slube [The Whole Adoption Book]. Bratislava: Návrat domov.

Schotsmans, P. (1996). Fertilizace In Vitro [Fertilisation in Vitro]. In: Medicína dnes a náš obraz člověka. 8. Evropský kongres FEAMC (Evropská federace Asociací katolických lékařů). Praha.

Schover, L.R., Collins, R.L., Richards, S. (1992). Psychological Aspects of Donor Insemiation: Evaluation and Follow-up of Recipient Couples. [Abstract]. [Electronic version]. Fertility and Sterility, 1992 57 (3), 583–90.

Shenfield, F., Sureau, C. (eds.) (2006). Contemporary Ethical Dilemmas in Assisted Reproduction. Abingdon, U.K.: Informa Healthcare.

Škapík, M., et al. (1994). Využití balneoterapie ve vnitřním lékařství [Using Balneotherapy in Internal Medicine]. Praha: Grada Publishing.

Slepičková, L. (2006). Nedobrovolná bezdětnost jako sociologické téma. Sociologický časopis no.05/2006, vol. 42. Sociologický ústav AV ČR.

Šmarda, J. (2000). Člověk v proudu dědičnosti [The Human Being in the Flow of Heredity]. Praha: Grada.

Sobotka, T. (2004). Postponement of Childbearing and Low Fertility in Europe. Doctoral thesis, University of Groningen. Amsterdam: Dutch University Press; http://dissertations.ub.rug.nl/faculties/rw/2004/t.sobotka/.

Solovjov, L. (1975). Nasreddinova dobrodružství [Nasreddin`s Adventures]. Praha: Svoboda.

Stark, V. (1974). Suppression of Ovulation by Emotional Factors and Its Restoration through Psychotherapy. In: The Family, 4th International Congress of Psychosomatic Obstetrics and Gynecology. Tel Aviv.

Strauss, A., & Corbinová, J. (1999). Základy kvalitativního výzkumu–postupy a techniky metody zakotvené teorie [The Basics of Qualitative Research]. Boskovice: Albert.

Sullerot, E. (1998). Krize rodiny [The Crisis of the Family]. Praha: Karolinum.

Šubrtová, A. (1989). Dějiny populačního myšlení a populačních teorií [A History of Population Thought and Population Theories]. Praha: Ústav československých a světových dějin ČSAV.

Tomek, D. (1998). Moře jangů [The Sea of the Jangs]. Olomouc: Fontána.

Trcalová, L. (1994). Patronství světců a světic v lidové tradici [The Patronage of the Saints in the Folk Tradition]. Slovácko.

Trnková, D. (2003). Ilegitimita a „nová ekonomie života v osvícenské Habsburské monarchii. Problém svobodných matek a nemanželských dětí mezi sociální kontrolou a sociální péčí na prahu občanské společnosti [Illegitimacy and the New Ecomy of Life in the Habsburg Monarchy of the Enlightenment]. Historická demografie, (27), 113–172. Praha: Sociologický ústav AV.

Ulčová-Gallová, Z. (1999). Diagnóza–neplodnost. Útok protilátek [Diagnosis—Infertility: The Attack of the Antibodies]. Praha: Petrklíč.

Úmluva o právech dítěte [Agreement On Children`s Rights], OSN 1989, Sbírka zákonů č. 104/1991, částka 22, str. 502. www.unhchr.ch/html/menu3/b/k2crc.htm

Uzel, R., Pekárková, M., Primusová, H., Salajka, M. (2000). Potrat ano–ne [Abortion Yes–No]. Praha: Grada.

Václavík, A. (1958). Genese obřadních plachet, koutnice a úvodnice. Příspěvky k lidovým obřadům rodinným, lidovému umění a kroji. [The Genesis of Ritual Scarfs, Koutnice and Úvodnice] Zvl. otisk ze sborníku Franku Wollmanovi k sedmdesátinám. Praha.

Váňa, Z. (1990). Svět slovanských bohů a démonů [The World of Slavic Gods and Demons]. Praha.

Vayena, E., Rowe, P.J., Griffin, P.D. (eds.) (2002). Current Practices and Controversies in Assisted Reproduction. Report of a meeting on "Medical, Ethical and Social Aspects of Assisted Reproduction" held at WHO

Headquarters in Geneva, Switzerland 17–21 September 2001. [Electronic version] Geneva: WHO.

Verbena, časopisy z let 1997–1998. [Verbena. Journals 1997–1998]. Praha: Sdružení nedobrovolně bezdětných párů.

Vogt-Frýba, B. (1991). Können und Vertrauen–Das Tovil Heilritual von Sri Lanka als kultureigene Psychotherapie [Skill and Trust–The Tovil Healing Ritual of Sri Lanka as Culture-Specific Psychotherapy]. Zürich: Verlag Rüegger.

Volejníková, H. (1992). Studie zur Objektivierung der Erfolgsraten nach der Behandlungsmethode von L. Mojžíšová bei weiblicher Sterilität infolge von Funktionsstörungen im Beckenbereich. Manuelle Medizin, 1992 (30), 96–98. Springer-Verlag.

Volejniková, H. (2001). Female Infertility: A Study of Physical Treatment by the Method of L. Mojzisova for Functional Disturbances of the Pelvic Region. The Journal of Orthopaedic Medicine 23 [2] 2001

Wendland, C., Byrn, F., Hill, C. (1996). Donor Insemination: A Comparison of Lesbian Couples, Heterosexual Couples and Single Women. [Abstract]. [Electronic version]. Fertility and Sterility, 1996 (65), 764–770.

Wilson, E.O. (1993). O lidské přirozenosti [On Human Nature]. Praha: Lidové noviny.

Wischmann, T. (2003). Psychogene Fertilitätstörungen. Mythen und Fakten [Psychogenic Fertility Disorders. Myths and Facts]. [Electronic version] Gynäkologische Endokrinologie, 2003 (1), 187–196.

Zákon o darování, odběrech a transplantacích tkání a orgánů č. 285/2002 Sb. [Act of Donating, Collecting, and Transplanting Tissues and Organs and of Changes in Certain Acts of Law (No. 285/2002 Coll.)]

Zákon o rodině č. 359/199 Sb. [Family Act (No. 94/1963 Coll.)]

Zákon o sociální a právní ochraně dětí č. 359/1999 Sb. [The Social and Legal Protection of Children Act (No. 359/1999 Coll.)]

Zeman, Z. & Doležal, A. (2000). Právní odpovědnost a právní vztahy v porodnictví [The Legal Responsibility and Legal Relations in Obstetrics]. Praha: Galén.

Zentrich, J. & Jonáš, J. (1990). Věčně zelené naděje [Eternal Hopes]. Ústí nad Labem: Severočeské nakladatelství.

Život moravských Slováků. [The Life of Moravian Slovaks] (1912). Obraz ze slovácké dědiny z Uh. Hradištska. Rkp. Javorovec 1912. Slovácké muzeum v Uherském Hradišti, inv. č. 118/77 H-260.